URINALYSIS AND BODY FLUIDS
A ColorText and Atlas

KAREN MUNSON RINGSRUD, BS, MT(ASCP)

Assistant Professor
Department of Laboratory Medicine and Pathology
University of Minnesota Medical School
Minneapolis, Minnesota

JEAN JORGENSON LINNÉ, BS, MT(ASCP)

Assistant Professor
Department of Laboratory Medicine and Pathology
University of Minnesota Medical School
Minneapolis, Minnesota

with 344 illustrations

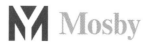
Mosby

St. Louis Baltimore Berlin Boston Carlsbad Chicago London Madrid
Naples New York Philadelphia Sydney Tokyo Toronto

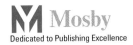

Dedicated to Publishing Excellence

Editor: James F. Shanahan
Assistant Editor: Anne Gleason
Project Manager: John Rogers
Senior Production Editor: Chris Murphy
Design: AKA Design Incorporated
Design Coordinator: Renée Duenow
Manufacturing Supervisor: Karen Lewis
Electronic Production Coordinator: Chris Robinson

Printed in the United States of America
Composition by Mosby Electronic Production
Printing/binding by Von Hoffmann Press, Inc.

Mosby–Year Book, Inc.
11830 Westline Industrial Drive
St. Louis, Missouri 63146

Library of Congress Cataloging-in-Publication Data

Ringsrud, Karen Munson.
 Urinalysis and body fluids: a colortext and atlas / Karen Munson
Ringsrud, Jean Jorgenson Linné.—1st ed.
  p. cm.
  Includes bibliographical references and index.
  ISBN 0-8016-7043-8
  1. Urine—Analysis. 2. Urine—Analysis—Atlases. I. Linné, Jean
Jorgenson. II. Title.
  [DNLM: 1. Urinalysis—atlases. 2. Body Fluids—atlases. QY 17
R582u 1994]
RB53.R53 1994
616.07'566—dc20
DNLM/DLC
for Library of Congress   94-35005
                                                                              CIP

95 96 97 98 99 / 9 8 7 6 5 4 3 2 1

Once Again To
Peter and Erik
David, David, Laura, and Jonathan

FOREWORD

or many years, the authors of this text have been involved with teaching in the health sciences always with great acclaim for their enthusiasm and their ability to innovate and stay in the forefront of technical subjects and educational methods.

Their communications and technical skills have been brought together in their text, *Basic Techniques in Clinical Laboratory Science,* now in its 3rd edition, and in this new *Urinalysis and Body Fluids: A ColorText and Atlas.*

Commonly performed tests such as urinalysis provide rapid, initial diagnoses of kidney and certain metabolic diseases—or help rule out disease—at relatively low cost. Recognition of synovial fluid crystals enables rapid initiation of appropriate therapy and relief of pain. The apparent simplicity of some of the procedures requires particular emphasis on quality performance without which many valuable qualitative and microscopic tests will be erroneously interpreted. This new book gives the reader a sound orientation to the basic principles of traditional and newer methods with an emphasis on quality assurance and test limitations. It also provides a practical bench-top atlas for microscopic findings in urine and body fluids. It will be useful in office practice, community and academic hospital laboratories, on wards, and in clinics.

G. MARY BRADLEY, MD
University of Minnesota Hospital and Clinic

PREFACE

The purpose of this textbook and atlas is to provide a basic resource for the study of urine and body cavity fluids for the many and varied persons working in the area of clinical laboratory science. The atlas section includes a substantial collection of full-color photomicrographs that serve to enhance the written information. We hope it will be of use to a varied level of persons, both as a textbook for students (including formal programs at technical, associate, and baccalaureate degree levels, on-the-job or cross-training programs, medical students and residents) and staff, and as a bench reference for new as well as experienced laboratorians in hospital laboratories, physicians offices and clinics.

Urinalysis and Body Fluids: A ColorText and Atlas is the result of more than 30 years of teaching a variety of students at the University of Minnesota. Our teaching experience began early in the 1960s while working with the University's Medical Laboratory Assistant Program. From this we moved on to teaching a course in Laboratory Medicine to second-year medical students at the University of Minnesota Medical School, which we have continued to do for more than 25 years. We also teach medical technology students in urine and body fluid analysis and pathophysiology, and Karen serves as a technical consultant to the University of Minnesota Hospital and Clinic (UMHC) Urinalysis, Body Fluid and Outpatient Laboratories.

As a result of this experience, we have accumulated an extensive collection of photomicrographs of the various constituents seen in the urine sediment and body cavity fluids. When new or unusual entities are encountered in the clinical laboratory, our collection of photomicrographs is expanded. This collection has been used in our hands-on, wet laboratory sessions for medical students, where actual case-related urine sediments are demonstrated microscopically with accompanying prints of photomicrographs. We have also developed in-house atlases of photographs of urine sediments and various body cavity fluid constituents

to help staff members when unusual entities are encountered, to instruct new staff members, and to teach new medical and medical technology students. This textbook and atlas is the result of this experience.

Although several multiple reagent strips are available for the chemical testing of urine, the three most commonly used products according to the College of American Pathologists' survey results are included in this text. Chemistry, sensitivities, and specificities are current at the date of publication of this text, but reagent strips are continually changed in a very competitive marketplace. Product inserts must be consulted for the most recent information, and manufacturer's directions must always be followed. Hopefully, the approach used to describe each of the chemical tests in this textbook will serve as a logical approach to future changes or additions to multiple reagent strips.

The order in which the chemical tests are described in this text is a pathophysiological approach, rather than the order encountered on any of the reagent strips described. Tests are grouped as outlined in Chapter 2, generally as tests related to kidney and urinary tract disease, and tests related to metabolic disorders.

We have not included all tests that are performed in urinalysis, rather the so-called "routine" urinalysis procedures plus the most common confirmatory tests. We have also chosen not to describe the various instruments that are available to read multiple reagent strips; the principle of reactions and interferences are the same as for visual readings, and details of instrument operation are beyond the scope of this text.

Information about required standards for the clinical laboratory—regulatory considerations, safety and quality assurance—is included in the first chapter. Study questions are included in each chapter. Case studies are included, where pertinent, to illustrate laboratory problems that may be encountered and common test patterns seen in disease states.

KAREN MUNSON RINGSRUD

JEAN JORGENSON LINNÉ

ACKNOWLEDGMENTS

We thank all of the clinical laboratory scientists at the UMHC who have saved innumerable interesting, unusual, unknown, and typical urine and body fluid specimens for teaching and photography. The photomicrographs in this text are the result of their intellectual curiosity and dedication to the learning process. We wish we could name them all, but hesitate to do so since we do not want to forget anyone in a long, much appreciated list of exceptional laboratorians.

We are particularly grateful for our association with Esther Mary Damron, MT, retired, and Dolores Harvey, MT, also retired. Mary, as Senior Medical Technologist in charge of the University of Minnesota Hospital Urinalysis laboratory for more than 20 years, and Dolores, as former director of the Division of Medical Technology Urinalysis and Clinical Chemistry course, were an inspiration to us and to countless students and staff members at the University of Minnesota.

Last, we must thank our mentor, Dr. G. Mary Bradley, without whose encouragement and extensive knowledge this project would never have begun. Her ideas, cases, and design of the University of Minnesota Medical School's Laboratory Medicine Course and her clinical laboratory experience are the basis of our knowledge and of this text. We thank her for the opportunities she has given us over these many years of our association—for her respectful friendship. We also appreciate the support of the Department of Laboratory Medicine and Pathology at the University of Minnesota, under the chairmanship of Leo T. Furcht MD.

Most of the photomicrographs in this atlas were taken by Karen Ringsrud. A few are very old slides used in teaching at the University of Minnesota, where the photographer is unknown. In addition, Figures 6-126 and 6-173 were photographed by Dr. G. Mary Bradley, Figures 6-75, 6-130 A, B, C, 6-159, 6-171, and 6-174 A, B, were photographed by Helen Louise Yates (now retired) of the UMHC Outpatient Laboratory, and Figures 6-7, 6-135, 6-189, 6-207, 6-209, 6-215, 6-219, 6-229, 6-230, and 6-232 were photographed by Dr. Patrick C.J. Ward, Professor and Head, Department of Pathology, School of Medicine, University of Minnesota, Duluth. We give special thanks to Dr. Ward for the use of Figures 6-135 and 6-230 as well and his photomicrographs as used in our textbook, *Basic Techniques in Clinical Laboratory Science*, ed 3.

We also thank Mosby–Year Book, Inc., for permission to use the following photomicrographs from our textbook: Fig. 6-7, Fig. 6-11, Fig. 6-22, Fig. 6-29, Fig. 6-30, Fig. 6-37, Fig. 6-39, Fig. 6-46, Fig. 6-58, Fig. 6-64, Fig. 6-69, Fig. 6-71, Fig. 6-79, Fig. 6-85, Fig. 6-86, Fig. 6-98, Fig. 6-100 A, Fig. 6-100 B, Fig. 6-101, Fig. 6-111, Fig. 6-112, Fig. 6-118, Fig. 6-126, Fig. 6-128, Fig. 6-133, Fig. 6-134, Fig. 6-136, Fig. 6-137 A, Fig. 6-137 B, Fig. 6-149, Fig. 6-150 A, Fig. 6-150 B, Fig. 6-151, Fig. 6-154, Fig. 6-155 A, Fig. 6-155 B, Fig. 6-160, Fig. 6-162, Fig. 6-164 A, Fig. 6-164 B, Fig. 6-189, Fig. 6-190, Fig. 6-192, Fig. 6-197, Fig. 6-200 A, Fig. 6-200 B, Fig. 6-202, Fig. 6-206, Fig. 6-207, Fig. 6-209, Fig. 6-215, Fig. 6-219, Fig. 6-229, Fig. 6-232, Fig. 6-233, Fig. 6-235 A, Fig. 6-235 B, Fig. 6-236, Fig. 6-241, Fig. 6-243.

Finally, and most importantly, there is need to acknowledge the support and dedication of our friends and family who truly suffered along with us while we were engaged in this project. Thank you, all of you, for maintaining your continual support and giving us the help and encouragement when we needed it.

KAREN MUNSON RINGSRUD

JEAN JORGENSON LINNE

CONTENTS

Urinalysis and Body Fluids
A ColorText and Atlas

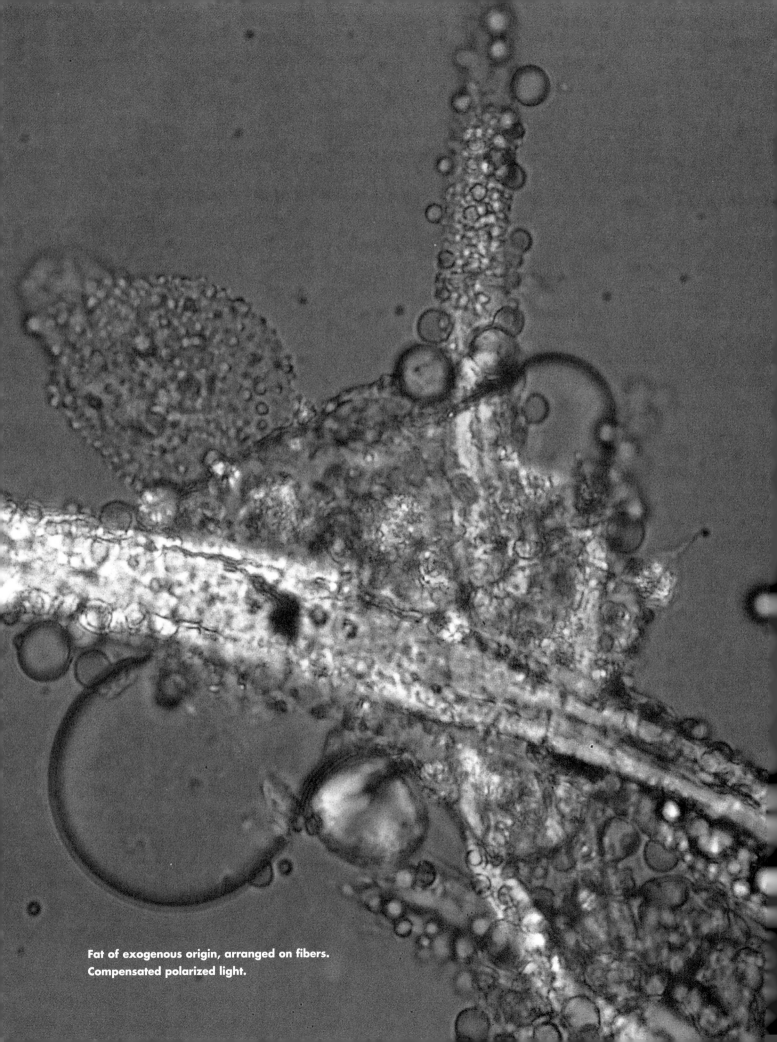

Fat of exogenous origin, arranged on fibers.
Compensated polarized light.

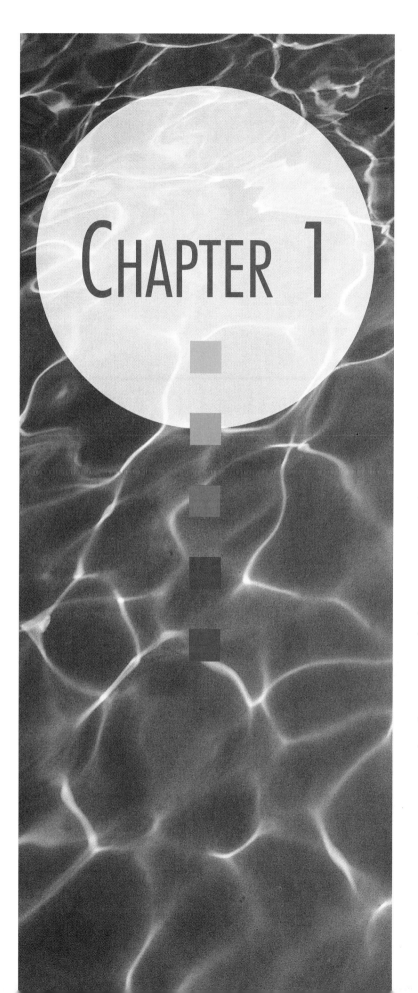

CHAPTER 1

REGULATIONS, SAFETY, AND QUALITY ASSURANCE:

STANDARDS FOR THE CLINICAL LABORATORY

CHAPTER OUTLINE

- **Federal Regulation of the Clinical Laboratory Under CLIA '88**
  Other Agencies and Organizations

- **Safety in the Clinical Laboratory**
  Safety Standards for the Clinical Laboratory
  Hazards in the Clinical Laboratory
  General Requirements and Policies for Safety of
      Personnel in the Clinical Laboratory
  First Aid
  Disposal of Laboratory Waste

- **Quality Assurance**
  Introduction
  Components of a Quality Assurance Program
  Commitment to Quality Assurance
  Facilities and Resources
  Technical Competence
  Quality Assurance Procedures
  The Quality Control Program
  Major Errors in Urine Testing

LEARNING OBJECTIVES

▶ Understand the importance of federal, state, and institutional **regulations** concerning the quality and reliability of work being done and safety of workers in the clinical laboratory.

▶ Understand the terms **OSHA, CLIA '88, HCFA, JCAHO, NCCLS, COLA,** and **CAP.**

▶ Understand the effects, significance, and purpose of **CLIA '88.**

▶ Understand the **concept of waived, moderately and highly complex test** with respect to laboratory testing.

▶ Understand **potential hazardous situations** in the laboratory workplace, including biohazards and chemical hazards.

▶ Understand **precautions to avoid exposure** to hazardous situations in the laboratory.

▶ Understand the basic aspects of **infection control policies.**

▶ Understand the appropriate use of **personal protective equipment/devices** and when to use them.

▶ Know the procedures for **workplace cleaning** and the proper procedure for **cleanup of spills** when necessary.

▶ Know the basic use of **first aid.**

▶ Understand the rationale for the separation or segregation of laboratory waste.

▶ Understand the rationale for **disposal of laboratory waste.**

▶ Understand **quality assurance (QA)** and **quality control (QC),** and how they relate to and differ from each other.

▶ List the components of a comprehensive quality assurance program.

▶ Understand the importance of quality assurance to diagnostic laboratories and patient care.

▶ Understand **proficiency testing,** how it relates to and differs from quality control, and obligations to participate in proficiency testing programs.

▶ Understand the concepts of **reliability, accuracy, precision,** and **variance** and how they relate to quality control, quality assurance, and proficiency testing.

▶ List the areas that must be monitored by an acceptable quality control program.

▶ Understand the term *quality control specimens,* and how they are to be used in the laboratory.

▶ List **10 major errors in urine testing** and understand how they relate to quality assurance.

■ INTRODUCTION

Many regulatory agencies or organizations are continually working to set standards and policies for different aspects of practice in the clinical laboratory. Many of these groups are working toward similar goals. Two primary ones are (1) ensuring that the quality of work being done in the laboratory is such that reliable results are reported to the physician treating the patient and (2) assuring the laboratory workers that the workplace is safe and healthful. Certain regulatory mandates have been issued externally, others are internal, and some are combinations of both.

Internal regulation comes from the need to ensure quality performance and reporting of results for the many laboratory tests being performed—a process of **quality assurance**. It is the responsibility of the clinical laboratory to both patient and physician to ensure that the results reported from that laboratory are reliable and to provide the physician with an estimate of what constitutes the reference range or "normal" for the analyte being measured. External standards have been set to ensure that all laboratories will provide the best, most reliable information to the physician and patient. It is to this end, primarily, that the **Clinical Laboratory Improvement Amendments of 1988** (CLIA '88) were enacted. Local, internal programs must be in place to carry out the external mandate. Internal monitoring programs are concerned with total quality management (TQM), quality assurance (QA), or continuous quality improvement (CQI)—all designed to monitor and improve the quality of services performed by the laboratory.

Externally, several federal agencies govern practices in the clinical laboratory. External regulatory agencies or organizations are primarily concerned with setting standards, conducting inspections, and imposing sanctions, when necessary. As discussed previously, standards have been set to ensure quality of results reported—quality assurance, as imposed by CLIA '88 administered by the **Health Care Financing Administration (HCFA)**.

From an external source, guidelines and standards also have been set governing safe work practices in the clinical laboratory. Through labor laws and environmental regulations, assurance has been given to laboratory workers that they are in a safe atmosphere and that every precaution has been taken to maintain that safe atmosphere. The **Occupational Safety and Health Administration (OSHA)** has been involved in setting these practices into motion, and it is through OSHA that the mandates have come to be a part of the daily life of the laboratory workplace. Other external controls include standards mandated by public health laws and reporting requirements via the **Centers for**

Disease Control and Prevention (CDC) via certification and licensure requirements issued by the **Food and Drug Administration (FDA)**. State regulations are imposed by Medicaid agencies, state environmental laws and state-specific public health laws, and licensure laws. Local regulations include those determined by building codes and fire prevention codes.

Independent agencies also influence practices in the clinical laboratory through accreditation policies or other responsibilites. These include groups such as the **College of American Pathologists (CAP)**, the **Joint Commission for the Accreditation of Healthcare Organizations (JCAHO)**, and other specific proficiency testing programs.

■ FEDERAL REGULATION OF THE CLINICAL LABORATORY UNDER CLIA '88

Regulation of clinical laboratories in general began at about the same time as the Medicare law in 1965. Since then, the federal government has been moving closer to regulating all types of clinical laboratories, from larger hospital and reference laboratories engaging in interstate commerce to **physician office laboratories (POLs)**. Until 1988, regulation applied only to hospitals and independent laboratories under the **Clinical Laboratory Improvement Act of 1967 (CLIA '67)**. This act provided for licensing of laboratories that tested specimens from across state lines (interstate commerce). In addition, Medicare law provided for inspection and accreditation of laboratories (hospital and independent) that performed tests on and billed for reimbursement of Medicare patients. These two laws generally did not apply to smaller laboratories, such as physician office laboratories.

On Oct. 31, 1988, Congress passed the **Clinical Improvement Amendments of 1988 (CLIA '88)** in response to a series of newspaper articles about poor PAP smear testing in the Washington, DC, area. As a result of CLIA '88, any entity that performs testing on material derived from humans for the purpose of diagnosis, assessment, or treatment is subject to federal regulation. Proposed regulations implementing CLIA '88 were published May 21, 1990. These were met with more than 60,000 comments and protests. On Feb. 28, 1992, the Secretary of the Department of Health and Human Services (HHS) published the final rules implementing CLIA '88. These regulations replaced the Medicare, Medicaid, and CLIA '67 standards and apply to almost all laboratory testing of human specimens. The administration of CLIA '88 is through the Health Care Financing Administration (HCFA), a division of the United States Department of Health and Human Services (HHS).

The regulations set standards for laboratory personnel, quality assurance and quality control, and proficiency testing, based on test complexity and risk factors. In addition, the regulations establish application procedures and fees for CLIA certification, plus enforcement procedures and sanctions if laboratories fail to meet standards. The regulations were generally effective (implemented) Sept. 1, 1992, although some parts of the regulations were effective at a later date, and modifications are ongoing. Although an important component of quality assurance, enrollment by previously unregulated laboratories in a proficiency testing program could be delayed until Jan. 1, 1994.

According to federal law, under CLIA '88, a laboratory is now defined as ". . . a facility for the biological, microbiological, serological, chemical, immunohematological, hematological, biophysical, cytological, pathological, or other examination of materials derived from the human body for the purpose of providing information for the diagnosis, prevention, or treatment of any disease or impairment of, or the assessment of the health of human beings." This means that virtually any entity that does laboratory testing on any person is included: hospital, independent and physician office laboratories, plus pharmacies, chiropractors, shopping mall health fairs, fitness centers, and weight reduction centers.

CLIA regulations divide laboratory tests into three groups based on "complexity" of the test. These are **waived, moderately complex,** and **highly complex.** Laboratories performing only waived tests must obtain a certificate of waiver. Laboratories performing moderately and/or highly complex tests must obtain a certificate of registration. Most tests are classified as moderately complex. An additional category, **physician performed microscopies (PPMs),** was added Jan. 19, 1993, for six specific microscopies (wet mounts) performed by a physician on his or her own patients. The federal government categorized tests based on the analyte tested and the method or instrumentation used to perform the test. As such, reagent strip or tablet urine tests are categorized as **waived tests** when results are read visually, but as moderately complex when results are read by instrumentation. The microscopic analysis of the urine sediment is categorized as a moderately complex test, unless performed by a physician (PPM).

Other Agencies and Organizations

Other agencies that regulate clinical laboratories and private accrediting organizations include the following:

The Occupational Safety and Health Administration (OSHA)
The Environmental Protection Agency (EPA)
The Food and Drug Administration (FDA)
State agencies

The College of American Pathologists (CAP)
The Commission on Office Laboratory Accreditation (COLA)
The Joint Commission for the Accreditation of Healthcare Organizations (JCAHO)
The National Committee for Clinical Laboratory Standards (NCCLS)

The Commission on Office Laboratory Accreditation (COLA). As of Dec. 29, 1993 HCFA approved the accreditation program developed by COLA for the physician office laboratory. This means that COLA accreditation requirements are recognized by HCFA as equivalent to those established by CLIA. The COLA accreditation established a peer-review option in place of the CLIA regulatory requirements. COLA-accredited laboratories are surveyed every 2 years to see that they meet requirements developed by their peers in family practice, internal medicine, or pathology.

The National Committee for Clinical Laboratory Standards (NCCLS). NCCLS is a nonprofit, educational organization created for the development, promotion, and use of national and international laboratory standards. It was founded in 1968 and accredited by the American National Standards Institute. It employs the use of voluntary consensus standards, which are intended to maintain the performance of the clinical laboratory at a high level necessary for quality patient care. Participants include individual laboratories, laboratory professional associations, industries, and agencies of the federal and state governments. NCCLS guidelines and standards are cited throughout this text when applicable.

■ SAFETY IN THE CLINICAL LABORATORY

Safety Standards for the Clinical Laboratory

Standards for regulation of the safety of workers in clinical laboratories are initiated, governed, and reviewed by several agencies or committees. Some of these are governmental agencies; others are educational or professional organizations. Examples are the U.S. Department of Labor's **Occupational Safety and Health Administration (OSHA),** the **Clinical Laboratory Improvement Amendments of 1988 (CLIA '88)—** regulated by the **Health Care Financing Administration (HCFA)**—the **National Committee for Clinical Laboratory Standards (NCCLS),** the **Centers for Disease Control and Prevention (CDC),** and the **College of American Pathologists (CAP).**

Standards have been designed on the federal, state, and local levels. The regulations and standards are designed specifically to protect people working in the laboratory, other healthcare personnel, patients being treated in the healthcare facility, and society as a whole. Federal regulations exist to meet these objectives. Many of the factors governing the standards and their resulting regulations are associated with laboratory-acquired infections or accidents involving hazards in the workplace. Noncompliance with the OSHA regulations, in particular, results in costly fines to the institution, as well as potential costly accidents to people working there.

In accordance with the **Americans with Disabilities Act**, specific plans should be developed that enable any known disabled laboratory personnel to work in a safe atmosphere.

Occupational Safety and Health Administration. The **Occupational Safety and Health Act** of 1970 created a system of safeguards and regulations to ensure that workers have a safe and healthful working environment. The **Occupational Safety and Health Administration (OSHA)**, under the direction of the U.S. Department of Labor, regulates all businesses with one or more employees, health care facilities included. The regulations deal with many aspects of safety and health protection, including compliance arrangements, inspection procedures, penalties for noncompliance, complaint procedures, duties and responsibilities for administration and operation of the system, and how the standards are set. The responsibility for compliance is placed on both the institution and the employee.

OSHA standards, where appropriate, include provisions for warning labels or other appropriate forms of warning to alert all workers of potential hazards, availability of suitable personal protective equipment, procedures for exposure control, and implementation of training and education programs. Two OSHA standards, one on bloodborne pathogens and the other on hazard communication, have the primary purpose of ensuring a safe and healthful working atmosphere for every American worker.

The **OSHA hazard communication standard**, issued in 1990, is designed to ensure that all laboratory workers are fully aware of possible hazardous situations present in their workplace that might be detrimental to their safety and well-being. With this standard in place, occupational exposures to hazardous chemicals should be minimized if the program is implemented according to its intent—a chemical hygiene plan must be in place for each laboratory site. This OSHA standard is also known as the employee "right to know" rule.

The **standard on exposure to bloodborne pathogens**, the final OSHA standard, was issued in late 1991 and declared that healthcare workers face a significant health risk in their workplace if their work is associated with the reasonable possibility of exposure to bloodborne pathogens. This final standard is called "Occupational Exposure to Bloodborne Pathogens." It was published in the Federal Register and combines

controls in engineering, general work practices, personal protective clothing and equipment, training and education of healthcare personnel, Hepatitis B vaccination of healthcare workers, and the use of warning signs and labels. The OSHA standard mandates the use of the **universal precautions** guidelines that had been recommended by the Centers for Disease Control and Prevention since 1987 (see under infection control). CLIA '88 regulations require that laboratories comply with national safety standards and practices.

SAFETY MANUAL. OSHA requires that each laboratory have a readily available safety manual that includes all safety practices and precautions. The manual must be frequently updated with additional or new information as it becomes available. Safety practices for the use and handling of all potentially hazardous chemicals, infectious materials, or equipment must be included, as well as current regulations concerning anything that might pose a potential safety hazard for persons working in the laboratory. It also must contain clear instructions about disposal of laboratory hazardous waste, directions for clean up of laboratory spills (blood or other body fluids), as well as information about safe work practices in general. All persons working in the laboratory must be familiar with the contents of the safety manual, through an ongoing educational program or systematic review process.

Hazards in the Clinical Laboratory

The person who understands the potential hazards in a given laboratory setting can usually take the necessary precautions to prevent most laboratory-related accidents. As emphasized by the scope of OSHA's final standard of 1991, there are unique problems in the clinical laboratory setting with respect to potential safety hazards, especially biological hazards. Other hazards can be chemical, fire- and/or explosion-related, electrical, or punctures and lacerations from glassware or blood/specimen collection equipment. Diseases or accidents associated with preventable causes are simply not acceptable. A safety program is required in every clinical laboratory, and identification of potential hazards is an important part of any such program.

Biological Hazards. A **biological hazard**, or **biohazard**, is a potential risk to the health of persons working in the area from contact, either directly or through the environment, with an infectious material or agent. The word or symbol for biohazard is posted throughout the laboratory to denote these potentially infectious agents (Fig. 1-1). Labels with the biohazard symbols are to be fluorescent orange or orange-red with the letters "biohazard" or the biohazard symbol in a contrasting color. Biological infections are frequently caused by accidental aspiration of infectious material, accidental inoculation with contaminated

Figure 1-1

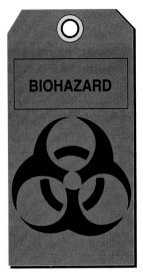

Biohazard symbol. (From Linne JJ, and Ringsrud KM: *Basic techniques in clinical laboratory science*, ed 3, St. Louis, 1992, Mosby, p 5.)

needles or syringes, sprays from syringes, aerosols from uncapping specimen containers, and centrifuge accidents. Cuts or scratches from contaminated glassware, cuts from laboratory instruments, and spilling or spattering of pathogenic samples on the workdesk or floors also can result in work-related infections if proper biohazard controls are not in place.

INFECTION CONTROL. One important aspect of biohazard control programs is that of **infection control.** Clinical specimens from patients present a potential hazard to laboratory personnel because of the infectious agents they might contain. Protection from **specimen-borne (bloodborne) pathogens** is of major importance. The Centers for Disease Control and Prevention (CDC) has recommended safety precautions for the handling of all patient specimens since 1987. These are known as **universal precautions (or universal blood and body fluid precautions)** and are published in the *Morbidity and Mortality Weekly Report (MMWR).* Universal precautions are a series of recommendations from the CDC to protect healthcare workers and others from acquiring infection with bloodborne pathogens. The final OSHA standards have made these recommendations mandatory. The National Committee for Clinical Laboratory Standards (NCCLS) has also issued guidelines for laboratory workers to offer protection from bloodborne diseases spread through contact with patient specimens.

The various agencies and committees are working to lessen the risk of exposure for healthcare workers to specimen-borne pathogens. Under OSHA, standards of practice have been developed to ensure the safety of people working in areas where patient specimens are being used. The CDC has issued guidelines for the implementation of these standards. The College of American Pathologists offers a voluntary accreditation program for clinical laboratories. The requirements include safe work practices, which in turn, include the implementation of safety measures to protect from exposure to biological hazards.

UNIVERSAL PRECAUTIONS. The term **universal precautions** designates a system of infectious disease control that assumes every direct contact with body fluids from any patient is potentially infectious. Controls include the use of **personal protective equipment (PPE)** or devices (such as specialized clothing or barriers worn for protection against a hazard), good work practices (altering the manner in which a task is performed to reduce exposure to a hazard), and the proper implementation of engineering controls (including practices that isolate or remove the bloodborne or specimen-borne hazards, such as sharps disposal containers or self-sheathing needles).

The policy requires that every employee exposed to direct contact with body fluids be protected as though such body fluids were infected with the most pathogenic of organisms, such as hepatitis B virus (HBV) or human immunodeficiency virus (HIV). Universal precautions are based on the recognition that different types of specimens carry different levels of risk, and that different types of exposure lead to different levels of risk.

Blood is the single most important source of possible transmission of HBV and HIV, but other body secretions such as semen and vaginal fluids can contain the viruses and transmissible agents, and can spread other diseases. Tissues, cerebrospinal fluid, synovial fluid, peritoneal fluid, or amniotic fluid all convey a risk of possible viral transmission. At the time of this writing, handling urine, feces, nasal secretions, sputum, saliva, sweat, tears, or vomitus specimens has not been implicated in the transmission of HIV, unless the specimens are bloody. Since not all patients carrying bloodborne pathogens are identified before the handling of their specimens, all persons handling patient specimens or who come in contact with patients in a healthcare setting must routinely exercise certain consistent precautions. The essence of any universal precaution policy is to **avoid direct contact with patient specimens in general.** These precautions recognize the infectious potential of any patient specimen. When contact with any patient specimen is anticipated, healthcare workers should use the appropriate barrier precautions to prevent cross-contamination and exposure of their own skin and mucous membranes to the potentially infected specimen.

Hepatitis B vaccine and the vaccination series of injections must be made available free of charge to any employee who has the likelihood of occupational exposure to blood or any other potentially HBV-infected material. Any worker involved in an accidental exposure to a potential pathogenic organism must be evaluated medically for any history, signs, or symptoms consistent with the concerned pathogen. Prompt medical attention is extremely important. The exposed worker must be advised of and alerted to the risks of infection from the pathogen involved.

SAFE WORK PRACTICES. Using techniques to reduce the likelihood of exposure to hazardous substances is included in the implementation of safe work practices. In this category is **handwashing**. Washing the hands frequently with soap and water is one of the most important ways of preventing transmission of most infectious agents. Use of **personal protective equipment** (PPE) is mandated by OSHA to provide laboratory personnel with safer working conditions. Protective equipment includes **barrier protection**, along with protective devices to prevent exposure to possible blood-borne pathogens. If compliance is strictly maintained, barrier protective devices will prevent the transmission of most infectious diseases. Protective clothing such as gloves, gowns, and masks are to be provided and maintained in a sanitary and reliable condition.

HANDWASHING. Handwashing interrupts the transmission of most infectious pathogens. Immediately after accidental exposure with blood, body fluids, or tissues, hands or other skin areas must be thoroughly washed. If the contact occurs through breaks in gloves, the gloves must be removed immediately and the hands thoroughly washed according to the established procedure for the laboratory. It is also good practice to wash the hands any time there is visible contamination with any body fluid specimen, after completion of laboratory work, and before leaving the laboratory, after removing gloves, and before any activities that involve contact with mucous membranes, eyes, or breaks in the skin.

Washing with soap and water is recommended (**Procedure 1-1**). Any standard detergent product acceptable to personnel may be used. No additional benefit has been seen from the use of antiseptic soaps or solutions and any product that disrupts the integrity of the skin should be avoided. Frequent skin washing is necessary, so the use of moisturizing creams or lotions should be considered to reduce skin irritation.

GLOVES. Protective gloves must be worn by all persons who engage in procedures that involve direct contact of skin with biological specimens. The implementation of universal precautions is recommended for handling all clinical specimens. Gloves must be manufactured from appropriate materials, usually intact latex or intact vinyl. The appropriate quantity of gloves in the correct sizes must be available for all persons working in the area where the patient specimens are directly handled. Since barrier protection is the goal, gloves must be discarded if they are peeling, cracking, or discolored (indicators of deterioration), or if they have tears or punctures. Proper discard of gloves into biohazard discard containers is necessary. After gloves are removed, hands must be immediately washed with soap and water.

Gloves must also be worn to protect the hands and arms from thermal burns or cuts resulting from exposure to chemicals where absorption through the skin or reaction with the surface of the skin may occur. Gloves are also required when working with any particularly hazardous substance to avoid possible transfer from hand to mouth.

GOWNS AND MASKS (INCLUDING EYE PROTECTION). Laboratory personnel should wear a long-sleeved laboratory coat or gown with a closed front while working in the laboratory. These gowns should be removed when the worker leaves the laboratory. Special protective apparel can be worn when splashes from biological specimens are likely to occur. These protective gowns or aprons must be manufactured from fluid-proof or fluid-resistant material and should protect all areas of exposed skin.

Procedure 1-1

HANDWASHING

1. Wet both hands and wrists with warm water only; do not use very hot or very cold water.

2. Apply soap from a dispenser to the palms first (about 1 teaspoonful).

3. Lather well and wash hands and wrists, fingernails, and between the fingers. Do this for a minimum of 5 seconds.

4. Rinse well with warm water and dry completely.

5. If the sink being used is not equipped with foot or knee-operated controls, use a paper towel to turn off hand faucets to avoid recontamination of clean hands.

When contamination of mucosal membranes (mouth, eyes, or nose) is likely to occur, the use of masks and protective eyewear or face shields is required. This contamination can occur with body fluid splashes or aerosolization. Eye protection is required when any potential exposure to physical, biological, or chemical hazards is possible. Side shields on safety glasses provide some protection against splashes or flying particles, but the use of safety goggles or face shields is recommended when there is a greater chance of potential damage to the eyes.

If there has been an acid or alkali splash to the eyes, the affected eye (or eyes) must be washed thoroughly with running water for a minimum of 15 minutes. It is important to assist the victim by holding the eyelid open so that the water can make contact with the eye. An eye fountain is recommended, but any running water will suffice. While the eye is being washed, a physician should be notified.

SPECIMEN PROCESSING PROTECTION. Specially constructed plastic splash shields are used for the processing of biological specimens. Tube and container tops are removed behind or under the protection of the shield, which acts as a barrier between the person and the specimen container with potentially infectious contents. This prevents aerosols from entering the nose, eyes, or mouth. Splash shields must be periodically decontaminated.

Tube or container caps should always be kept on when centrifuging specimens. Centrifuge covers must be used and left on until the centrifuge has come to a complete stop. The centrifuge should be allowed to stop by itself and not be manually stopped.

DECONTAMINATION. The laboratory workplace must be kept clean and sanitary. Cleaning and disinfecting the working surfaces after contact with blood or other potentially infectious body fluids is of primary importance. Spilled fluids should be absorbed as completely as possible with disposable towels or other absorbent material before actual disinfection. The materials used to absorb the spill must be discarded as biohazardous waste. After absorption, the spill site should be cleaned with an aqueous detergent solution and then disinfected with an approved hospital disinfectant such as a dilution of household bleach—sodium hypochlorite.

Sodium hypochlorite is often used as an intermediate-level disinfectant. Undiluted bleach is a 5.25% solution. A dilution of the bleach—an approximate 1% solution made from the 5% solution (1 part sodium hypochlorite and 4 parts water), a 1:5 solution, or as an alternate, a 1:10 solution—should be made up fresh weekly to ensure that it maintains its germicidal activity. Prolonged storage can reduce the activity of the disinfectant. A strong solution of bleach can be used for spills of biological solutions. Daily cleaning of the work area can be done using a dilute solution of

bleach. When a spill has occurred, the spill site should be flooded with the disinfectant solution using an ample amount—enough so the surface "glistens." The solution should be left on the site for a period of time; 20 minutes is usually long enough for most average spills. The disinfectant solution should then be absorbed with disposable toweling or other absorbent material, the site rinsed well with water to remove noxious chemicals or odors, and allowed to dry. All materials used in the cleanup process must be properly discarded into a biohazardous waste container.

Chemical Hazards. Many **chemical hazards** are present in the clinical laboratory. Poisonous, caustic, volatile, or corrosive chemicals are used in various assays or are constituents of reagents used in the assays. Good work practice minimizes all chemical exposures because few laboratory chemicals are without some hazardous components. Chemicals and reagents can present different kinds of hazards. Some are dangerous when inhaled (sulfuric acid), some are corrosive to the skin (phenol), some are caustic (acetic acid), some are volatile (many solvents), and some offer a combination of hazards. Proper storage of all chemicals and reagents is necessary. All reagents and chemicals must be properly labeled.

HAZARD IDENTIFICATION SYSTEM. The system, developed by the National Fire Protection Association, provides, at a glance, information on the presence of potential health, flammability, and chemical reactivity for potential hazards from materials used in the laboratory. The identification uses symbols, colors, and words on a special label provided on all containers for hazardous chemicals (such as on reagent storage cabinets or refrigerators) (see Fig. 1-2).

The identification system consists of four diamond-shaped symbols grouped into a larger diamond shape (Fig. 1-2). The top diamond is red and indicates a flammability hazard. The diamond on the left is blue and indicates a possible health hazard. The diamond on the right is yellow and indicates a reactivity-stability hazard. The diamond on the bottom is white and indicates specific unique hazard information such as radioactivity, specific biological hazards, or other potentially dangerous elements. The identification system also uses a numbering designation from 4 to 0, in which 4 is extremely dangerous and 0 is considered no hazard.

RIGHT TO KNOW RULE/CHEMICAL HYGIENE PLAN. OSHA is also involved in setting standards for minimizing occupational exposure to hazardous chemicals in the workplace. The OSHA hazard communication standard, the employee "right to know" rule, is designed to ensure that all laboratory workers are fully aware of possible hazardous workplace situations that might be detrimental to their safety and well-being. The **"right to know" rule** is also included in the CLIA '88 regulations.

Figure 1-2

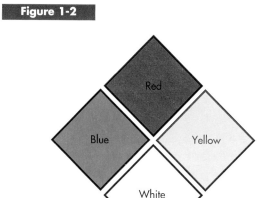

Identification system of the National Fire Protection Association. (From Bauer JD: *Clinical laboratory methods*, ed 9, St. Louis, 1982, Mosby, p 19.)

A chemical hygiene plan for each laboratory must be in place to inform workers and carry out implementation of safety practices necessary to protect workers from any chemical health hazards. Laboratory workers must not be exposed to substances in excess of the permissible exposure limits (PEL). Any worker who uses hazardous chemicals must be informed about the potential hazards and be given the proper information about protective practices to employ in their use. OSHA has designated "permissible exposure limits" or "action levels" for many of the chemicals used in the clinical laboratory. **Action levels** are exposures below the permissible exposure limit that still require certain actions take place. These actions require that medical surveillance or monitoring of the workplace be done under specific conditions.

For hazardous chemical spills, the area should be evacuated and secured, the supervisor notified, and the spill evaluated. The pertinent **Material Safety Data Sheets** must be consulted for proper handling of the spill or for any chemical cleanup needed (see under Material Safety Data Sheets).

The individual states also have enacted "right to know" laws to ensure that available information is disseminated at the local level.

Measures to limit exposures to hazardous chemicals must be implemented. Appropriate work practices, emergency procedures, and use of personal protective equipment are to be employed by all persons in the laboratory. Many of these measures are the same as described for protection from biological hazards— gloves, eye protection (see under Biological Hazards, Safe Work Practices).

Other protective devices include the use of fume hoods, respiratory equipment, eye protection, and eye-washing devices. Keeping the work area clean and uncluttered, labeling all chemicals and reagents properly and completely, and managing disposing of hazardous chemical waste in appropriately labeled receptacles are all important in preventing accidental exposures to workplace hazards.

Containment devices, such as glove boxes or gas cabinets, may be required when the standard fume hood does not provide adequate assurance that overexposure to a hazardous chemical will not occur. Ventilated chemical storage cabinets or rooms should be used when the chemicals being stored generate toxic, flammable, or irritating levels of airborne contamination.

The chemical hygiene plan for a clinical laboratory mandates that the healthcare facility provide any person working with hazardous chemicals the opportunity to receive medical attention, including any follow-up examinations that the examining physician determines to be necessary, when the exposure to the hazardous chemical (a spill, leak, or other occurrence) has occurred as a result of working in the laboratory. Information about signs and symptoms associated with exposures to hazardous chemicals used in the laboratory must be communicated and be accessible to all persons in the workplace. One source of information about hazardous chemicals are material safety data sheets (MSDS).

MATERIAL SAFETY DATA SHEETS (MSDS). OSHA requires information be provided by all chemical manufacturers and suppliers about each chemical. This information must accompany the shipment of all chemicals and should be available for anyone to review. Each laboratory must have available all MSDSs for the hazardous chemicals used in the laboratory. The health care facility, in turn, is required to provide the information to its personnel working with the chemicals.

Each material safety data sheet contains basic information about the specific chemical or product. Trade name, chemical name and synonyms, chemical family, manufacturer's name and address, emergency telephone number for further information about the chemical, hazardous ingredients, physical data, fire and explosion data, and health hazard and protection information are to be included for each chemical.

Electrical Hazards. Electrical equipment used in the clinical laboratory can be a source of injury if one is not aware of the potential hazard. All electrical instruments must be grounded. Electrical current will flow when a difference in potential exists between two points. This knowledge is used in determining the approach to safety in the use of electrical equipment. Grounding all electrical equipment is essential. Serious injury can result if there is no path to ground and if such a path can be established through the person contacting the apparatus. Serious shocks or burns can result from an electrical apparatus not handled properly. Do not attempt to directly touch a victim who is still in contact with an electrical current. The rescuer also will become part of the circuit and may be electrocuted. Medical assistance should be summoned while first aid is being administered.

Fire Hazards. Various types of fire-extinguishing agents must be available for fire hazards. Their proper use must be understood by all persons in the workplace. Fire in clothing must be smothered with a fire blanket or heavy toweling, or the flame should be beaten out; it should not be flooded with water. The correct use of the fire alarm and its location must be known by all. The specific procedure devised by the healthcare facility to be used in case of fire must be understood and practiced through drills and ongoing educational sessions.

First aid for heat burns includes applying cold running water to relieve the pain and to stop further tissue damage, using a wet dressing of 2 tablespoons of sodium bicarbonate in 1 quart of warm water, and bandaging the burned area securely, but not tightly. If it is a third-degree burn—the skin is burned off—do not use ointment or grease; consult a physician immediately.

Glassware Hazards. The use of many kinds of glassware is the source of another potential laboratory hazard—cuts or lacerations because of accidental handling of broken glassware. Caution must be taken to prevent unnecessary or accidental breakage of glassware. Any broken or cracked glassware must be discarded in a container for sharps to prevent custodial or other personnel from being injured accidentally when disposing of laboratory waste. Common sense should be used when storing glassware, placing heavier pieces on lower shelves and taller pieces behind shorter, smaller pieces. Laboratory shelves should be placed at reasonable heights; glassware must not be stored out of reach. Lacerations or cuts from broken glassware must be tended to without delay. Minor cuts should be carefully and thoroughly washed with soap and water. All foreign material should be removed from the wound and a clean bandage applied, if necessary. Bleeding from serious cuts should be stopped by application of direct pressure to the cut area, using the hand over a clean compress covering the wound. A physician should be consulted immediately.

General Requirements and Policies for Safety of Personnel in the Laboratory

The purpose of the many safety regulations and recommendations described is to protect the people working in the laboratory, as well as other healthcare personnel and patients in the facility. The great variety of potential hazards present in the clinical laboratory already have been discussed. A thorough understanding of the various specific potential hazards must be instilled in each person working in the area. There are, however, some general practices/policies that must be included in any laboratory's safety program.

1. Everyone in the laboratory must comply with the laboratory safety policies and procedures.
2. Smoking, eating, and drinking are not permitted in the laboratory area.
3. Food must not be stored in laboratory refrigerators or any other laboratory area where potential infectious, chemical, or hazardous possibilities exist. Refrigerators designated for food must be available in a "clean room" such as a storage area or lounge.
4. Application of cosmetics in the laboratory work area is not permitted.
5. Contact lenses are discouraged for laboratory work. Lenses should never be inserted while in the laboratory. If a spill or splash occurs to someone wearing contact lenses, the eyes should be flushed with water immediately and the lenses removed, even if irritation is not evident initially.
6. Eye and face protection are important. Safety glasses or goggles should be worn routinely while working in the laboratory.
7. Clothing policies will vary from laboratory to laboratory. Generally, laboratory coats worn in the laboratory are to be removed when leaving the laboratory.
8. Shoes with closed toes must be worn in laboratories and in patient areas.
9. Personal articles such as glasses, purses, or articles of clothing must not be placed on work surfaces where infectious materials are handled.
10. Pens and pencils used in the laboratory must be left in the laboratory. They should not be put to the face, into the mouth, or behind the ear.
11. Hair must be worn in a style that does not impair vision, cause distractions, or come in contact with work surfaces, flames, moving equipment, or contaminate sterile working areas or specimens.
12. Long beards on men should also be styled to avoid the same hazards as listed in No. 11 above.
13. Handwashing must be done frequently during the day—after accidental exposure to any hazardous substance, after removing gloves, or before leaving the laboratory.
14. Cuts or lacerations on hands must be bandaged, before gloves are put on.
15. Mouth pipetting is prohibited. Pipetting devices must be available to all laboratory workers for any pipetting task.

16. Glassware requires special precautions: broken glassware must not be used and must be discarded into specific containers for broken glass or sharps, broken glassware must be cleaned up carefully to prevent injury to personnel and to prevent spread of contamination—a brush and/or forceps and dustpan is recommended—and heated glassware should be handled with a heat-resistant nonasbestos glove.

17. Step stools must be used to reach items on shelves and other hard-to-reach places; chairs should not be used as step stools.

18. Centrifuges must not be operated without being covered and latched. All tubes of specimens should be covered during the centrifugation process. The centrifuge's interior surfaces should be disinfected at least weekly with a phenolic detergent solution and must be cleaned and disinfected immediately if a breakage or a spill occurs.

19. Exits and aisles must not be obstructed by equipment, chairs, supplies, or trash. Exit doors must not be blocked, locked, or obstructed in any way. The doors to the laboratory should be kept closed.

20. All equipment must be used following the instructions of the manufacturer for safe operation. Anytime a piece of laboratory equipment must be moved to another location—sent out to be repaired or moved to another laboratory area—it must be decontaminated first. Equipment that cannot be decontaminated must be labeled with a biohazard label.

First Aid

Since there are so many potential hazards in a clinical laboratory, any educational program for workers must include a basic understanding of **first aid** procedures. Each facility will have its own specific protocol to follow. The first emphasis must be to remove the victim of the accident from further possible injury. The next step is to take definitive action to begin first aid to the victim. By definition, *first aid* is "the immediate care given to a person who has been injured or suddenly taken ill." First aid is only a stopgap—emergency treatment to be followed until the physician arrives: stop bleeding, prevent shock, and then treat the wound, in that order. Application of the proper first aid procedures is most critical and should be understood by all in the workplace.

In the event of a serious laboratory accident such as a burn, medical assistance should be summoned while first aid is being administered. For general, less serious accidents, competent medical assistance should be sought as soon as possible after first aid treatment has been completed. In many instances, fast reactions are essential, especially so in the case of chemical or physical injury to the eyes.

Disposal of Laboratory Waste

Standards from OSHA provide for a laboratory waste management program. The proper techniques to use are directed by the OSHA guidelines. The Environmental Protection Agency also has regulations pertaining to the management of laboratory waste. The purpose of any waste disposal program is to confine or isolate any possible hazardous material from laboratory personnel and custodial and housekeeping personnel.

Containers for laboratory waste should always be easily accessible to persons needing them and located in areas where they are commonly used. They should be constructed so that their contents will not be spilled if the container is tipped over accidentally. The containers used for collection of laboratory waste should be manufactured from leakproof materials and be maintained in a clean and sanitary condition.

Waste should be separated into categories by specific type. Types will vary as to their potential hazard to others. Waste separation, or segregation, can be by paper and domestic waste, hazardous nonchemical solid waste (sharps, glass, needles), biohazardous waste (infectious or potentially infectious specimens, blood-contaminated products, or microbiologic cultures), and chemical waste (by-products of laboratory diagnostic reactions or drainage from equipment). Paper and domestic waste can be placed into the local trash disposal containers and buried in a landfill or incinerated as local policy dictates. Materials normally excreted by patients (for example, urine and feces) can be disposed of into the sewer system of the facility.

Disposal of medical waste should be done by licensed organizations that can ensure that no environmental damage or anything aesthetically displeasing is done. The Environmental Protection Agency carries on a continuing process to ensure that this is done in the most prudent fashion.

Infectious/Biohazardous Waste. **Infectious** or **biohazardous** waste products include blood or other body fluid specimens containing potentially pathogenic organisms. Elimination of organisms is by incineration or autoclaving. Other infectious waste such as contaminated gloves, gowns, specimen containers, slides, and other equipment must be incinerated or first decontaminated and then handled as domestic waste. Infectious waste must be packaged for disposal in color-coded containers labeled with the universal biohazard symbol. Red bags or red containers may be substituted for labels. Cultures of infectious agents may be autoclaved and then discarded as domestic waste.

SHARPS CONTAINERS. Contaminated **sharps** (needles, glassware, or other sharp items) must be placed in a closable, puncture-resistant, labeled, or red color-coded container; the container must be leak-proof on the sides and bottom. These precautions are necessary to prevent accidental injuries to persons using and handling the containers. The purpose of these containers is to provide a quick, convenient, safe place for the disposal of all needles or other sharps without having to look for a place to put them. They must be located in all patient areas and throughout the laboratory where they may be needed. Use of sharps containers permits quick disposal without having to recap or resheath the needle. This supports the recommendations against recapping, bending, breaking, or otherwise handling any sharp needle or lancet-device by hand. If a needle does need recapping, it should be done using one hand, with one hand held behind the back to prevent needle-stick accidents. The sharps containers are incinerated or autoclaved and sent to a landfill, depending on local regulations.

■ QUALITY ASSURANCE

Introduction

Quality assurance (QA) is a continuing process that includes all aspects of the laboratory (technical and nontechnical) to prevent errors and ensure accuracy of test results. It applies to the management and treatment of the whole patient. Quality control (QC) is only part of many elements in a quality assurance program. These include preanalytical (patient preparation and specimen acquisition), analytical (test analysis or examination), and postanalytical (test result reporting) factors. Quality assurance includes the interaction and responsibility between the laboratory and patients, physicians, and other departments of the organization. Quality assurance includes evaluation, monitoring, documentation, and communication to remove obstacles to quality patient testing.

As described in the College of American Pathologists' *Physician Office Laboratory Policy and Procedure Manual*, "All laboratories must have a quality assurance program with the proper documentation defining the goals of the program, the procedures necessary to achieve the goals, and specific records showing that procedures have been carried out. A comprehensive quality assurance program must be designed to monitor and evaluate the ongoing and overall quality of the total testing process (preanalytic, analytic, and postanalytic). The laboratory's quality assurance program must evaluate the effectiveness of its policies and procedures; identify and correct problems; assure the accurate, reliable, and prompt reporting of test results; and assure the adequacy and competency of the staff."[2] All quality assurance activities must be documented according to CLIA regulations.

Components of a Quality Assurance Program

According to the College of American Pathologists, a comprehensive quality assurance program should include the following components:
  Patient test management
  Procedure manuals
  Quality control assessment
  Proficiency testing
  Comparison of test results
  Relationship of patient information to test results
  Personnel assessment
  Communications
  Complaint investigations
  Quality assurance review with staff
  Quality assurance records

Commitment to Quality Assurance

It is essential that all persons working in the clinical laboratory be committed to the concepts of the quality assurance process as it is defined by their institution. The importance of sufficient planning time dedicated to the topic of quality assurance and the priority given to attention to the program implemented in the total laboratory operation is critical. All persons working in the clinical laboratory must be willing to work together to make quality patient service their top priority. Quality assurance should be appreciated as a tool to ensure reported results are of the highest quality. It is not a system meant to check up on the laboratory staff but a means of giving self-confidence to the persons performing tests. Because the total laboratory staff must be involved in carrying out any quality assurance process, it is important to develop a comprehensive program to include all levels of laboratorians.

Facilities and Resources

The physical location and layout of the laboratory is an important aspect of quality assurance. It is vital that the physical laboratory site be conducive to good performance by the persons working there. A safe working site with adequate, properly maintained equipment and supplies is essential to ensure quality results (see also under Safety in the Clinical Laboratory).

Technical Competence

Competence of personnel is an important determinant of the quality of the laboratory result. Crucial to any quality assurance process is the maintenance of high-level performance by the persons doing the analyses. Only well-trained, competent personnel should be carrying out the testing processes. Competent laboratory personnel also must be able to perform quality control activities, maintain instruments, and keep accurate and systematic records of reagents and control specimens, equipment maintenance, and patient and analytic data. For new laboratory personnel, a thorough orientation to the laboratory procedures and policies is vital.

Periodic opportunities for personal upgrading of technical skills and for obtaining new relevant information should be made available to all persons working in the laboratory. This can be accomplished through in-service training classes, opportunities to attend continuing education courses, and by encouraging independent study of scientific journals and audiovisual materials.

Personnel performance should be monitored with periodic evaluations and reports. Quality assurance demands that the results of daily work be monitored by a supervisor and that all analytic reports produced during a particular shift be evaluated for errors and omissions. Quality control measures (one aspect of quality assurance) are used to monitor possible human error in performing laboratory analyses.

Quality Assurance Procedures

Quality assurance programs monitor test requesting procedures, patient identification, specimen procurement, and labeling; specimen transportation and processing procedures; laboratory personnel performance; laboratory instrumentation, reagents, and analytic test procedures; turnaround times; and accuracy of the final result. Complete documentation of all procedures involved in obtaining the final analytic result for the patient sample must be maintained and monitored in a systematic manner.

Test Ordering. Laboratory tests may be performed only at the request of an authorized person (the definition of which varies from state to state). The request form for each patient must include the following: patient's name (or other unique identifier); sex; name and address of person ordering the test (or other unique identifier); date of collection; time of collection (when applicable), source of the specimen (if pertinent), test name or identifying code, and any other relevant and necessary information for a specific test to ensure accurate and timely testing and reporting of results.

The complete request form must accompany the specimen to the laboratory. The request form must be clean and legible. The information on the accompanying specimen container must match exactly the patient identification on the request slip.

Patient Identification, Specimen Procurement, and Labeling. A process of educating all health care personnel involved in collecting clinical specimens is extremely important. A handbook or electronic database of specimen requirement information, in an easily accessible format and location, is one of the first steps in establishing a quality assurance program for the clinical laboratory. This information must be made available where patient specimens are collected and must be kept current. Information about obtaining appropriate specimens, special collection requirements for special kinds of tests, ordering tests correctly, and transporting and processing specimens appropriately should also be included.

Patients must be carefully identified by name and unique identification number before the specimen is collected.

Once it has been obtained from the patient, the specimen must be properly labeled or identified. All containers must be labeled by the person doing the collection to make certain that the specimen has been collected from the patient whose identification is noted on the label.

The laboratory should have written guidelines for the acceptance and rejection of specimens and authority to implement these guidelines. Reasons for rejection of a urine specimen, for example, might include:

Visible signs of contamination of the specimen;
Submission of inappropriate specimen type for the tests requested;
Use of the wrong preservative;
Incorrect labeling of the specimen or requisition;
Transportation delay in delivery of the specimen to the laboratory.

Specimen Transportation and Processing. Specimens must be transported to the laboratory in a safe, timely, and efficient manner. The documentation of specimen arrival times in the laboratory as well as other specific test request data is an important aspect of laboratory organization and an essential part of the quality assurance process. It is important that the specimen status can be determined at any time; that is, where the specimen is in the laboratory processing and testing system at all times. **Turnaround time** is an important factor, and specimen processing, analyses, and reporting of results within an acceptable time frame is a part of the whole quality assurance process.

Laboratory Procedure Manuals. A complete procedure manual for all analytic procedures performed with the laboratory must be maintained. According to NCCLS guidelines, the following should be included:

Title (test name)
Principle
Specimen (including patient preparation, specimen requirements, collection and handling, storage and transportation, and acceptability requirements)

Reagents
Calibration
Quality control
Procedure
Calculations
Reporting
Procedure notes and comments
Limitation of procedure
References
Review and update

Quality Control. Quality control activities include monitoring the performance of laboratory instruments, reagents, products, and equipment. The quality assurance process requires documenting the performance of quality control measures. The written record of quality control activities for each procedure or function also should include details of deviation from the usual results, problems, or failures in functioning or in the analytic procedure, as well as any corrective action taken in response to these problems.

Elements of quality control can include preventive maintenance records, temperature charts, and other records of performance, such as quality control charts for specific analytic procedures. All products and reagents used in the analytic procedures must be carefully checked before actual use in testing patient samples. Use of quality control specimens, proficiency testing, and standards depends on the specific requirements of the accrediting agency of the health care facility.

External quality control activities include periodic inspections by the various accrediting agencies involved in the regulation of clinical laboratories. Well-monitored, well-documented quality assurance records are essential for these inspections.

Problem Solving Mechanisms. Since an important aspect of quality assurance is **documentation**, any problem or situation that might affect the outcome of a test result must be recorded and reported. All such incidents must be documented in writing, including the changes proposed and implemented, and follow-up monitoring. These incidents can involve specimens that are improperly collected, labeled, or transported to the laboratory, or problems concerning prolonged turnaround times for test results. Errors in procedure are the responsibility of laboratory personnel. Quality control measures are used to ascertain the confidence level for the specific analytic result obtained. There must be a reasonable attempt to correct problems or laboratory impropriety, and all steps in this process must be documented.

Test Results and Information Processing. The laboratory must maintain a written record of all patient test results. These records should include the patient's name, identification number, accession number or other unique specimen identifier, date and time of analysis, test results, and initials of individuals performing the test. General laboratory result records are retained and should be readily retrievable by the laboratory for at least 2 years. Blood bank records are kept for at least 5 years, and surgical pathology/cytology reports for at least 10 years.

All test results should be accurately reported to the ordering physician or authorized person in a timely manner. **Critical (panic) values** must be established and should be reported immediately. Confidentiality of results should be maintained.

A written record of results should be maintained in the patient's medical record in the form of handwritten results or a paper report. In general, the test results should be located in and retrievable from two locations: the patient's medical record and the laboratory.

Proficiency Testing. Proficiency testing (PT) is a means of establishing quality control between laboratories. Each laboratory enrolled in a specific proficiency testing program tests samples for specified analytes and sends its results to a center for tabulation. The results of each laboratory are graded according to designated evaluation limits and the results compared with those of other laboratories using the same instrument-reagent methods.

Proficiency testing is an important aspect of the Clinical Laboratory Improvement Amendments of 1988 (CLIA '88). As of Jan. 1994, essentially all laboratories must participate in a proficiency testing program. The program must provide at least three mailings of samples per year (testing events) with each mailing containing five challenges for each analyte tested.

Proficiency testing programs must be approved by CLIA. Programs approved for 1993 included the American Association of Bioanalysts, American Association for Clinical Chemistry, the American Proficiency Institute, and Accutest. State health departments with CLIA-approved proficiency programs included Idaho, New York, New Jersey, Ohio, Puerto Rico, and Wisconsin. Physician professional societies with CLIA-approved proficiency programs included the College of American Pathologists (CAP), American Society of Internal Medicine, American Academy of Family Physicians, and the American and California Thoracic Societies.

Only the **waived tests** under CLIA '88 are exempt from proficiency testing regulations. These are:
Urinalysis by reagent strip or tablet test (nonautomated)
Fecal occult blood
Ovulation tests (visual color comparison tests for human luteinizing hormone)
Urine pregnancy tests (visual color comparison tests)
Erythrocyte sedimentation rate (nonautomated)
Hemoglobin, copper sulfate (nonautomated)

Hemoglobin by single analyte instruments with self-contained or component features to perform specimens/reagent interaction, providing direct measurement and readout (e.g., Hemocue)

Blood glucose by glucose monitoring devices approved by the FDA specific for home use

Spun microhematocrit

If a laboratory performs only waived tests, it is not required to participate in a proficiency testing program. However, it must have a Certificate of Waiver from the United States Department of Health and Human Services (HHS).

If a laboratory performs moderate or high **complexity** tests for which no proficiency testing is available, it must have a system for verifying the accuracy and reliability of its test results at least twice a year.

The Quality Control Program

Some type of control system to ensure reliable results in the clinical laboratory is essential, a fact that has been proven by numerous laboratory accuracy surveys. A means of ensuring that a particular procedure is performed in such a way that the day-to-day results are within the established precision for the procedure and that the values reported to the physician represent the true clinical condition of the patient is essential for quality assurance. Control of laboratory error is influenced and maintained by several factors. The laboratory must be sure that the results it reports for any analysis is clinically correct. This is done primarily through the use of a quality control program.

According to CLIA '88, "The laboratory must establish and follow written quality control procedures for monitoring and evaluating the quality of the analytical testing process of each method to assure the accuracy and reliability of patient test results and reports."[1]

Reliability: Accuracy and Precision

When describing **reliability**, two terms are commonly used: **accuracy** and **precision**. The reliability of a procedure or test depends on a combination of these two factors. *Accuracy* refers to the closeness of a test result to the true or actual value, while *precision* refers to repeatability or reproducibility; that is, the ability to get the same value in subsequent tests on the same sample. It is possible to have great precision, where all laboratory personnel performing the same procedure arrive at the same answer, but without accuracy if the test result does not represent the actual value being tested for. On the other hand, a procedure may be extremely accurate, yet so difficult to perform that individuals are unable to arrive at values that are close (precise) enough to be clinically meaningful.

In very general terms, accuracy can be aided by the use of properly standardized procedures, statistically valid comparisons of new methods with established reference methods, and the use of samples of known values (controls), and participation in proficiency testing programs.

Precision can be measured by the proper inclusion of standards, reference samples, or control solutions; statistically valid replicate determination of a single sample; or duplicate determinations of sufficient numbers of unknown samples. Day-to-day and between-run precision is measured by inclusion of blind samples and control specimens.

Variance (error). **Variance** is another general term that describes the factors or fluctuations that affect the measurement of the substance in question. In general it is impossible to obtain the same result each time a determination is performed on a particular sample. This may be described as the variance (or error) of a procedure. Variance includes limitations of the procedure itself and limitations related to the sampling mechanism used.

General Quality Control Requirements. CLIA regulations regarding quality control are very complicated, with many variables depending on complexity level of tests performed in a laboratory, whether the equipment or test system has been cleared by the FDA or meets CLIA requirements for general quality control, and whether the manufacturer's instructions have been modified in any way by the laboratory. The material that follows refers to quality control in general and does not attempt to describe all CLIA regulations. However, it should be remembered that an acceptable quality control program must monitor all of the following areas:

Facilities
Test methods and equipment
Reagents, materials, and supplies
Procedure manual
Method verification
Equipment maintenance
Calibration and calibration verification
Control procedures
Remedial actions
Quality control records

In controlling the reliability of laboratory results, the objective is to reject results when there is evidence that more than the permitted amount of error has occurred.

Control Specimens. The quality control program for the clinical laboratory makes use of a control specimen whenever possible. This control specimen is similar in composition to the unknown specimen and is included in every batch or run. According to CLIA '88, a minimum of two control specimens (negative or normal and positive or increased) must be run in every 24-hour period when patient specimens are run. The control must be carried through the entire test procedure, treated in the same way as any unknown specimen, and is therefore affected by any or all of the variables that affect the unknown specimen.

For the control specimen to have meaning in terms of the reliability of all results reported by the laboratory, it must be treated exactly like any unknown specimen. The use of quality control specimens is an indication of the overall reliability (both accuracy and precision) of the reported result.

If the value of the control specimen for a particular method is not within the predetermined acceptable range, it must be assumed that the values obtained for the unknown specimens are also incorrect. After the procedure has been reviewed for any indicator of error, and the error has been found and corrected, the batch must be repeated until the control value falls within the acceptable range.

If the control value in a determination is out of the acceptable range (out of control), one or more of the following factors may be responsible: (1) deterioration of reagents or standards (e.g., outdated or otherwise deteriorated urine reagent strips or tablets), (2) faulty instrument or equipment, (3) dirty glassware, (4) lack of attention to timing or incubation temperature, (5) use of a method not suited to the needs and facilities of the laboratory, (6) use of poor technique by the person doing the test because of carelessness or lack of proper training, and (7) statistics; a certain percentage of all determinations will be statistically out of control.

COMMERCIAL CONTROL SPECIMENS. Commercially prepared control specimens can be purchased for most analytes, including specimens for the chemical screening of urine by reagent strips and tablets. These controls are obtained in small samples, called **aliquots**, prepared originally from a large pooled supply. Commercial controls are usually obtained in a lyophilized (or dried) form. Care must be taken in reconstituting the material to add exactly the correct amount of diluent (usually deionized or distilled water) and then to make certain that the material is completely dissolved and well mixed.

Commercial control solutions generally have an expiration date to ensure reliable results. Controls should not be used after the expiration date. Reconstituted control solutions must be used within a relatively short period of time, specified by the manufacturer. The control material may be purchased either assayed or unassayed. Assayed control preparations have been tested by the manufacturer, and stated values are given for each constituent. The manufacturer should provide information concerning the analytic method and statistical procedures used in arriving at the stated values, so that the laboratory can determine the appropriateness of the material for its particular methods and practices. If unassayed control preparations are used, the laboratory will have to establish its own range of acceptable results for each constituent being measured. Statistical parameters must be established over time through concurrent testing with calibration materials or control materials with previously determined statistical parameters. Control results must meet the laboratory's criteria for acceptability before reporting any patient results.

Other Components of Quality Control

SPECIMEN APPEARANCE. First, consider the specimen itself—how it is collected, transported to the laboratory, received, identified, processed, and stored. The specimen should be visually inspected for hemolysis or lipemia in the case of serum or plasma, for signs of contamination in the case of urine.

VALIDATION OF NEW PROCEDURES. A laboratory that introduces a new FDA-approved instrument, kit, or test system for patient testing must demonstrate that the method can obtain the performance specifications for accuracy, precision, and reportable range of patient test results comparable to those of the manufacturer, before patient test results are reported. The appropriateness of the manufacturer's reference range to the laboratory's patient population is also required. Methods not cleared by the FDA, modified by the laboratory, or developed in-house require much more effort in verification.

CONTROL OF HUMAN ERROR. The quality control program should include a means of independent monitoring to minimize bias on the part of the person doing the tests. This may be done by using blind controls, such as commercial control solutions labeled as patient unknowns, or dividing patient specimens into different aliquots to be processed blindly and independently on the same day, or carried over to another day if the constituent is stable. In institutions with more than one laboratory setting such as an inpatient and outpatient laboratory, specimens such as urine may be split and processed by both laboratories. This is especially useful in evaluating accuracy and precision in the microscopic analysis of the urine sediment where control solutions representing the full range of constituents that might be encountered are not available.

CORRELATION OF TEST RESULTS. Another valuable quality control technique is to look at the data generated for each patient and inspect them for relationships between results obtained by the laboratory. This is especially useful in the complete urinalysis where there is a correlation between physical, chemical, and microscopic findings. If urine specimens are analyzed in batches, where the chemical and microscopic analysis are done as different steps, the results should be visually inspected, and abnormal findings explained by common correlations whenever possible before results are released. Examples are the presence of protein in the chemical screen with the presence of casts in the urine; or an abnormal urine color (pink or red), a positive chemical test for blood, and the presence of red blood cells in the urine sediment. Such correlations are discussed throughout this text.

EVALUATION OF PROCEDURES. Each laboratory must have an assessment routine for all procedures to be done on a daily, weekly, and monthly basis to detect problems such as trends and shifts of the established mean value. When such problems are indicated, it is most important that they be corrected and corrective action documented as soon as possible. Many of the components of the quality control program are the responsibility of the laboratory supervisor or director. However, every person working in the laboratory has an important role in ensuring reliable laboratory results, either by running the control specimen or by calling potential problems to the attention of the supervisor or technical advisor.

Major Errors in Urine Testing. The following major errors in urine testing, from the Pennsylvania Department of Health, Physician Office Laboratory Series, are examples of errors that result from failure to adhere to the principles of quality assurance:[3]

1. Failure to test fresh urine
2. Use of unclean collection containers
3. Inadequate care of reagents such as failure to keep reagent strip bottle or vial tightly capped
4. Poor technique in testing—failure to follow directions
5. Failure to mix the urine specimen (this is critical when testing for blood and when doing a microscopic examination of the sediment)
6. Inadequate understanding of interfering substances
7. Improper recording of results (clerical errors are the most common cause of error in the laboratory)
8. Failure to recognize implications of a result, especially in emergency testing
9. Disregard for a result (rarely, a result may be so unusual, the test should be repeated if the specimen is available before the result is reported)
10. Failure to recognize that the result is only part of the picture (a diagnosis should not be made, nor treatment changed, on the basis of only one test result).

REVIEW QUESTIONS

1 Which of the following acts, agencies, or organizations is primarily responsible for safeguards and regulations to ensure a safe and healthful workplace?
   a. Healthcare Finance Administration (HCFA)
   b. Occupational Safety and Health Administration (OSHA)
   c. Clinical Laboratory Improvement Act (CLIA)
   d. Centers for Disease Control (CDC)

2 Which of the following acts, agencies, or organizations was designed to make certain the quality of work done in the laboratory is reliable?
   a. Healthcare Finance Administration (HCFA)
   b. Occupational Safety and Health Administration (OSHA)
   c. Clinical Laboratory Improvement Amendments of 1988 (CLIA '88)
   d. Centers for Disease Control (CDC)

3 Name the three groups of laboratory tests based on the complexity of the test performed as established by CLIA '88.

4 The OSHA hazard communication standard, the "right to know" rule, is designed for what purpose?

5 To comply with various federal safety regulations, each laboratory must have which of the following? (more than one of the answers may be correct)
   a. A chemical hygiene plan
   b. A safety manual
   c. Biohazard labels in place
   d. An infection control plan

6 What is the essence of any Universal Precautions policy?

7 If an employee has the likelihood of exposure to blood or any other potentially HBV-infected material, what preventive measure is the employee entitled to free of charge?

8 What is the single most important procedure that can be performed to prevent the transmission of most infectious agents?

9 If a chemical spill occurs, what is one important source of information about the potential hazards due to exposure to that chemical? Explain how this source is used?

10 What is the main purpose of any waste disposal program in place in the laboratory?

11 Laboratories performing which of the following types of tests must be enrolled in a CLIA-approved Proficiency Testing Program? (More than one of the answers may be correct.)
   a. waived
   b. moderately complex
   c. highly complex
   d. physician performed microscopies

12 Match the following terms to the statements that follow:
   ___ accuracy
   ___ control specimen
   ___ precision
   ___ proficiency testing (PT)
   ___ quality assurance (QA)
   ___ quality control (QC)
   ___ reliability
   ___ variance
   a. A continuing process that includes all aspects of the laboratory to prevent errors and ensure accuracy of test results.
   b. Quality control is only a part of this process that applies to the management and treatment of the whole patient.
   c. A means of evaluating the quality of the analytical testing process of each test method to ensure accuracy and reliability.
   d. A means of establishing quality control between laboratories.
   e. The closeness of a test result to the true or actual value.
   f. Repeatability or reproducibility.
   g. A combination of accuracy and precision.
   h. The factors or fluctuations that affect the measurement of a substance (method error).
   i. Must be carried through the entire test procedure and treated exactly like any unknown specimen.

13 What is the minimum CLIA '88 requirement for the use of control specimens?

REFERENCES

1. Clinical Laboratory Improvements of 1988, final rule, *Federal Register*, Feb. 28, 1992. Clinical Laboratory Improvements of 1988, Final Rule. 42 CFR. Subpart K, 493.1201.
2. *Physician office laboratory policy and procedure manual*, Northfield, Ill, 1993, College of American Pathologists, Section 4, p 1.
3. *Physician office laboratory series*. Commonwealth of Pennsylvania, Department of Health, Bureau of Laboratories, 1988.

BIBLIOGRAPHY

Clinical Laboratory Improvement Amendments of 1988, final rule. *Federal Register* 1992; 42 (Feb. 28).
Clinical laboratory waste management, tentative guidelines. Villanova, Pa., 1991, National Committee for Clinical Laboratory Standards, GP5T.
Linne JJ, Ringsrud KM: *Basic techniques in clinical laboratory science*, ed 3, St. Louis, 1992, Mosby.
National Fire Protection Association: *Hazardous chemical data*. Boston, Mass., National Fire Protection Association, 1975, No. 49.
OSHA Standard, 1910.1030, Occupational exposure to bloodborne pathogens, final rule, *Federal Register* 1991; 56 (Dec. 6).
OSHA Standard, 1910.1450, Occupational exposure to hazardous chemicals in laboratories, *Federal Register* 1990; 55 (Jan 31).
Physician office laboratory policy and procedure manual, Northfield, Ill, 1993, College of American Pathologists.
Physician's office laboratory guidelines, tentative guidelines, ed 2, June 1992, Villanova, Pa., National Committee for Clinical Laboratory Standards, 12(5) POL1-T2.
Protection of laboratory workers from infectious disease transmitted by blood, body fluids, and tissues, tentative guidelines. Villanova, Pa., 1989, National Committee for Clinical Laboratory Standards, 9 (January):M29-T
Recommendations for prevention of HIV transmission in health-care settings. Centers for Disease Control. MMWR 1987; 36 (suppl):3s.
Routine urinalysis and collection, transportation, and preservation of urine specimens, tentative guidelines, Villanova, Pa., Dec. 1992, National Committee for Clinical Laboratory Standards, 12(26) GP16-T.
Schweitzer SC, Schumann JL, Schumann GB: Quality assurance guidelines for the urinalysis laboratory, *J Med Technol*, 3:11, Nov. 1986.
Self-Instruction manual for today's physician office laboratory, Northfield, Ill. 1992, College of American Pathologists.

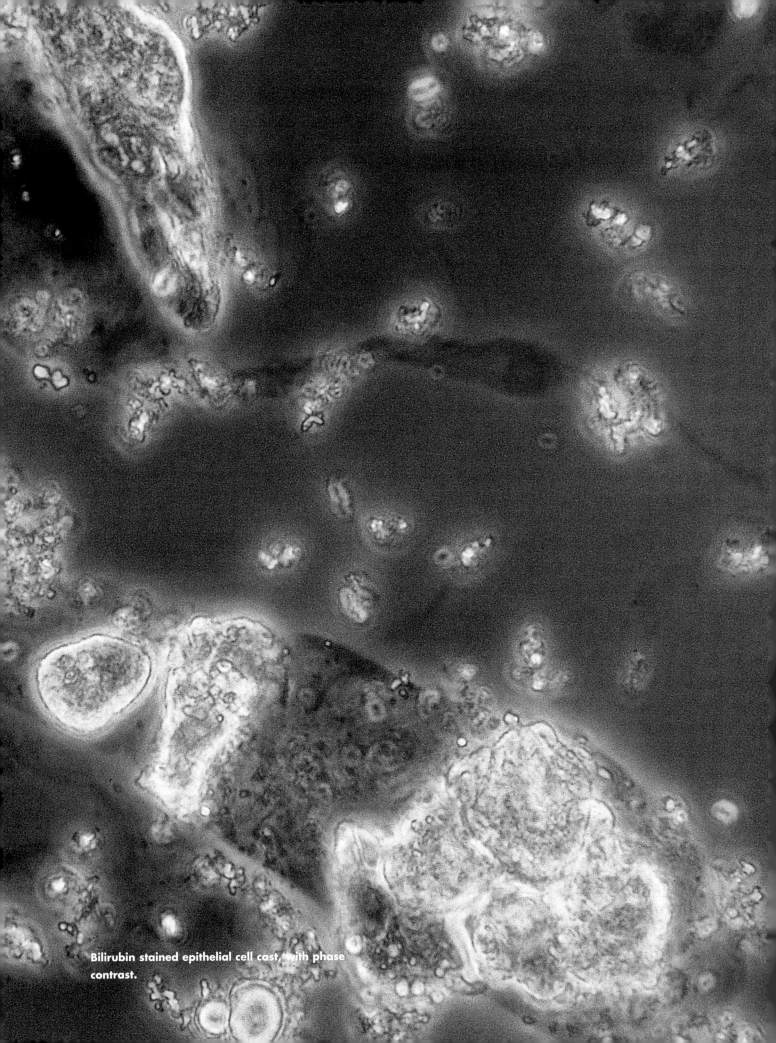

Bilirubin stained epithelial cell cast, with phase contrast.

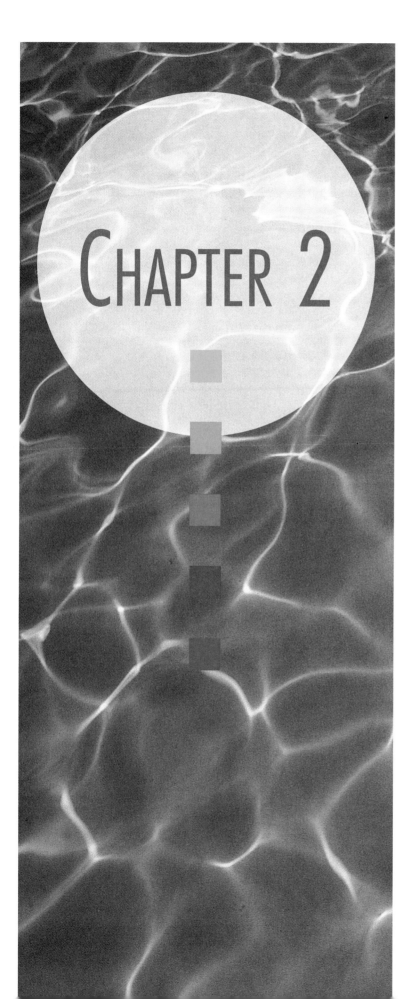

CHAPTER 2

INTRODUCTION TO URINALYSIS

CHAPTER OUTLINE

- **Historical Background**

- **Definition**
  Clinical Usefulness of Urinalysis
  Considerations in Performing the Urinalysis

- **Renal Anatomy and Physiology**
  The Urinary System
  Renal Physiology
  Histology

- **Urine Composition**
  Normal Urine (Reference Values)
  Identification of Urine

- **Collection and Preservation**
  Specimen for Routine Urinalysis
  Types of Urine Collections
  Urine Volume for Routine Urinalysis
  Urine Container

LEARNING OBJECTIVES

▶ Understand the purposes for urinalysis.

▶ Describe the three main components of a urinalysis.

▶ Understand the clinical usefulness of urinalysis and indicators of kidney and urinary tract or metabolic disease.

▶ List the considerations necessary in the performance of the urinalysis.

▶ Describe the basic anatomical components of the urinary system and the function of each.

▶ Describe five main functions of the kidney.

▶ Understand filtration, reabsorption, and secretion as it occurs within the nephron and state where each occurs.

▶ State the main chemical composition of urine.

▶ Describe the preferred urine specimen for urinalysis and storage requirements.

▶ Describe observed changes and mechanism of change in the improperly stored urine specimen.

▶ Describe requirements for urine containers used for urinalysis specimen collection.

At first glance, routine urinalysis appears to be a relatively simple process. Most urine specimens are easily obtained and tested by using readily available chemical reagent strips. The reagent strip (a plastic strip with one or more chemically impregnated test sites on an absorbent pad) is immersed into the urine specimen, and a color reaction is observed by comparison with a color chart at an appropriate time. As an alternative, urine may be tested with a commercially available tablet test. This apparent testing simplicity may account for the classification of chemical urinalysis by reagent or tablet test as a waived test according to the Clinical Laboratories Improvement Amendments of 1988 (**CLIA '88**) regulations.

The information contained within this text will give the reader a realistic appreciation for the complexity and utility of the routine urinalysis and the importance of the technical ability and knowledge of the person performing the procedure.

▪ HISTORICAL BACKGROUND

As stated by G. Mary Bradley, M.D., and Ellis S. Benson, M.D., in the 15th edition of the textbook, *Todd-Sanford Clinical Diagnosis by Laboratory Methods,*[1] the analysis of urine—urinalysis—for the purposes of diagnosis has been used for centuries and is one of the oldest of the laboratory procedures used in the practice of medicine. In the earliest times, a careful examination of all excreta from the sick person—including the urine—was used as a basis for estimating the course of the disease.

In the fifth century BC, Hippocrates described the relationship between fluid intake and urine output. He was an early advocate for urinalysis as an important diagnostic tool. In medieval times, probably too much emphasis was placed on the examination of urine—physicians and apothecaries might observe the urine and not observe the patient. In the earliest days, the color of the specimen, especially reddish urine, was noted and used in the evaluation of the patient's condition. Several early paintings and woodcuts depict examinations of urine as part of the practice of medicine in medieval times.

The polyuria of diabetes was noticed by the ancient physicians and, as early as 600 BC, the sweet taste of diabetic urine was noted. The significance of these observations was not understood until much later.

The relationship between edema, protein in the urine, and abnormal kidney autopsy findings was described by Richard Bright in 1827. John Bostock, a physician-chemist doing much of Bright's work on urinalysis, reported low specific gravity and large amounts of protein in the urine of patients with renal disease. Many handbooks on urinalysis were published near the end of the nineteenth century. One of the earliest was issued by William Prout, a colleague of Bright's. Routine tests in Prout's urinalysis included daily measurement of urine volume, color, specific gravity, and reaction to litmus paper. Urine protein was detected by heat and sugar either by taste or by noting a specific gravity higher than 1.030. By the mid 1800s, textbooks of medicine recommended that a routine urinalysis be included in the examination of all patients.

Development of urinalysis methodology benefited greatly from the work of chemists. The biuret test for protein was developed in 1833. Urine sugar was identified as glucose in 1838, and the Fehling test for sugar was described in 1848. As chemical tests were being developed, the use of medical microscopy was also evolving. One of the earliest medical microscopy courses was taught by Alfred Donne in Paris in 1837.

As part of Donne's teaching, white blood (pus) cells were identified in cloudy urine and differentiated from crystals and amorphous substances. Golding Bird, a pathologist in London, observed casts in the urine of patients with Bright's disease. Techniques for the quantitation of sediment in urine were developed by Thomas Addis in the early twentieth century.

The concepts of urinalysis have changed very little over the years, but chemical tests have become easier to perform with the advent of reagent-impregnated test strips and tablets. New technology has allowed the many specific methodologies to give fast, concise, accurate results for the constituents being analyzed as part of today's urinalysis protocol.

■ DEFINITION

The National Committee for Clinical Laboratory Standards (**NCCLS**) has defined routine urinalysis as, "the testing of urine with procedures commonly performed in an expeditious, reliable, and cost-effective manner in clinical laboratories."[3]

NCCLS continues to state that urinalysis should not be ordered indiscriminately, even if called "routine." These NCCLS guidelines further define the following as purposes for urinalysis:

1. To aid in the diagnosis of disease;
2. To screen a population for asymptomatic, congenital, or hereditary diseases (to monitor wellness);
3. To monitor the progress of disease;

Box 2-1

ROUTINE URINALYSIS PROTOCOL

PHYSICAL PROPERTIES
Color
Transparency
Odor
Foam
Specific gravity

CHEMICAL SCREENING TESTS
(reagent strips and/or tablets)
pH   Glucose
Specific gravity (strip)   Ketones
Protein   Bilirubin
Blood   Urobilinogen
Nitrite
Leukocyte esterase

MICROSCOPIC EXAMINATION
Red blood cells
White blood cells
Epithelial cells
Casts
Bacteria and other microorganisms
Crystals
Other components

Modified from Linne JJ, *Ringsrud KM: Basic techniques in clinical laboratory science*, ed 3, St. Louis, 1992, Mosby, p 324.

4. To monitor the effectiveness or complications of therapy.

Each laboratory needs to determine the exact components and protocol of their routine urinalysis procedure and whether or when to include a microscopic examination of the urine sediment. Routine urinalysis generally includes a physical, chemical, and microscopic analysis of urine. These are outlined in Box 2-1.

Clinical Usefulness of Urinalysis

When the urinalysis is performed in an orderly fashion and the results recorded accurately, the combination of observations and test results gives an overview of the patient's general health pattern.

In general the urinalysis will provide information concerning (1) the state of the kidney and urinary tract, and (2) information about metabolic or systemic (nonrenal) disorders. These are summarized in Boxes 2-2 through 2-4.

Considerations in Performing the Urinalysis

Factors that must be kept in mind and understood when performing the routine urinalysis include:
1. The basic principle upon which the test is based;
2. Limitations of the test. This includes specificity for the substance being measured together with the sensitivity (minimum detectable concentration) and range of detectable substance being measured;
3. Knowledge of common interfering substances; false-negative and false-positive reactions;
4. Knowledge of any critical steps or considerations in the procedure;
5. A general idea of the clinical application of the substance being tested for and its correlation to other findings in the urinalysis: physical, chemical, and microscopic;
6. The need for additional or confirmatory tests based on results of the physical and chemical screen and microscopic examination.

Box 2-2

INDICATORS OF DISEASE OF THE KIDNEY OR URINARY TRACT

Appearance (color, transparency, odor, and foam)
Specific gravity

Chemical tests for protein, blood, nitrite, leukocyte esterase
Urinary sediment for cells, casts, and certain crystals

Box 2-3

INDICATORS OF METABOLIC AND OTHER DISEASE

pH	(mainly for crystal identification— occasionally for acid-base status)	Glucose and ketones	(for diabetes mellitus)
Appearance	(pigments, concentration, and/or dilution)	Bilirubin	(jaundice and liver disease)
		Urobilinogen	(hemolytic anemias and some liver diseases)

Box 2-4

INDICATORS OF OTHER (RARE) CONDITIONS OR DISEASE

Hemoglobin	(intravascular hemolysis)	Light chain proteins	(multiple myeloma or other gammaglobulinopathies)
Myoglobin	(rhabdomyolysis)	Porphobilinogen	(some porphyrias)

Most of this information is contained within the product inserts that are supplied with the reagent strip in use. Testing factors change as products evolve, and current knowledge of the product in use is essential. The previously mentioned considerations will be described in the sections that follow for each portion of the urinalysis.

■ RENAL ANATOMY AND PHYSIOLOGY

The Urinary System

This consists of two kidneys and ureters, the **bladder** and the **urethra**. The working unit of the kidney is the **nephron** where urine is formed. The formed urine flows from the kidney into the ureter and is passed to the bladder for temporary storage. It is eliminated from the body through the urethra (Fig. 2-1).

The nephron consists of the **glomerulus** (made up of a tuft of blood vessels) and the renal tubules, which include the glomerular (Bowman's) capsule, the proximal convoluted tubule, the Loop of Henle, and the distal convoluted tubule. Several nephrons flow into the collecting duct that combine to form the renal papilla and eventually the ureter (see Fig. 2-1). Each kidney consists of about 1.2 million nephrons, and the total length of the tubules in each nephron is 30 to 40 mm. The kidney itself has two anatomical portions: the outer **cortex**, which is made up of the glomerular portions of the nephron and the proximal convoluted tubules, and the central **medulla**, consisting of the Loop of Henle, the distal convoluted tubules, and the collecting tubes.

Blood enters the kidney through the renal artery. This branches into smaller and smaller units, finally becoming the afferent arterioles entering the glomerular tuft. Blood leaves the glomerulus via the efferent

Figure 2-1

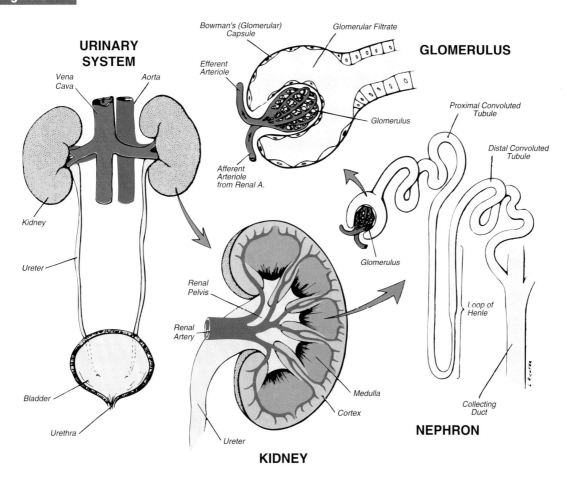

The urinary system. (From Linne JJ, Ringsrud KM: *Basic techniques in clinical laboratory science,* St. Louis, 1992, Mosby, p. 320.)

arterioles. These arterioles run close to the corresponding renal tubules of the nephron so that reabsorption and secretion between the blood and glomerular filtrate can occur. The kidney is a highly vascular organ. Normally, one fourth of the cardiac output is contained within the kidneys at a given time.

Renal Physiology

The kidney may be described as having the following main functions:
1. Removal of waste products—primarily nitrogenous wastes from protein metabolism and acids;
2. Retention of nutrients such as electrolytes, protein, water, and glucose;
3. Acid-base balance;
4. Water and electrolyte balance;
5. Hormone synthesis such as erythropoietin, renin, and vitamin D.

These functions are carried out by means of filtration, reabsorption, and secretion.

Glomerulus

The glomerulus consists of a small knot or tuft of blood capillaries. Blood enters the glomerulus from the renal circulation through the afferent arteriole and leaves through the efferent arteriole. Urine formation begins with the glomerulus, the structure that delivers the blood to the nephron—the working portion of the kidney.

Glomerular (Bowman's) Capsule

As blood circulates through the glomerulus, it is filtered into Bowman's capsule. The glomerular capillaries are covered by the inner layer of Bowman's capsule, forming a semipermeable membrane that allows passage of all substances with molecular weights less than about 70,000 daltons. The fluid that passes through this membrane is basically blood plasma without proteins and fats. It is an ultrafiltrate of blood called the glomerular filtrate. Because it has most of the solutes of plasma, the **glomerular filtrate** is **iso-osmolar** with plasma. That is, it has about the same osmolality as plasma—232-300 mOsm/L with a specific gravity of ~1.008. The formation of the glomerular filtrate is the first step in urine formation. Approximately 180 liters of glomerular filtrate are produced daily, yet only 1 or 2 liters of urine are eliminated from the body. Therefore most of the glomerular filtrate is reabsorbed into the blood.

Proximal Convoluted Tubule

Reabsorption begins at the proximal convoluted tubule where about 80% of the fluid and electrolytes filtered by the glomerulus are reabsorbed.

Reabsorption may be **active reabsorption** with an expenditure of energy required for the analyte to be reabsorbed, usually against a concentration gradient from a region of lower to one of higher concentration. The **reabsorption** may be **passive**, in which an analyte

moves passively down a concentration gradient from a region of higher to a region of lower concentration. In addition, an analyte can move passively along with another analyte that may be actively reabsorbed.

Most of the water in the glomerular filtrate is passively reabsorbed along with sodium ions that are actively reabsorbed by the sodium pump mechanism. Chloride, bicarbonate, and potassium ions, together with 40%-50% of the urea present in the filtrate, are passively reabsorbed with water at the proximal tubules. Other analytes that are actively reabsorbed in the proximal convoluted tubules include glucose, protein (albumin), amino acids, uric acid, calcium, potassium, magnesium, and phosphate.

The proximal tubule has a limit to how much analyte will be completely reabsorbed from the glomerular filtrate. This is referred to as the **renal plasma threshold**, which differs with each analyte. When the plasma concentration of an analyte is greater than its renal plasma threshold, it will remain in the glomerular filtrate and be excreted in the urine. For example, the renal plasma threshold for glucose is about 180 mg/dL. When a patient with diabetes mellitus has a blood glucose concentration greater than 180 mg/dL, excess glucose will be eliminated in the urine.

The proximal convoluted tubules are also a site of active secretion of body wastes. The secretion includes hydrogen ions, phosphate, organic acids, and certain drugs such as penicillin. Hydrogen ions are secreted in exchange for sodium ions that are reabsorbed with bicarbonate into the plasma. This exchange is dependent on the enzyme carbonic anhydrase, which is present in proximal and distal renal tubular cells and red blood cells.

Solutes and water are reabsorbed in equal proportions at the proximal tubules; therefore the tubular fluid is still iso-osmolar with plasma when it leaves the proximal tubules.

Loop of Henle

The descending and ascending loops of Henle function to reduce the volume of the urine while reabsorbing or recovering sodium and chloride. The descending portion of the loop is the concentrating portion. The interstitial fluid outside the tubules in the medulla becomes hypertonic because of increased concentrations of sodium, chloride, and urea in the tubules. This occurs because the descending portion is freely permeable to water but not to solutes. As the loop passes farther into the medulla, water moves from the loop into the interstitium, additionally concentrating the urine in the tubule. The water released into the interstitium is then reabsorbed into the blood vessels that accompany the tubules. In other words, as the fluid (to be urine) moves down the descending loop, water moves out and into the bloodstream in a so-called **countercurrent mechanism**.

The ascending loop of Henle serves as the diluting segment because of its ability to actively secrete sodium and chloride, but prevent water loss. Therefore the fluid within the tubule loses sodium and chloride and eventually is either hypertonic or isotonic compared with plasma when it reaches the distal convoluted tubule.

Distal Convoluted Tubule

There are two main functions of the nephron at the distal tubule: the final reabsorption of sodium (maintaining water and electrolyte balance), and the removal of excess acid from the body (acid-base balance).

Sodium is actively reabsorbed with some bicarbonate at this point. However, the primary mechanism for sodium reabsorption is by the sodium/potassium pump under the control of the hormone **aldosterone**. Aldosterone is released from the adrenal medulla in response to angiotension 2, which is a product of the renin response to either hypotension or low plasma sodium. Aldosterone stimulates active absorption of sodium ions in exchange for potassium, which is excreted by tubular cells (the sodium/potassium pump). Overall there is an increase in plasma sodium and water with a decrease in body potassium levels.

When it is necessary to retain more sodium ion, ammonia is formed from glutamine and combines with hydrogen ions to form ammonium ion. This allows for a greater exchange of hydrogen ions for sodium ion. The pH of the final urine is affected by the distal tubules, especially by an excretion of hydrogen and ammonium ions in exchange for sodium. In general, the blood pH is maintained within very narrow limits at about 7.4, whereas urine commonly has a pH of 5 or 6. Water is also reabsorbed under the influence of **antidiuretic hormone (ADH)**.

Collecting tubules

This is the site of the final concentration of urine. The fluid that eventually will be urine is still isotonic when it leaves the distal tubule and enters the collecting ducts. Although permeable to water, reabsorption is under the control of ADH or vasopressin, a hormone produced by the pituitary gland. ADH is produced in response to increased plasma osmolality and has the effect of preventing excess excretion of water (anti-diuresis). A lack of ADH results in production of a more dilute urine (diuresis).

Ureter

The fluid that leaves the collecting ducts and enters the ureters is now urine. It is temporarily stored in the bladder and eliminated from the body through the urethra.

Histology

All structures that make up the urinary system, from the glomerular capsule to the terminal portion of the urethra, are lined with epithelial cells. Each of these portions is characterized as having a specific type of epithelial cells, generally classified as renal (meaning from the kidney or nephron itself), transitional, or squamous. These will be described in the section on the microscopic examination of the urinary sediment. A few of these cells are constantly sloughed off into the urine. However, it should be remembered that increased numbers or cytologic changes of any of these cells may have clinical significance and may be important in determining the cause of renal dysfunction.

URINE COMPOSITION

Urine is a complex mixture consisting of about 96% water and 4% dissolved substances that generally come from foods eaten or waste products of metabolism. Urine is essentially a solution of salt (sodium and some potassium chloride) and urea (the primary end product of protein metabolism). The actual composition of urine varies, depending on such factors as diet, nutritional status, metabolic rate, the general state of the body, and the state of the kidney or its ability to function normally.

Besides urea, the principal normal organic substances include uric acid and creatinine. These are nitrogenous waste products of protein metabolism, which must be eliminated from the body since increased levels are toxic. Urea accounts for about one half of the dissolved substances in urine. It is the end product of amino acid and protein breakdown. Creatinine excretion is related to the muscle mass of the body, not diet. A constant amount is excreted daily by each individual; therefore creatinine measurements are used to assess the completeness of timed urine collections. Since creatinine is normally filtered through the glomerulus and none reabsorbed, an increased concentration of creatinine in the blood indicates impaired glomerular filtration, and blood creatinine levels are used to indicate renal function.

In addition to sodium and chloride, the main inorganic substances present in urine include potassium, calcium, magnesium, and ammonia plus phosphates and sulfates.

Normal Urine (Reference Values)

Any of the substances tested for in routine urinalysis may be present in various disease states. However, normal urine contains a few cells from the blood and lining of the urinary tract but little or no protein and no casts (although a few hyaline casts may be present). Each laboratory must establish its own reference values for normal urine based on its particular methodology and patient population.

The following reference values are those established for the University of Minnesota Hospital and Clinic and are included as an example of what may be "normally" encountered when the urine is examined for physical and chemical properties.

Color	yellow
Transparency	clear
pH	5-7
Specific Gravity	1.001–1.035 (adult-random urine)
Protein, Albumin	negative–trace (in a concentrated specimen)
Blood	negative
Nitrite	negative
Leukocyte esterase	negative
Glucose	negative
Ketones	negative
Bilirubin	negative
Urobilinogen	≤1Ehrlich Unit/dL

Reference values for the urine sediment are given in Chapter 5.

Identification of Urine

It sometimes is necessary to determine if a specimen is urine or a body fluid such as drainage fluid formed after abdominal or pelvic surgery. This is done by measuring urea, creatinine, sodium, and chloride levels that are significantly higher in urine than in such fluids.

■ COLLECTION AND PRESERVATION

Specimen for Routine Urinalysis

NCCLS recommends the preferred urine specimen for routine urinalysis be a well-mixed, first-morning (eight-hour concentrated), uncentrifuged specimen, which is tested at room temperature. Ideally the specimen should be tested within 30 minutes of voiding—within 2 hours of collection, according to NCCLS. Specimens should not be accepted if left at room temperature for more than 2 hours.

Although the first specimen voided in the morning is preferred, any fresh **random** urine **specimen** is acceptable for chemical analysis.[4] If it is impossible to test the specimen within 1 or 2 hours, it should be refrigerated at 4° C as soon as possible after collection. Specimens can be maintained for 6 to 8 hours with refrigeration with no gross alterations (with the possible exception of bilirubin and urobilinogen, which are also susceptible to exposure to light). Refrigeration will reduce the growth of bacteria, the primary cause for decomposition of urine after it is voided. The growth of bacteria will cause an increased pH as urea is converted to ammonia, increasing the hydroxyl ion concentration. Cells, casts, and chemical constituents are lost if the urine is allowed to stand at room temperature. These changes are summarized in Table 2-1.

Refrigeration may cause precipitation of amorphous urates or amorphous phosphates and confusion

Table 2-1

CHANGES IN URINE LEFT AT ROOM TEMPERATURE OVER 24 HOURS

Constituent	Observed Change	Mechanism Of Change
pH	increased (alkaline)	breakdown of urea to ammonia
Cells	disappear (number decreased)	lysis
Casts	disappear (number decreased)	dissolved
Sugar	decreased	glycolysis (bacterial action)
Acetone	decreased	evaporation
Acetoacetic acid	decreased	converted to acetone
Bilirubin	decreased (color changed from yellow to green)	oxidized to biliverdin
Urobilinogen	decreased (changed from colorless to orange-red)	oxidized to urobilin

in the microscopic analysis of the specimen. Refrigerated specimens must be returned to room temperature before testing, since many of the chemical reactions on the reagent strips employ enzymatic reactions that are temperature dependent. Specimens that have been left at room temperature for more than 2 hours should not be accepted for testing. The use of chemical preservation is sometimes necessary, especially for 24-hour collections of urine. However, a preservative that does not interfere with the analyte in question must be used.

Types of Urine Collections

Although the random or first-morning voided urine specimen is generally the specimen of choice for routine urinalysis, several other types of urine specimens are obtainable. These are described in NCCLS Physician's Office Laboratory Guidelines Vol. 12 No. 5, June 1992 (POL1-T2), and include the following:

Random specimens

First-morning or eight-hour specimens

Timed specimens (such as complete 24-hour collections)

Double-voided specimens (such as for glucose testing where blood and urine concentrations are compared)

Midstream-voided specimens (either random or first morning—used for routine urinalysis)

Clean-catch (midstream) specimens (for bacterial culture)

Catheterized specimens

Suprapubic specimens

In any case, the patient should receive oral and detailed written instructions for the desired urine collection technique. Collection of catheterized and suprapubic specimens requires the active participation of clinical personnel from outside the laboratory.

Urine Volume for Routine Urinalysis

The minimum volume for routine urinalysis is usually 12 mL, but 50 mL is preferable. Twelve mL is the minimum amount necessary for the usual specimen processing procedure in which 12 mL of urine is placed in a disposable centrifuge tube, centrifuged, and concentrated 12:1, so that 1 mL of sediment is retained for the microscopic analysis of the sediment. This volume also allows for a convenient, standardized volume of urine for assessment of physical properties, such as color and transparency, which are often observed in the centrifuge tube.

Smaller volumes may be accepted for chemical analysis from certain oliguric patients or from infants, when it is impossible to obtain even 12 mL. For example, if only 3 mL of urine is collected, a 12:1 concentration of sediment may still be made. A drop placed on the desired portion of the reagent strip or observed microscopically may be all that is possible in some situations.

Urine Container

The urine container is an important consideration in the collection of urine. NCCLS Physician's Office Laboratory Guidelines, June 1992 recommend the following:[2]

1. Collection containers must be clean and made of inert disposable plastic and should not be reused. Containers should generally have a capacity of 50 to 100 mL with a round opening at least 2 inches in diameter.

2. If the specimen is to be transported, the container should have a lid [sealable or screw-top] to prevent leakage of the specimen.

3. Sterile containers with lids or sterile urine transport tubes with no preservatives are required if the specimen is to be used for microbiological studies.

4. The container must have a label that will adhere under refrigeration. The label must include the patient's identification and the date and time of specimen collection, and the labels must be placed on the container, not on the lid.

5. Chemical preservatives must be added to the container or the urine specimens if the specimen is to be preserved because of delayed analysis or an unstable analyte. Labels should contain a warning if caustic substances are used as preservatives.

REVIEW QUESTIONS

1 List four main reasons for performing a urinalysis.
   a.
   b.
   c.
   d.

2 What are the three main parts of a urinalysis?
   a.
   b.
   c.

3 Urinalysis will provide information concerning what two general areas of knowledge?
   a.
   b.

4 List six factors that must be kept in mind and understood when performing a routine urinalysis.
   a.
   b.
   c.
   d.
   e.
   f.

5 Name the main anatomical parts of the urinary system.
   a.
   b.
   c.
   d.

6 The working unit of the kidney is the:
   a. Bowman's capsule
   b. glomerulus
   c. nephron
   d. Loop of Henle
   e. proximal and distal tubule

7 What are the two major chemical constituents in urine?
   a.
   b.

8 Which of the following substances is used as a measure of the completeness of collection of a timed urine specimen?
   a. creatinine
   b. salt
   c. urea
   d. urea nitrogen
   e. uric acid

9 What is the primary cause of decomposition of urine after it is voided?

10 What is the preferred method of preservation of the urine specimen if it cannot be examined immediately after it is voided?

REFERENCES

1. Davidsohn I, Henry JB, eds: *Todd-Sanford clinical diagnosis by laboratory methods*, ed 15, Philadelphia, 1974, WB Saunders, pp 15-16.
2. *Physician's office laboratory guidelines, tentative guidelines*, ed 2, Villanova, Pa., June 1992, National Committee for Clinical Laboratory Standards, 12(5), POL1-T2, pp 24-25.
3. *Routine urinalysis and collection, transportation, and preservation of urine specimens, tentative guidelines*, Villanova, Pa., Dec. 1992, National Committee for Clinical Laboratory Standards, 12(26) GP 16-T, p. 1.
4. *Routine urinalysis and collection, transportation, and preservation of urine specimens, tentative guidelines*, Villanova, Pa., Dec. 1992, National Committee for Clinical Laboratory Standards, 23(26) GP 16-T p 8.

BIBLIOGRAPHY

Kaplan LA: *Renal physiology and water and electrolyte balance.* In Tilton RC, Balows A, Hohnadel DC, Reiss RF: *Clinical laboratory medicine,* St. Louis, 1992, Mosby.

Linne JJ, Ringsrud KM: *Basic techniques in clinical laboratory science,* ed 3, St. Louis, 1992, Mosby.

Physician's office laboratory guidelines, tentative guidelines, ed 2, Villanova, Pa., June 1992, National Committee for Clinical Laboratory Standards, 12(5) POL1-T2.

Routine urinalysis and collection, transportation, and preservation of urine specimens, tentative guidelines, Villanova, Pa., Dec. 1992, National Committee for Clinical Laboratory Standards, 12(26) GP16-T.

Schumann GB, Schweitzer SC: *Examination of urine.* In Henry JB, ed: *Clinical diagnosis and management by laboratory methods,* ed 18, Philadelphia, 1991, WB Saunders.

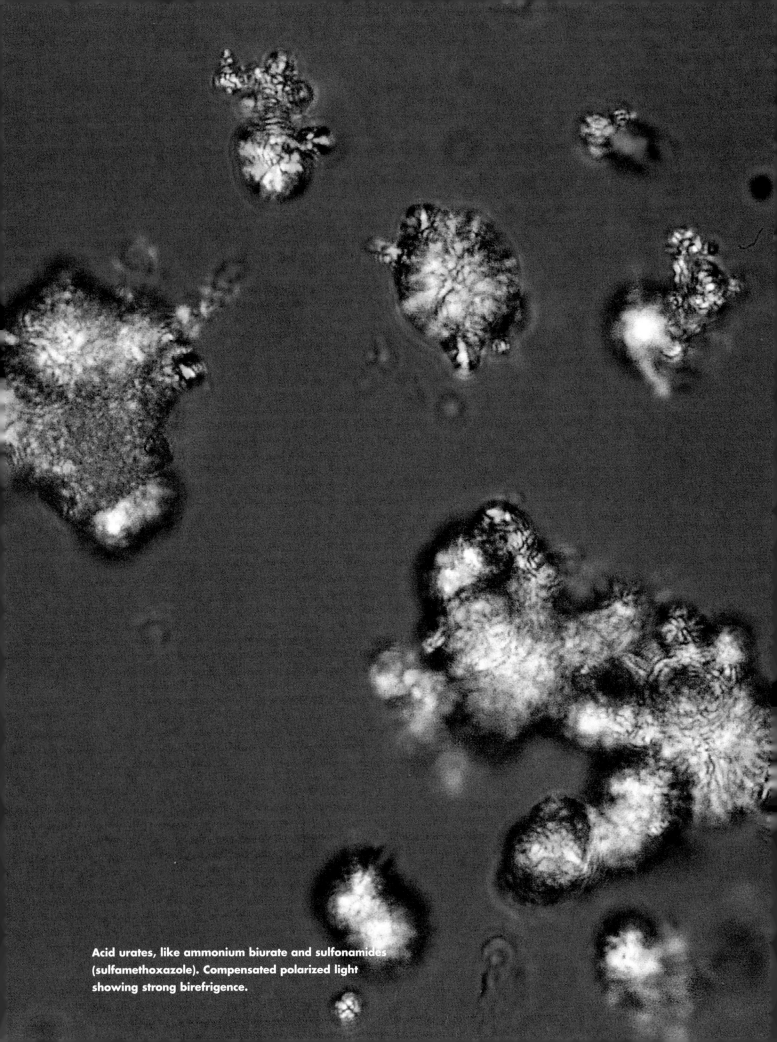

Acid urates, like ammonium biurate and sulfonamides (sulfamethoxazole). Compensated polarized light showing strong birefrigence.

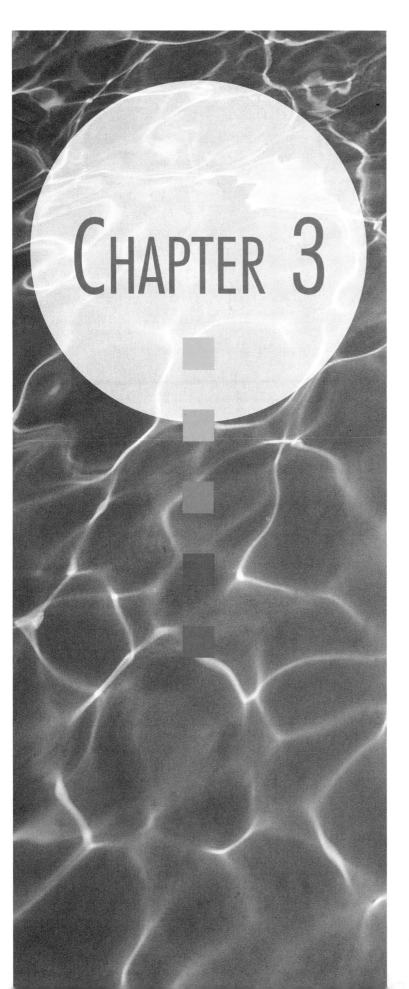

CHAPTER 3

EXAMINATION OF PHYSICAL PROPERTIES OF URINE

CHAPTER OUTLINE

● **Introduction**

● **Color**
Normal Color
Abnormal Color

● **Transparency (clarity)**

● **Odor**

● **Foam**

● **Specific Gravity**
Introduction
Measures of Urine Solute Concentration
Use of the Refractometer

LEARNING OBJECTIVES

▶ Recognize and describe normal color and transparency (clarity) of urine specimens.

▶ Recognize and describe abnormal color and transparency (clarity) of urine specimens and the significance of each.

▶ Recognize and describe normal and abnormal odor and foam of urine specimens and the significance of each.

▶ Know the relationship between urine volume, urine color, and solute concentration (specific gravity and osmolality).

▶ Understand the difference between the various measures of solute concentration referred to as specific gravity and osmolality and how they are measured.

▶ Correct specific gravity values measured by refractometer and hydrometer for glucose, protein, and radiopaque media.

■ INTRODUCTION

Urinalysis begins with an examination of the physical properties of urine. This includes an assessment of color and transparency (clarity). The presence of abnormal odor should be noted. The volume of urine is not measured routinely, although it is a physical property. Specific gravity is another physical property, related to volume of the urine, which may be measured by refractometer, urinometer, or reagent strip.

Assessment of color and transparency of the urine specimen is an essential component of the urinalysis. This is especially important if a microscopic examination of the urinary sediment is not part of every urinalysis, but included on the basis of other findings. In such cases, abnormalities in color or transparency may be the only indicator of pathologic findings in the urine sediment. For example, increased cloudiness may be the only indication of the presence of yeast or abnormal epithelial cells. Or the presence of bilirubin might be detected by performing a special tablet test for bilirubin when the reagent strip is negative, based on observation of an abnormal color and foam. In general, abnormalities in physical properties

must be explained by other results in the urinalysis, and correlation of physical, chemical, and microscopic findings are part of a good quality assurance program. Physical properties are summarized in Table 3-1.

■ COLOR

Normal Color

The normal **color** of urine varies considerably, even between specimens from the same person in a given day. It is generally some shade of yellow and has been described by various terms, most commonly yellow, straw, and amber. As such, normal urine color has been described as varying from light straw to dark amber. Straw implies a lighter-colored urine with normal yellow pigment, amber a darker color with red or orange pigments in addition to yellow. Most importantly, the person performing the urinalysis must be able to recognize what constitutes normal color so abnormal colors may be noted and explained in the urinalysis. Use of the term *yellow* may suffice to describe all normal color encountered.

Table 3-1

PHYSICAL PROPERTIES OF URINE

Physical Property	Description	Possible Cause
Normal color	Yellow (straw to amber)	Urochrome, the chief pigment in normal urine with uroerythrin and urobilin
Abnormal color	Pale	Dilute urine
	Amber (dark yellow or orange-red)	Concentrated urine or bilirubin
	Brown (yellow-brown or green-brown)	Bilirubin or biliverdin
	Orange (orange-red or orange-brown)	Urobilin (excreted colorless as urobilinogen)
	Bright orange	Phenazopyridine (aminopyrine drugs)
	Red	Blood or heme-derived pigment, urates or uric acid, drugs, foodstuffs
	Clear red	Hemoglobin
	Cloudy red	Red blood cells
	Dark red-brown	Myoglobin
	Dark red or red-purple	Porphyrins
	Black (dark brown and black)	Melanin, homogentisic acid, phenol poisoning
	Green, blue, orange	Drugs, medications, foodstuffs
Transparency (Clarity)	Clear	Normal or dilute
	Hazy Cloudy Turbid	Mucus, phosphates, urates, crystals, bacteria, pus, blood, fat, casts
Odor	Aromatic	Normal, volatile acid
	Ammoniacal	Breakdown of urea by bacteria on standing
	Putrid or foul	Urinary tract infection
	Sweet or "fruity"	Ketone bodies
Foam	White, small amount	Normal
	White, large amount	Protein
	Yellow, large amount	Bilirubin

Modified from Linne JJ, Ringsrud KM: *Basic techniques in clinical laboratory science*, ed 3, St. Louis, 1992, Mosby, p 327.

The color of normal urine probably results from the presence of three pigments: urochrome, uroerythrin, and urobilin. Urochrome is a yellow pigment. It is the primary pigment in normal urine. Uroerythrin is a red pigment, and urobilin is an orange-red pigment; they are normally present in lesser concentrations.

According to NCCLS, "The specimen should be examined under a good light looking through the container against a white background . . . Laboratories should establish standard terminology to reduce ambi-guity and subjectivity of reporting. Examples of descriptive terminology pertaining to color include red, yellow, green, and brown."[1]

In general, an inverse relationship exists between the intensity of urine color and volume. The greater the volume of urine, the less the concentration of normal waste products and therefore the paler the color. In contrast, the darker the color of the urine, the greater the concentration of normal waste products and the smaller the volume of urine produced.

Abnormal Color

Abnormal colors may be seen in urine as the result of pathologic conditions or as the result of various dyes, medications, or foodstuffs. The ability to recognize normal color is necessary to ensure recognition of abnormal color. Very vivid, highly colored urine specimens are often the result of various medications, chemicals, dyes, vitamins, fruits, or vegetables. Although these substances have little clinical significance, they are a problem in the laboratory since they may interfere with or mask the various chemical reactions on reagent strips that depend on color development to indicate the presence and concentration of abnormal constituents. Azo dyes, such as phenazopyridine, a drug commonly used for urinary tract infection, result in an intense orange-colored specimen that looks very much like bilirubin and interferes with several of the reagent strip tests.

Pale. A pale or colorless urine specimen suggests the urine is dilute. When urine volume is increased, there is usually a correspondingly lower concentration of normal urine constituents. Clinically pale urine may be associated with diabetes mellitus or diabetes insipidis. Diabetes mellitus produces a very high glucose content with a high specific gravity when measured by refractometer or hydrometer together with a large urine volume. Pale urine specimens are also seen in kidney and urinary tract disease where there is a loss of the ability to concentrate urine.

Amber (Dark Yellow or Orange-red). Amber urine indicates a very concentrated specimen, usually with a correspondingly low volume. It is often seen in conditions such as fever or dehydration. The color may be similar to specimens containing the pigments bilirubin or urobilin (the oxidation product of urobilinogen).

Brown (Yellow-brown or Green-brown). Brown indicates the presence of bilirubin, a highly colored bile pigment related to the clinical condition **jaundice**. The color is a characteristic vivid yellow or yellow-brown, also referred to as "beer brown." On standing, bilirubin may oxidize to biliverdin, a green pigment resulting in a green-brown specimen. Urine specimens containing bilirubin will foam considerably when shaken and the foam will be vivid yellow. Specimens should be tested chemically for bilirubin when its presence is suspected from visual observation.

Orange (Orange-red or Orange-brown). This color is very similar to that of urine containing bilirubin and results from urobilin, a related pigment that is an oxidation product of urobilinogen. Urine specimens tested for bilirubin on the basis of color should also be tested for urobilinogen. The presence or absence of both urobilinogen and bilirubin are used in determining the cause of clinical jaundice.

Orange (Bright Orange). This is very similar to the color of urine containing bilirubin or urobilinogen;

however, the color is more vivid and represents a substance that interferes with many of the reagent strip tests. The color is caused by an azo-containing compound, phenazopyridine (Pyridium) or other aminopyrine drugs, given to the patient as a urinary analgesic. Similar colors may be seen with certain azo-containing antibiotics such as Azo Gantrisin, a sulfonamide containing sulfisoxazole and phenazopyridine.

Red or Pink. There are many causes of red or pink urine; however, when this color is seen, the presence of blood or a heme-related pigment is suspected, and the presence of such pathologic constituents should be ruled out. Red-colored urine caused by the presence of red blood cells, hemoglobin, and myoglobin will all show a positive reagent strip test for blood. A concentrated urine specimen such as that voided in persons with dehydration or fever may show a characteristic precipitate and color caused by the presence of amorphous urates or uric acid. The precipitate is a pink to red color referred to as "brick dust." An unusual beet red colored urine may be voided by genetically susceptible individuals after eating beets. Many other drugs and foodstuffs may cause a red or pink urine specimen. These include rhubarb, red or pink dyes, such as congo red, bromsulphthalein (BSP), phenolsulfonphthalein (PSP), ethoxazene (Serenium), anthraquinone laxatives (senna, cascara), levodopa, methyldopa (Aldomet), and azo-containing compounds.

CLEAR RED. Urine that is clear and red characteristically contains hemoglobin, the color pigment of red blood cells. The hemoglobin may result from intravascular hemolysis or from lysis of red cells in the urine specimen or urinary tract. The specimen may be pink, red, red-brown, or even black, which is a result of the conversion of hemoglobin to methemoglobin.

CLOUDY RED. Urine that is cloudy and red suggests the presence of red blood cells. The intensity of red will depend on the number of red cells present. It may range from barely pink to smoky red, reddish-brown to a frankly bloody specimen. The possibility of menstrual contamination should be considered in urine from a female patient.

DARK RED-BROWN. Urine that shows a color similar to cola is characteristic of myoglobin. It is associated with cases of extensive muscle injury from trauma or extreme exercise.

DARK RED OR RED-PURPLE. Urine described as being the color of port wine is characteristic of the presence of porphyrins (porphobilin) in urine. The urine may be colorless when voided but darkens upon standing.

Brown or Black. Urine containing melanin or homogentisic acid may be normally colored when voided but become brown or black upon standing. Phenol poisoning may also result in an olive-green to black urine. All represent serious pathologic conditions that require prompt diagnosis and treatment.

Blue or Green. These colors are most likely caused by the presence of dyes, drugs, or other ingested substances. For example, the ingestion of chlorophyll in mouth deodorants may color the urine green. Pathologic findings include indicans produced from infections of the small intestine and *Pseudomonas* infections that may result in blue or green specimens.

■ TRANSPARENCY (CLARITY)

Urine is normally clear when voided but often becomes cloudy when it stands. This may be due to precipitation of amorphous crystals (urates in acid urine, phosphates in alkaline urine) or mucus. Growth of bacteria in an improperly stored specimen also will result in loss of clarity of the urine specimen. The degree of cloudiness should be observed and supported by the microscopic analysis of the urine sediment. Lack of clarity may be the only indicator that the sediment should be examined microscopically.

The degree of transparency (clear to turbid) should be assessed on a well-mixed urine specimen by looking through the specimen in an optically clear container held in front of a light source. All specimens should be assessed for color and **transparency** in similar containers to ensure uniform results. The specimen may be held against printed material (newsprint or other appropriately printed material). According to NCCLS, standardized terms such as clear, hazy, cloudy, and turbid should be used to reduce ambiguity and subjectivity of the report. These have been defined by Schweitzer et al as follows:[4]

Clear   No visible particulate matter present.

Hazy   Some visible particulate matter present; newsprint is not distorted or obscured when viewed through the urine.

Cloudy   Newsprint can be seen through the urine but letters are distorted or blurry.

Turbid   Newsprint cannot be seen through the urine.

Common constituents that cause cloudiness in urine are summarized in Table 3-2. As shown, these may be generally normal, or possibly significant or pathologic. See the section on the microscopic analysis of the urine sediment for descriptions of each.

■ ODOR

Normal urine has a characteristic, faintly aromatic odor because of the presence of certain volatile acids. Although the odor of the urine specimen should be observed as part of the urinalysis, it is commented on or reported only if abnormal. See Table 3-1, **Physical Properties of Urine**, for a summary of abnormal odors and possible causes.

Abnormal odor occurs most often as the result of improper handling and storage of the urine specimen. If allowed to stand, urine acquires a strong ammoniacal odor because of the breakdown of urea by bacte-

Table 3-2

COMMON CONSTITUENTS CAUSING CLOUDINESS IN URINE

Generally Normal	Possibly Pathologic
Amorphous phosphates	Amorphous urates (also normal)
Normal crystals	Abnormal crystals
	Red blood cells
	White blood cells (pus)
	Casts
	Fat (lipids)
Epithelial cells (squamous, transitional)	Epithelial cells (renal, transitional, malignant)
Bacteria (old urine)	Bacteria (fresh urine)
	Other microorganisms (yeast, fungi, parasites)
Mucus	
Sperm, prostatic fluid	Chyluria (lymph, rare)
Powders, antiseptics	Fecal matter (from fistula)

Modified from Linne JJ, Ringsrud KM: *Basic techniques in clinical laboratory science*, ed 3, St. Louis, 1992, Mosby, p 330.

ria, resulting in the formation of ammonia. The odor indicates the urine specimen is probably unsuitable for examination because clinically significant components present when voided may have decomposed to undetectable levels.

If the urine specimen is known to be freshly voided, the observation of a **foul** or **putrid** odor may be significant. With urinary tract infection, the presence of large numbers of bacteria acting on urea will result in the formation of ammonia which, together with decay of protein, will result in a particularly unpleasant odor. However, it is practically impossible to distinguish the odor of an infection from the smell of an old, unacceptable urine collection, so knowledge of the time of collection of the specimen is essential.

The urine of patients with increased ketone bodies in the blood and urine will produce a characteristic odor referred to as **fruity** or **sweet**. This is an especially important observation in a diabetic patient who is in or at risk of diabetic coma.

Various other abnormal urine odors have been observed and described. The more important are those associated with extremely rare disorders of amino acid metabolism. Specific odors have been described for specific amino acid disorders. These distinctive odors are usually observed by the mother or caretaker of a baby when changing diapers. Finally, ingestion of certain foodstuffs such as asparagus will result in a characteristic odor of no clinical significance.

FOAM

Normal urine will foam slightly when stoppered and shaken, and the foam will be white. Like odor, foam should be observed but reported only if abnormal. See also Table 3-1, Physical Properties of Urine.

Urine containing the bile pigment bilirubin will show a characteristic **abundant vivid yellow foam** when shaken. When large concentrations of protein are present, the urine will show an **abundant white foam** when the container is closed and shaken. The foam resembles beaten egg white and is caused by the presence of albumin in both cases. This finding is associated with significantly increased protein in the chemical screen plus significant findings (especially casts) in the microscopic analysis of the sediment.

SPECIFIC GRAVITY

Introduction

Specific gravity is a measure of dissolved substances present in a solution. Urine is a mixture of substances dissolved in water. These are primarily urea and sodi-

um chloride; however, any substance dissolved in urine will contribute to the specific gravity of the specimen.

Specific gravity is defined as the mass of a solution compared with the mass of an equal volume of water. Specifically, it is the ratio of the density (mass per unit volume) of a solution compared with the **density** (mass per unit volume) of an equal volume of pure, solute-free water at a constant temperature. Therefore the specific gravity of water is always 1.000. Since it is a ratio, specific gravity has no units. In urine, specific gravity is always reported to the third decimal place. Specific gravity is dependent both on the mass (density) and the number of particles in solution.

Clinically, specific gravity is used to obtain information about the state of the kidney and the state of hydration of the patient. (See also Chapter 4, Specific Gravity, for more information on the clinical importance of specific gravity.) Assuming a constant amount of waste products (solutes) is produced daily by a normal kidney, the organ is able to concentrate or dilute urine depending on the amount of water (fluid) taken in or lost. Normally an inverse relationship exists between urine volume and urine concentration. The greater the volume, the lower the specific gravity and vice versa. Although normal specific gravity may range from about 1.003 to 1.035, the diseased kidney gradually loses the ability to concentrate and dilute urine and eventually the specific gravity becomes fixed at about 1.010 (approximately the specific gravity of plasma and initial glomerular filtrate).

Measures Of Urine Solute Concentration

Osmolality by Osmometer. Although specific gravity is a convenient measure of urine solute concentration, others are available. For critically significant values, measurement of urine and plasma **osmolality** is preferred to specific gravity as a measure of solute concentration. Osmolality is a measure of the number of solute particles per unit of solvent and dependent only on the number of particles in solution. It is measured with an **osmometer** by measuring the freezing point depression of a solution. In healthy persons with a regular diet and fluid intake, the urine will contain about 500 to 850 mOsm/kg of water.

Specific Gravity By Urinometer. Specific gravity in urine may be measured with a urinometer, a specialized hydrometer calibrated to measure specific gravity in urine at a given temperature. The urinometer is a glass float weighted with mercury, with an air bulb above the weight and a graduated stem on the top (Fig. 3-1). It is weighted to float at the 1.000 graduation in pure water. Specific gravity by urinometer has generally been replaced by the refractometer or reagent strip method. It has the disadvantage of being

Figure 3-1

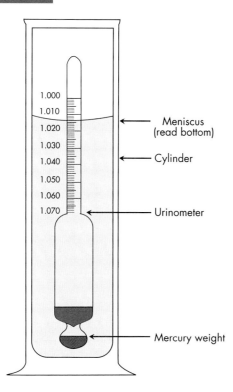

1.000
1.010
1.020 ← Meniscus (read bottom)
1.030
1.040 ← Cylinder
1.050
1.060
1.070 ← Urinometer

← Mercury weight

Urinometer and urinometer cylinder. (From Linne JJ, Ringsrud KM: *Basic techniques in clinical laboratory science*, ed 3, St. Louis, 1992, Mosby, p 334)

Figure 3-2

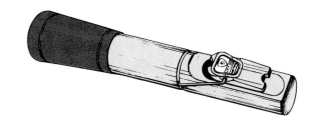

The refractometer. (From Linne JJ, Ringsrud KM: *Basic techniques in clinical laboratory science*, ed 3, St. Louis, 1992, Mosby, p 336)

time-consuming and requires a relatively large volume of urine. NCCLS considers specific gravity measurement by urinometer an inaccurate method and discourages its use.

Refractive Index by Refractometer. The **refractive index** of a solution is the ratio of the velocity of light in air to the velocity of light in solution. It varies directly with the number of particles in solution. Although not identical to specific gravity, refractive index varies and corresponds with specific gravity. Refractive index is measured with a **refractometer**, calibrated to give results in terms of specific gravity, and results agree well with urinometer readings (Fig. 3-2). However, it should be noted that the specific gravity scale by refractometer is valid only for urine. The refractometer cannot be used to determine the specific gravity of salt or glucose solutions, which have much lower readings on the urine specific gravity scale by refractometer than by urinometer.[3]

The refractometer has the advantage of requiring only a drop of urine, whereas the urinometer requires at least 15 mL of specimen. Pass through models are available that are generally used with automated instruments; however, they require a larger volume of

urine. The refractometer is simple to operate and gives reliable results rapidly. Results are valid up to 1.035. Above this, results should be reported only as greater than 1.035. Values greater than 1.035 suggest the presence of unusual solutes such as glucose or radiopaque compounds. The procedure for measurement of specific gravity with a hand-held refractometer is given in Procedure 3-1.

Ionic Concentration by Reagent Strip. Reagent strips indicate they measure specific gravity but actually measure ionic concentration that relates to specific gravity. Values are reported as specific gravity, but are not identical to results obtained with either the urinometer or refractometer. Substances dissolved in urine must **ionize** in order to be measured by this method. The waste products that constitute normal urinary constituents and indicate the concentration and dilution ability of the kidney do ionize. However, certain substances present in urine may not ionize yet contribute to the specific gravity when measured by urinometer or refractometer. Two important examples are glucose and certain radiopaque dyes. If present, they will give significantly higher values with the urinometer or refractometer than with the reagent strip. See Chapter 4, Specific Gravity, for clinical importance, principle, interferences, and additional comments of reagent strip specific gravity determinations.

Use Of The Refractometer

Since the development of the Goldberg refractometer—a temperature-compensated small hand-held instrument—measurements of refractive index have become common in routine urinalysis (see Fig. 3-2). NCCLS states: "Refractometers are often the instrument of choice to determine specific gravity because they are temperature corrected, require only a small volume of urine, and are easy to operate."[2] They go on to say reagent strips can be used to determine specific

Procedure 3-1

SPECIFIC GRAVITY BY REFRACTOMETER

1. Clean surface of instrument prism and cover by rinsing with water. Wipe dry.
2. Close the coverplate of the instrument.
3. Apply a drop of urine to the exposed portion of the measuring prism, at the notched bottom of the cover, using a disposable pipette. The liquid will be drawn into the space between the prisms by capillary action.
4. Hold the instrument up to a light source or position in the refractometer stand so that light passes over the chanber.
5. Looking through the eyepiece, make the reading on the specific gravity scale at the point where the dividing line between the bright- and dark-fields crosses the scale.
6. Rinse the chamber and cover with water and wipe dry.

From Linne JJ, Ringsrud KM: *Basic techniques in clinical laboratory science*, ed 3, St. Louis, 1992, Mosby, p. 337.

gravity by ionic concentration but urinometers are not considered to be an accurate method for determining specific gravity.

Quality Control

According to NCCLS, the refractometer should be checked each day with deionized or distilled water and with a solution of known specific gravity. The water should read 1.000 ± .001. In addition to commercial control urine, examples of solutions of known specific gravity include:

NaCl	0.513 mol/L	3% w/v	SG = 1.015
NaCl	0.856 mol/L	5% w/v	SG = 1.022
Sucrose	0.263 mol/L	9% w/v	SG = 1.034

Correction for Abnormal Dissolved Substances. As mentioned, specific gravity represents the amount of dissolved substances present in urine, and unlike reagent strip tests that measure only ionizable substances, any dissolved substance will be measured as specific gravity by refractometer or urinometer. Substances such as glucose, protein, or radiopaque dyes will act to raise the specific gravity when mea-

sured with the refractometer as compared with reagent strips. Since specific gravity is used to determine the concentrating ability of the kidney, it is sometimes desirable to correct refractometer or urinometer readings for abnormal dissolved substances.

CORRECTION FOR GLUCOSE. Subtract 0.004 from the refractometer value for each gram of glucose per 100 mL urine.

CORRECTION FOR PROTEIN. Subtract 0.003 from the refractometer value for each gram of protein per 100 mL urine.

RADIOPAQUE MEDIA. When specific gravity values greater than 1.035 by refractometer are seen and cannot be explained by the presence of large quantities of glucose or protein, radiopaque media or certain antibiotics should be suspected. These may be associated with the presence of unusual crystals in the microscopic analysis of the urine sediment and/or the occurrence of a delayed false-positive sulfosalicylic acid test for urine protein (See also Chapter 4, Protein Tests and Chapter 5, Crystals).

REVIEW QUESTIONS

❶ The color of normal urine is primarily caused by which of the following pigments?
   a. bilirubin
   b. hemoglobin
   c. urobilin
   d. urochrome
   e. uroerythrin

❷ What is the relationship between urine color and urine volume?

3 Match the following urine colors and possible causes of the color:
- a. amber
- b. brown or black on standing
- c. brown (yellow-brown or green-brown)
- d. clear red
- e. cloudy red
- f. dark red or red-purple
- g. dark red-brown
- h. orange (orange-red or orange-brown)
- i. pale
- j. red or pink

___ blood or heme-related pigment
___ concentrated urine
___ dilute urine
___ hemoglobin
___ homogentisic acid, melanin
___ jaundice/bilirubin
___ myoglobin
___ porphobilinogen (porphyrin)
___ red blood cells
___ urobilinogen (urobilin)

4 The observation of a strong ammoniacal odor when performing the urinalysis is most often caused by:
- a. diabetes mellitus
- b. improper handling and storage
- c. ingestion of certain foodstuffs
- d. urinary tract infection

5 Match the appearance of the foam that appears when the urine specimens containing the following constituents are stoppered and shaken:
- a. bilirubin
- b. normal urine
- c. protein

___ abundant vivid yellow foam
___ abundant white foam
___ small amount of white foam that dissipates

6 What is the relationship between urine volume and specific gravity in normal healthy persons?

7 Loss of the ability of the kidney to concentrate and dilute urine will result in a fixed specific gravity of:
- a. 1.005
- b. 1.010
- c. 1.015
- d. 1.020
- e. 1.025

8 Match the following concerning measurement of specific gravity. Responses may be used more than once.
- a. Urinometer
- b. Refractometer
- c. Reagent Strip

___ measures all dissolved substances
___ measures ionizable substances only
___ values affected by temperature of the urine specimen
___ values affected by the presence of protein
___ values affected by the presence of glucose
___ values affected by the presence of radiographic contrast media
___ measurement requires relative large urine volume

REFERENCES

1. *Routine urinalysis and collection, transportation, and preservation of urine specimens, tentative guideline,* Villanova, Pa., Dec. 1992, National Committee for Clinical Laboratory Standards, 12(26), GP 16-T, p 6.
2. *Routine urinalysis and collection, transportation, and preservation of urine specimens, tentative guideline,* Villanova, Pa., Dec. 1992, National Committee for Clinical Laboratory Standards, 12(26), GP 16-T, p 7.
3. Schumann GB, Schweitzer SC: *Examination of urine.* In Henry JB (ed): *Clinical diagnosis and management by laboratory methods,* ed 18, Philadelphia, 1991, WB Saunders, p 397.
4. Schweitzer SS, Schumann JL, Schumann GB: Quality assurance guidelines of the urinalysis laboratory, *J Med Technol,* 3:11, Nov. 1986, p. 569

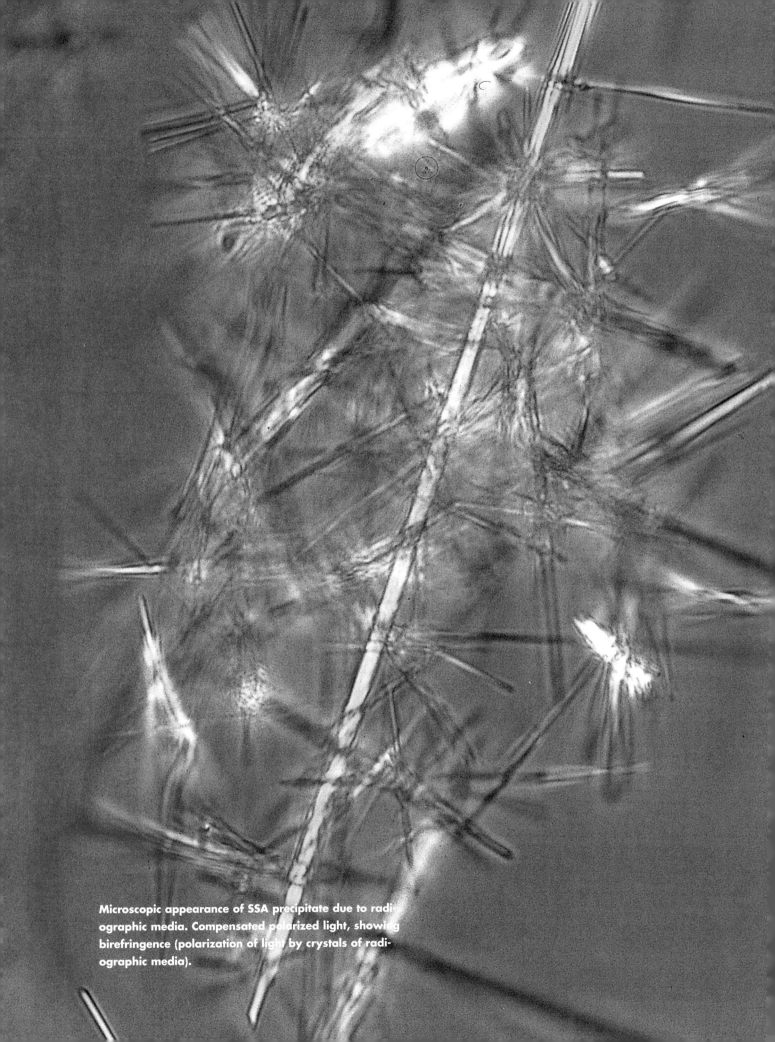

Microscopic appearance of SSA precipitate due to radiographic media. Compensated polarized light, showing birefringence (polarization of light by crystals of radiographic media).

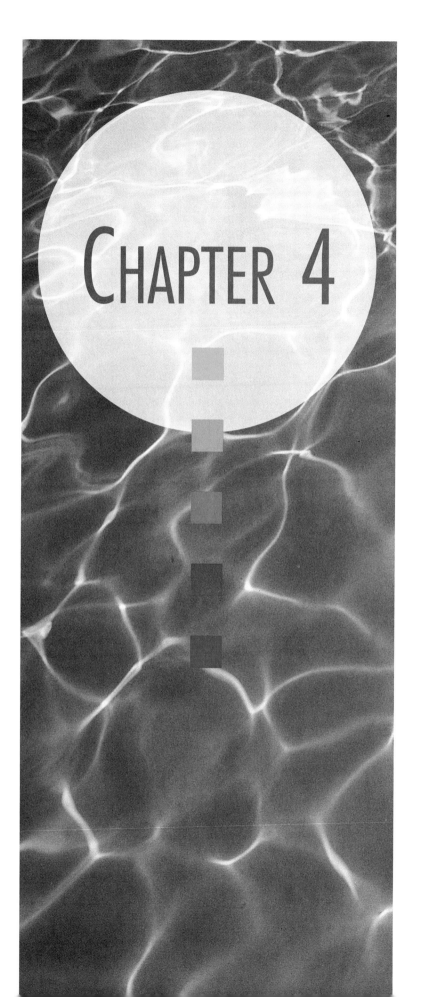

CHAPTER 4

CHEMICAL EXAMINATION OF URINE

CHAPTER OUTLINE

● **General Procedure and Precautions**
Manufacturer's Directions
Specimen Requirements
Wetting the Strip (Sampling)
Storage and General Precautions
Stability
Timing
Results—Color Comparison
Control Solutions

● **pH**
Clinical Importance
Principle
Interferences
Precautions
Confirmatory Tests

● **Specific Gravity**
Clinical Importance
Principle
Specificity
Interferences
Additional Comments

● **Protein**
Clinical Importance
Principle of Tests for Urinary Protein
Specificity
Sensitivity (Minimum Detectable Level)
Reagent Strip Tests for Urine Protein
Principle
Interferences
Additional Comments
Confirmatory Tests
Sulfosalicylic Acid Test for Urine Protein
Principle
Reagent—Sulfosalicylic Acid (7% w/v)
Interferences
Additional Comments

● **Blood (Hemoglobin and Myoglobin)**
Clinical Importance
Principle and Specificity
Sensitivity (Minimum Detectable Level)
Interferences
Additional Comments
Confirmatory Tests

● **Nitrite**
Clinical Importance
Principle
Specificity

Results
Sensitivity (Minimum Detectable Level)
Interferences
Additional Comments

● **Leukocyte Esterase**
Clinical Importance
Principle
Sensitivity (Minimum Detectable Level)
Interferences
Additional Comments

● **Glucose (Sugar)**
Clinical Importance
Reagent Strip Tests for Glucose
Principle
Specificity
Sensitivity (Minimum Detectable Level)
Range of Values
Interferences
Confirmatory and Follow-up Tests
Clinitest Copper Reduction Test for Reducing
   Sugars
Principle
Specificity
Sensitivity
Interferences
Additional Comments
Additional Tests

● **Ketone Bodies**
Clinical Importance
Principle
Specificity and Sensitivity
Interferences
Additional Comments

● **Bilirubin**
Clinical Importance
Reagent Strip Tests for Bilirubin
Principle
Specificity
Sensitivity (Minimum Detectable Level)
Interferences
Additional Comments
Confirmatory and Related Tests
Ictotest Tablet Test
Principle
Specificity
Sensitivity
Interferences
Additional Comments

- **Urobilinogen and Porphobilinogen**
  Clinical Importance of Urobilinogen
  Clinical Importance of Porphobilinogen
  Principle of Reagent Strip Tests
  Specificity and Sensitivity
  Interferences
  Additional Comments
  Confirmatory and Additional Tests

- **Watson-Schwartz Qualitative Test for Urobilinogen and Porphobilinogen**
  Principle
  Reagents
  Interferences
  Additional Comments

- **Hoesch Test for Porphobilinogen**
  Principle
  Reagents
  Interferences
  Additional Comments

- **Ascorbic Acid**
  Clinical Importance
  Reagent Strip Tests
  Principle
  Specificity
  Additional Comments

LEARNING OBJECTIVES

▶ Test a urine specimen for chemical constituents using a multiple reagent strip with correct technique and knowledge of the general procedure and precautions necessary for valid results.

▶ Know and understand the importance of each of the following when testing urine with reagent strips:
  following manufacturer's directions
  specimen requirements
  sampling
  storage and general precautions
  stability
  timing
  color comparison
  reporting of results
  use of control solutions

▶ For each of the 10 analytes described in detail in this chapter, describe and understand each of the following:
  clinical importance (pathophysiology)
  principle of the test
  specificity
  sensitivity
  interferences (false-positive and false-negative reactions)
  additional considerations
  confirmatory and related or follow-up tests

▶ Recognize interferences when they occur and know how to resolve discrepant results from the presence of interfering substances such as ascorbic acid, radiographic media, mesna, and azo dyes such as phenazopyridine.

▶ For each of the 10 analytes, recognize the relationship between analytes and know when discrepant results are obtained.

▶ For protein, understand the pathophysiology of proteinuria caused by glomerular damage, tubular damage, prerenal disorders, lower urinary tract disorders, asymptomatic proteinuria, and consistent microalbuminuria.

▶ For blood, understand the pathophysiology of hematuria, hemoglobinuria, and myoglobinuria, and how to differentiate between these analytes when a positive reagent strip test for blood is seen.

▶ Understand the difference between reagent strip tests for glucose and copper reduction tests for reducing sugars.

▶ Understand metabolism and pathophysiology of bilirubin and urobilinogen and laboratory findings in various types of jaundice.

▶ Understand the difference between reagent strip tests for Ehrlich reactive substances and urobilinogen and how to differentiate the presence of urobilinogen from porphobilinogen.

▶ Understand the significance of the presence of ascorbic acid in urine, how to recognize its presence, and how to resolve discrepancies when they exist.

■ INTRODUCTION

After an assessment of physical properties, urine is tested for a variety of chemical constituents. This chemical analysis is usually done with dry reagent strips, available both as single tests for a specific chemical substance and as combinations, referred to as **multiple reagent strips.** Multiple strips are available in various combinations, and the exact product chosen for the routine testing of urine depends on a variety of factors including the patient population of the individual laboratory. The maximum number of different tests presently contained on a single multiple reagent strip is 10; these are the substances listed under Chemical Screening Test in Box 2-1. Three commercially available products will be described in the sections that follow. These are the Multistix reagent strips and other tablet tests formerly Ames products (Miles, Inc., Diagnostics Div., Tarrytown, NY), the Chem-strip products (Boehringer Mannheim Diagnostics, Indianapolis, Ind.), and the Rapignost products (Behringwerke AG Marburg, Germany, distributed by Behring Diagnostics Inc., Somerville, NJ). Other products exist; however, the three described are by far the most commonly used in the CAP Interlaboratory Comparison Program (College of American Pathologists, 325 Waukegan Rd., Northfield, Ill).

Reagent strips are plastic strips or supports that contain one or more chemically impregnated test sites on an absorbent pad. When the dry reagents come in contact with urine or a suitable control solution, the reagents are activated and a chemical reaction occurs. The chemical reaction is a specific color change. This may be observed visually and compared with a special color chart provided by the product manufacturer (usually printed on the bottle of reagent strips), or the color intensity may be measured electronically, usually by reflectance, by an instrument designed to be used with the product in question.

The intensity of the color formed is generally proportional to the amount of substance present in the specimen or control solution when observed at a specific time. Some test areas are used as screening tests and reported as only positive or negative. Others are used to estimate (semiquantitate) the amount of substance present and are reported in a plus system or in numerical values (e.g., mg/dL, g/dL). The method of reporting results will vary from laboratory to laboratory but must be consistent for a given laboratory.

Advantages of dry reagent strips over more traditional chemical tests upon which they are based include:
1. Convenience and greater speed with fewer personnel needed
2. Cost effectiveness
3. Stability
4. Relative ease in learning to use
5. Disposability
6. Smaller sample volume
7. Space savings

Although easy to use and reliable, reproducible results with reagent strips depend on correct technique. Manufacturer's directions must be followed and will differ for the same substance tested with different products. Any person using reagent strips should understand the principle and specificity of each chemical test area, be aware of precautions or limitations and interferences that occur, and know the sensitivity and significance of positive or negative results. A knowledge of appropriate confirmatory tests when a positive reaction is obtained on the reagent strip test is also needed. These may be in the form of commercially available tablet tests, more traditional chemical tests, or correlations with other parts of the urinalysis such as physical properties and the microscopic analysis of the sediment. According to NCCLS, confirmatory tests will confirm the presence or absence of a substance by another method or procedure. They may be more sensitive, more specific, or both. Appropriate confirmatory tests will be described in this section.

■ GENERAL PROCEDURE AND PRECAUTIONS

See also Procedure 4-1.

Manufacturer's Directions

Although there are general directions that apply to all reagent strip tests, the specific manufacturer's directions must be followed for any strip used. Reagent strips are continually changed and reformulated, and laboratory protocol must reflect these changes. Each test product is supplied with a product insert containing the most up-to-date information. Inserts include directions for use, warnings, procedure limitations, specimen handling information, storage, and expected values together with information about interfering substances that give false-positive or false-negative reactions. Product inserts must be compared for each new lot number of reagent strips and laboratory procedures adjusted accordingly.

Specimen Requirements

The specimen must be fresh (tested less than 2 hours after collection) or adequately preserved (usually by refrigeration), completely mixed, uncentrifuged, and tested at room temperature.

Procedure 4-1

GENERAL PROCEDURE FOR URINE REAGENT STRIPS

1. Test fresh, well-mixed, uncentrifuged urine.
2. Completely immerse all chemical areas of the reagent strip briefly—not over 1 second.
3. Remove excess urine from the reagent strip by drawing the strip along the lip or rim of the urine container as it is removed.
4. Avoid possible mixing of chemicals from adjacent reagent areas.
5. Read each chemical reaction at the time stated. Timing is critical for semiquantitation of results.

6. Use adequate light. Hold the strip close to the color block on the chart supplied by the manufacturer and match carefully for each chemical test. Be sure the strip is properly oriented to the color chart: horizontal for Multistix, vertical for Chemstrip and Rapignost products.
7. Record the results in consistent units as established for your laboratory.

Modified from Linne JJ, Ringsrud KM: *Basic techniques in clinical laboratory science*, ed 3, St. Louis, 1992, Mosby, p 339.

Wetting the Strip (Sampling)

The strip must be completely moistened so that all test areas are in contact with the sample. However, the strip must be removed immediately (within 1 second) so that chemicals do not leach out of the strip. To avoid runover between chemicals on adjacent pads, the strip is drawn along the edge of the urine container as it is removed and the edge of the strip may be touched to absorbent paper or gauze. To further avoid runover, the strip is then placed in a horizontal position while waiting for and reading results.

Storage and General Precautions

Reagent strips must be kept in tightly capped or stoppered containers. Strips will deteriorate when exposed to moisture, direct sunlight, heat, or volatile substances. Containers are provided with a desiccant to protect strips from moisture. Do not remove the desiccant from the container. Strips should be stored as recommended by each manufacturer, generally at room temperature, under 30° C but not refrigerated or frozen. Keep strips in their original container; do not mix strips from different containers. Remove only the number of strips needed at a time, and keep the container tightly closed at all times. Do not touch test areas. Keep reagent strips away from contaminating substances such as chlorine bleach (hypochlorite) that may be present in the work area.

Stability

Unopened reagent strips are stable until the expiration date printed on the bottle. Do not use reagent strips after the expiration date. Write the date on each container when it is opened and use within 6 months of opening. Monitor possible deterioration by com-

paring the color of the dry reagent with a negative test block on the color chart. Discard the entire bottle of strips if any reagent pads are discolored or when quality control is consistently out of range.

Timing

Read results of each chemical test at the time stated by the manufacturer. Use a timing device with a second hand. Timing is essential for semiquantitation of results. In general, the Miles products are read during the kinetic phase of the chemical reaction, and timing is absolutely critical. However, the Chemstrip and Rapignost products are generally read at an end point or stable phase of the reaction, allowing most results to be read within 1 to 2 minutes. Automated or semiautomated instruments have the advantage of reading each analyte at an exact and specific time determined by the manufacturer.

Results—Color Comparison

Whenever results depend on visual comparison of color, individual interpretation is a possible source of error. Adequate light is essential. Hold the reagent strip next to the most closely matched color block for each chemical test. Be sure to correctly orient the reagent strip to the color chart when reading results. Miles products are held horizontally with respect to the bottle; Chemstrip and Rapignost products should be held vertically.

Automated or semi-automated instruments will eliminate differences in individual visual interpretation of color and improve reproducibility of results. However, certain interfering pigments may be more easily recognized by visual assessment. Some instruments utilize an area on the reagent strip that compensates for the color of the urine specimen.

Reporting Results. Results may be reported as positive or negative, graded in a plus system, or semiquantitated and reported in units such as mg/dL, g/dL. Any method used must be consistent for each analyte as established by the institution (laboratory). Semiquantitation is preferred since it allows for better comparison of values between products and laboratories, although it may imply better precision than is obtainable.

Control Solutions

Part of quality assurance in urinalysis involves the use of control solutions to test the reactivity of the reagent strip being used. NCCLS recommends that multiconstituent control solutions be used to validate the performance of each chemical test at two distinct levels. One of these should be a negative control solution. Reagent strips should be tested with control solutions at least once each day that the test is performed and whenever a new bottle of reagent strips is opened. Control solutions are available commercially either lyophilized or as a liquid. Manufacturer's directions for reconstitution and use should be followed. Larger laboratories may find it cost effective to prepare their own control solutions. Acceptable results are generally ± one color block of the assigned target. However, the only acceptable result for a negative control solution is a negative reaction.

■ pH

Clinical Importance

Although the kidney is essential in controlling the **pH** of blood and extracellular fluid, measurement of urinary pH is limited in assessment of acid base status. However, measurement of urinary pH is included in the routine urinalysis for several reasons.

Freshly voided urine usually has a pH of 5 or 6. When allowed to stand at room temperature, urea is converted to ammonia by bacterial action, resulting in increased urinary pH (increased hydroxyl ion concentration). Therefore a very alkaline urine pH often indicates that the sample has been improperly stored or handled after collection. This type of specimen is not suitable for testing, and a new specimen should be requested.

However, persistently alkaline urinary pH in a freshly voided urine specimen may indicate a urinary tract infection. Other typical findings in infection include positive chemical tests for nitrite, and leukocyte esterase, plus the presence of bacteria and white blood cells in the urinary sediment.

The urine pH helps in the identification of crystals of certain chemical compounds that may be seen in the urine sediment. Certain crystals are associated with acid urine (pH below 7), and others with alkaline urine (pH 7 and above). Knowledge of the urine pH is of great importance in the identification of crystals and should be known whenever the urine sediment is examined microscopically.

If the urine specimen is dilute (specific gravity <1.0l0) and alkaline, various formed elements such as casts and cells will rapidly dissolve. Thus discrepant results in the chemical screen and microscopic examination may be explained by knowledge of the urine pH.

Acidosis with an acid urinary pH is seen in cases of starvation, severe diarrhea, diabetes mellitus, and respiratory disease. Paradoxical aciduria (urine pH <7) occurs in potassium-depleted, chloride-depleted alkalosis.

Alkalosis with an alkaline urine pH is seen with excess alkali, severe vomiting, and respiratory hyperventilation. In renal tubular acidosis, the urine pH is relatively alkaline with metabolic acidosis.

Finally, it is sometimes necessary to control the urinary pH in the management of kidney infections, in cases of renal calculi (stones), and during the administration of certain drugs. This is done with the administration of certain drugs or by regulating the diet. Meat diets generally result in acidic urine and vegetable diets in alkaline urine.

Principle

Reagent strip tests utilize a methyl red and bromthymol blue double indicator system that measures urine pH in a range from 5 to 9. The methyl red is used to indicate a pH change from 4.4 to 6.2 with a color change from red to yellow. Bromthymol blue indicates a pH change from 6.0 to 7.6 as seen by a color change from yellow to blue.

Interferences

None are known. The pH value is not affected by the buffer concentration of the urine or protein concentration.

Falsely Elevated Results. Urine left standing at room temperature becomes more alkaline because of the growth of bacteria and formation of ammonia from the breakdown of urea.

Precautions

Take care not to wet the reagent strips excessively so that highly acidic adjacent test pads do not run into the pH pad causing falsely acidic readings.

Follow-up or Confirmatory Tests

For more accurate measurements, a pH meter may be used. This is rarely clinically necessary but may be useful in suspected renal tubular acidosis.

If the reagent strip value is greater than 9.0 or if results are uncertain, the specimen may be tested with special pH indicator strips.

SPECIFIC GRAVITY

Clinical Importance

The **specific gravity** of urine is used to obtain information about the state of the kidney and the state of hydration of the patient (see also Specific Gravity in Chapter 3, Physical Properties). The normal kidney can produce urine with a specific gravity ranging from about 1.003 to 1.035. If dysfunctional, the kidney loses its ability to concentrate and dilute urine, and the urinary specific gravity will be fixed at about 1.010. Normal specific gravity reflects sodium, potassium, chloride, and urea content, and generally parallels osmolality.

If the kidney is known to function adequately, the specific gravity is a reflection of the state of hydration of the body. Although normal specific gravity may range from about 1.001 to 1.035, it is usually between 1.016 and 1.022 in adults with normal fluid intake. Since specific gravity is a reflection of the amount of dissolved substances present in solution, it varies inversely with the volume of urine which is normally about 600 to 1600 ml per day. If the urine volume increases because of increased water intake, the specific gravity of urine decreases. If the urinary volume is high, the specific gravity is low, assuming the kidney is functioning normally. In some renal diseases such as glomerulonephritis, pyelonephritis, and various anomalies, a combination of low specific gravity and low urine volume results since the renal epithelium is unable to either excrete normal amounts of water or concentrate the waste products. Loss of concentrating ability is also seen in diabetes insipidus, an impairment of antidiuretic hormone (ADH). This rare condition results in the voiding of extremely large volumes of urine with very low specific gravity, ranging from 1.001 to 1.003.

With a restricted fluid diet for 12 hours, the normal kidney is capable of concentrating urine to a specific gravity of 1.022 or more—after 24 hours to 1.026. On a very high fluid diet, the normal kidney is capable of diluting the urine to a specific gravity of about 1.003. The first urine specimen passed in the morning should have a specific gravity greater than 1.020 if the kidney is functioning normally.

Principle

Although specific gravity is a measure of the amount of dissolved substances present in a solution, the reagent strip tests for specific gravity actually measure ionic concentration. Both Multistix and Chemstrip products have a test area for specific gravity; Rapignost does not. Reagent strip tests are based on a pKa change of certain pretreated polyelectrolytes in relation to the ionic concentration of urine. Acid groups of polyelectrolytes in the reagent strip dissociate in proportion to the numbers of ions in solution. Hydrogen ions produced reduce the pH, which is reflected by the color change of a pH indicator. The system is buffered so that any change in color is related to pKa change, and not pH of the urine itself. Readings are made at 0.005 intervals from 1.000 to 1.030 by comparison with a color chart.

Specificity

Reagent strip tests measure only ionizable substances unlike the urinometer or refractometer, which measure any dissolved substances.

Interferences

Nonionizable substances such as urea, glucose, and radiographic contrast media do not affect the reagent strip but contribute to the urinometer or refractometer readings.

Increased Values

- With moderate quantities of protein, the reagent strip specific gravity may be elevated 1 block (0.005) because of protein anion.
- The presence of ketone bodies may give elevated values with reagent strip methods.

Decreased Values

- Highly buffered alkaline urine may cause low readings, and 0.005 may be added to readings from urines with pH equal to or greater than 6.5. Automatic reagent strip instruments make the calculation automatically.
- The presence of nonionizable substances such as glucose, radiopaque dyes, and certain antibiotics will not affect the reagent strip values for specific gravity but will show significant increases with the urinometer and refractometer.
- Specimens containing urea at concentrations greater than 1 g/dL will show low readings relative to more traditional methods since urea does not ionize.

Additional Comments

In general the reagent strip test correlates to within 0.005 of the refractometer or urinometer test. However, urines with specific gravity greater than 1.025 are not reliably measured with ionic concentration methodology and should be tested with the refractometer.

■ PROTEIN

Clinical Importance

In the detection and diagnosis of renal disease, the presence and relative concentration of protein is probably the most significant single finding. This together with chemical tests for blood, nitrite, and leukocyte esterase and microscopic evidence of casts and cells will help in the final diagnosis.

The presence of detectable protein in the urine is termed **proteinuria**. It is not normal unless the urine is highly concentrated. In general, proteinuria may be classified as prerenal, glomerular, tubular, lower urinary tract, and asymptomatic. The amount (quantity) or degree of proteinuria may be referred to as small (mild or minimal), moderate, or large (heavy) proteinuria. These are roughly defined as:

Degree of proteinuria	Grams protein excreted per day
Mild (minimal)	<1.0 g/day
Moderate	1.0 to 3 or 4 g/day
Large (heavy)	>3 to 4 g/day

Normal glomerular filtrate is an ultrafiltrate of blood plasma. It is essentially blood plasma without cells, larger protein molecules, and certain fatty substances.

As a result of hydrostatic pressure, the glomerular membrane generally allows the passage of molecules of molecular weight of 50,000 to 60,000 or less. Albumin has a molecular weight of about 67,000. This is a fairly small molecule, and some albumin is normally filtered through the glomerulus. However, this is normally reabsorbed into the blood at the convoluted tubules. Therefore two mechanisms for proteinuria are increased permeability of the glomerulus and decreased reabsorption by the convoluted tubules.

Another type of protein that may be in the urine is **Tamm-Horsfall** protein. This high molecular weight glycoprotein (mucoprotein) is normally secreted by renal tubular cells and is not present in the blood plasma. It is important in that it forms the basic matrix of most urinary casts, an important pathologic urinary finding associated with proteinuria.

Glomerular Damage and Proteinuria. Proteinuria (generally **albuminuria**) is consistently present in glomerular disease. When the glomerular membrane is damaged, because of disease or other reasons, it allows passage of larger molecules including protein. Initially, only smaller albumin molecules pass through the glomerular membrane, whereas larger globulin protein molecules remain in the plasma.

Glomerular damage with increased filtration may result from a variety of causes such as toxins, infections, vascular disorders, and immunologic reactions. An example of glomerular proteinuria is poststreptococcal **acute glomerulonephritis (AGN)**. This immuno-

logic sequele of a bacterial infection, usually Group A beta-hemolytic streptococcus, is seen in the urinalysis as proteinuria accompanied by the presence of red blood cells (**hematuria**) and casts (red blood cell, blood, or granular) in the urine sediment.

In early stages of glomerular damage, only the smaller protein molecules such as albumin are filtered through the glomerulus. Later, virtually all proteins present in the plasma are filtered through the glomerulus and found in the urine. The nephrotic syndrome can result from very heavy or massive proteinuria (>3 or 4 g/day). In this syndrome, so much protein is lost from the body via the urine, the liver is unable to synthesize enough albumin to maintain the blood albumin concentration, resulting in **albuminemia**. This decreased blood albumin results in generalized swelling or edema throughout the body caused by loss of osmotic pressure. Besides massive proteinuria, the nephrotic syndrome is associated with the finding of fat, fatty casts, and tubular epithelial cells containing fat (oval fat bodies) in the urine sediment.

Tubular Damage and Proteinuria. As mentioned previously, a small amount of protein (albumin) is normally filtered through the glomerulus. Normally, all this protein is reabsorbed into the blood through the renal convoluted tubules. Failure to reabsorb the albumin into the bloodstream will result in measurable protein in the urine (proteinuria). The degree of proteinuria in tubular damage is generally mild to moderate. Examples of tubular proteinuria include pyelonephritis, acute tubular necrosis, polycystic kidney disease, heavy metal and Vitamin D intoxication, phenacetin damage, hypokalemia, Wilson's disease, galactosemia, Fanconi's syndrome, and posttransplantation syndrome.

Acute pyelonephritis is an infection of the upper urinary tract or kidney. Besides moderate proteinuria, other urinalysis findings may include the presence of **nitrite** and **leukocyte esterase** in the chemical screen plus white blood cells (neutrophils) and casts (white cell, cellular, granular, or bacterial) in the urine sediment.

Proteinuria with drug-induced acute interstitial disease (an allergic response) may be seen along with the presence of eosinophils in addition to neutrophils, red cells, and cellular or granular casts in the urine sediment.

Acute renal failure or acute tubular necrosis may show only mild proteinuria. However, the sediment may contain renal tubular epithelial cells and epithelial cell, granular, or waxy casts.

Prerenal Disorders and Proteinuria. Proteinuria may be seen as the result of disorders in body sites other than the kidney. These may result from excessive production of low–molecular weight proteins such as hemoglobin, myoglobin, or immunoglobulins that overflow into the urine. An example is the presence of light chain immunoglobulins (Bence Jones protein) associated with multiple myeloma.

Another general mechanism for prerenal proteinuria is caused by a change in the hydrostatic pressure in the kidney glomerulus. As a result of increased blood pressure, proteins normally retained in the blood plasma are forced through the glomerulus and eventually found in the urine. Therefore conditions associated with mild proteinuria in the absence of renal disease include hypertension, congestive heart failure, and dehydration.

Lower Urinary Tract Disorders and Proteinuria. A mild proteinuria may be seen in infections of the lower urinary tract. In this case, proteinuria may result from infection of the ureters or bladder with exudation through the mucosa (lining). Other signs of such infections include positive chemical tests for nitrite (depending on the infecting organism) and leukocyte esterase together with the presence of white blood cells (neutrophils) in the urine sediment. Casts are not present in a lower urinary tract infection since they originate in the kidney tubules.

Asymptomatic Proteinuria. These are conditions in which small amounts of protein may appear transiently in normal persons. Such proteinuria may be found after excessive exercise or exposure to cold. Another example is orthostatic proteinuria, which occurs in persons engaged in normal activity but disappears when they lie down. Tests for orthostatic proteinuria are made on urine collections obtained both when the patient is at rest (first-morning collected immediately after rising) and after the patient has been walking and standing, but not sitting for about 2 hours.

In general, proteinuria associated with renal disease is consistent, whereas that found in normal persons is transient. Long-term significance of asymptomatic proteinuria is unclear. A quantitative protein determination on a 24-hour collection may be necessary to determine the cause of proteinuria.

Consistent Microalbuminuria. Screening tests for urine protein are not sensitive enough to detect the very small amount of protein that might be present in normal urine. However, it is sometimes desirable to detect microalbuminuria, which is the consistent passage of very small amounts of protein as albumin. In cases of diabetes mellitus, the development of renal complications can be predicted and altered or delayed by the early detection of consistent microalbuminuria. This may be measured by means of nephelometry, radial immunodiffusion, and radioimmunoassay. Reagent strip and tablet tests have been developed to screen for microalbuminuria. Micro-Bumintest (Miles Inc, Diagnostics Div.) is a tablet test similar to the reagent strip test for protein, but with a sensitivity of 4 to 8 mg albumin/dL urine. Micral (Boehringer Mannheim Diagnostics Div. of Boehringer Mannheim

Corp.) is a reagent strip immunoassay specific for very small amounts of human albumin. It has a sensitivity of about 0 to 10 mg albumin/dL urine.

Principle of Tests for Urinary Protein

Tests for urinary protein are of two major types:
Reagent Strip Tests (protein, albumin). These tests are based on the principle of protein error of pH indicators and are more sensitive to the presence of albumin than to other proteins.

Precipitation Tests (protein, total). These are tests for protein based on precipitation of all proteins by a chemical or coagulation by heat.

In some laboratories, all urine specimens are tested both with reagent strips and precipitation tests; in others, urine specimens are screened with reagent strips for albumin and confirmed with a precipitation test such as the sulfosalicylic acid test, which is referred to in this text.

Specificity

Reagent Strip Tests	Sulfosalicylic Acid Test
Albumin	All proteins including:
(more sensitive)	albumin
	glycoproteins
	globulins
	(light-chain immunoglobulin or Bence Jones protein, hemoglobin)

Sensitivity (Minimum Detectable Level)

	Test	Sensitivity (mg/dL)
Reagent strip test	Multistix/Albustix	15-30 mg/dL*
	Chemstrip	6 mg/dL* (in 90% tested)
	Rapignost	15 mg/dL* (S_{90})
Sulfosalicylic acid test		5-10 mg/dL

*Manufacturer's values; see product profiles for details.

■ REAGENT STRIP TESTS FOR URINE PROTEIN

Principle

Reagent strip tests for protein are based on the protein error of pH indicators. At a fixed pH, certain pH indicators will show one color in the presence of protein and another color in its absence. Urine pH is held constant by means of a buffer to pH 3, so that any color change indicates the presence of protein, especially albumin. In general, reagent strips detect albumin and will not detect abnormal proteins such as light-chain immunoglobulins (Bence Jones protein) seen in multiple myeloma or other gammaglobulinopathies.

Interferences

Strongly pigmented urine interferes with the color reaction. This may be seen with pigments such as bilirubin and drugs such as phenazopyridine (Pyridium), and other azo-containing compounds, which give a vivid orange color.

False-Positive Results
- Highly buffered or alkaline urines raise the reagent pH and may show a positive color reaction in the absence of protein.
- Contamination of the urine container or specimen with residues of disinfectants containing quaternary ammonium compounds or very small amounts of chlorohexidine may show a positive reaction because of increased alkalinity.
- Loss of buffer caused by exposure of the urine to the reagent strip for an excessive period of time will result in the formation of a blue color whether protein is present or not.

False-Negative Results
- When proteins other than albumin are present.

Additional Comments

Reagent strips are unaffected by turbidity, radiographic contrast media, most drugs and their metabolites, and urine preservatives that occasionally affect protein precipitation tests.

When reading results, color must be matched closely with the color chart. The protein portion of the reagent strip is difficult to interpret, especially at the trace level. When in doubt, the slightly more sensitive SSA protein test or a test for microalbuminuria such as Micro-Bumintest (Miles, Inc.) or Micral (Chemstrip) might be helpful.

Confirmatory Tests

The sulfosalicylic acid test or another protein precipitation method may be used to confirm the presence of protein or when reagent strip results are in doubt. See Table 4-1 for comparison of urine protein test results with different methods.

■ SULFOSALICYLIC ACID TEST FOR URINE PROTEIN

Principle

This precipitation test for urine protein is based on cold precipitation with a strong acid. Various concentrations of **sulfosalicylic acid** have been described. In the procedure described in this text, which is used at the University of Minnesota Hospital and Clinic, a 7 g/dL (7% w/v) solution of SSA is employed so that 11 mL of cleared urine, resulting from the routine 12:1 concentration of the urinary sediment, can be used. Other procedures using equal amounts of cleared urine and SSA reagent employ a 3% (3 g/dL) solution of SSA. See Procedure 4-2.

Reagent - Sulfosalicylic Acid (7% w/v)

Dissolve 70.0 g of 5-sulfosalicylic acid ($C_7H_6O_6S \cdot 2 H_2O$) in deionized or distilled water and dilute to exactly 1 L.

Interferences

False-Positive Results
- Turbidity (cloudiness) in the urine specimen itself would be interpreted as a positive reaction.

COMPARISON OF URINE PROTEIN TEST RESULTS WITH DIFFERENT METHODS							
Test or Method	Results						
	Grade compared with approximate mg/dL per color block						
	Neg	Trace	1+	2+	3+	4+	
SSA	Neg	5-20	30	100	300 to 500	>500	
Multistix	Neg	Trace	30	100	300	≥2000	
Chemstrip	Neg	Trace	30	100	≥500	No color block	
Rapignost	Neg	No color block	30	100	≥500	No color block	

SULFOSALICYLIC ACID TEST FOR PROTEIN

1. Centrifuge a 12 mL aliquot of urine.

2. Decant 11 mL of the supernatant urine into a 16 × 125 mm tube. Note clarity of the supernatant urine.

3. Add 3 mL of 7% sulfosalicylic acid reagent.

4. Stopper the tube and mix by inverting twice.

5. Let stand exactly 10 minutes.

6. Invert tube twice.

7. Observe the degree of precipitation and grade the results according to the descriptions in Table 4-2. To avoid making the test too sensitive, examine negative and trace reactions in ordinary room light. If available, use an agglutination viewer to grade results higher than a trace. To observe the degree of precipitation, tilt the test tube while simultaneously viewing the quality and quantity of precipitate in the mirror.

Urine must be clear before testing. This is usually done by centrifugation.

- Organic iodides in radiographic contrast media such as meglumine diatrizoate (Renografin, Hypaque) used for diagnostic procedures may give a delayed positive reaction. The precipitate in this case is rather crystalline in appearance, unlike the granular protein precipitate, and the solution remains clear for a short time after addition of the SSA reagent, unlike the immediate precipitation seen when protein is present.

- Interference by radiographic media is suggested by specific gravity values greater than 1.035 by urinometer or refractometer, with a normal specific gravity by reagent strip. It may be confirmed by checking the patient's history for the use of diagnostic radiographic procedures. The precipitated material in the SSA tube also may be observed microscopically for the presence of crystals, which polarize light, as opposed to the amorphous precipitate, which does not polarize light, characteristic of true protein precipitation (Fig. 4-1).

Table 4-2

SSA PROTEIN TEST RESULTS

SSA result	Description	Approximate protein concentration in mg/dL by reagent strip*
Negative	No turbidity, or no increase in turbidity	<5 mg/dL
	Clear ring is visible at bottom of tube when viewed from above (top to bottom)	
Trace	Barely perceptible turbidity in ordinary room light	5-20 mg/dL
	Printed material distorted but readable through the tube	
	Cannot see a ring at bottom of tube when viewed from above	
1+	Distinct turbidity but no distinct granulation	30 mg/dL
2+	Turbidity with granulation but no flocculation	100 mg/dL
3+	Turbidity with granulation and flocculation	300-500 mg/dL
4+	Clumps of precipitated protein or solid precipitate	>500 mg/dL

*Based on a comparison of SSA values by reagent strip (Multistix) and Cobas protein results UMHC Jan. 1993. Unpublished.

Figure 4-1

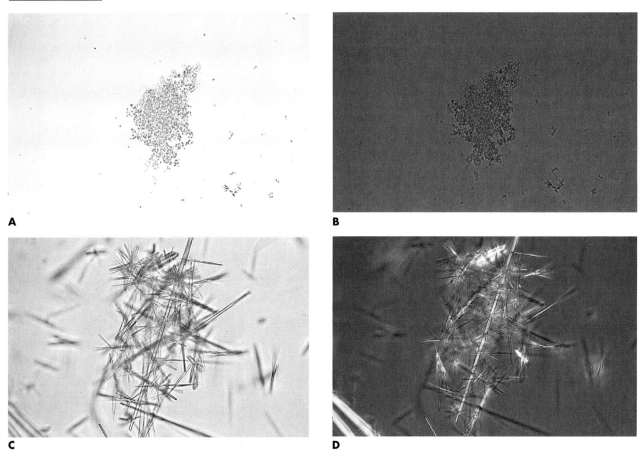

Microscopic appearance of SSA precipitate due to protein and radiographic media.
A, Amorphous appearing SSA precipitate of protein, brightfield, ×400. B, Same
field as A with compensated polarized light, ×400, showing lack of polarization of
light. C, Crystals of radiographic media (Hypaque meglumine) precipitated by SSA,
brightfield, ×400. D, Same field as C with compensated polarized light, ×400,
showing birefringence (polarization of light by crystals of radiographic media).

• Other drugs causing false-positive reactions include the following: high levels of penicillin, sulfonamides, or cephalosporin; Tolbutamide metabolites—an oral insulin substitute; Tolmetin (Tolectin)—an anti-inflammatory agent. The presence of drug interference should be confirmed by checking the patient history and observing the SSA precipitate microscopically for the presence of crystals. Reagent strip results would be negative or more than one grade lower than the SSA result in cases of drug interference.

False-Negative Results

• Rarely, a highly buffered alkaline urine contains enough buffer to neutralize the sulfosalicylic acid reagent and cause falsely low or negative protein results. Such specimens might also give a false-positive reaction with the reagent strip test. To resolve this discrepancy, acidify the urine specimen to pH 5 or 6 and retest with reagent strip and SSA. Results should be similar on the acidified urine.

Additional Comments

If specimens show a positive SSA protein test with a negative reagent strip test or value more than one grade less than the SSA value, suspect the presence of a protein other than albumin, such as the light-chain immunoglobulins (Bence Jones protein) seen in multiple myeloma. This may be confirmed by electrophoresis or immunoelectrophoresis.

Patients who have received a pancreas transplant with anastomosis may excrete nonalbumin pancreatic fluid proteins into the urine, which is seen as a negative reagent strip and positive SSA protein reaction.

BLOOD (HEMOGLOBIN AND MYOGLOBIN)

Clinical Importance

Tests for blood in the urine, in addition to tests for protein and the microscopic analysis of the urinary sediment, are used to assess the condition of the kidney and urinary tract. **Hematuria,** which is the presence of blood in the urine, may indicate bleeding at any point in the urinary system from the glomerulus to the urethra. The actual location of the bleeding and its cause is important in the diagnosis and treatment of the patient. Blood in the urine may be an early sign of kidney or bladder tumor (benign and malignant) or result from stone formation in the kidney or bladder. Hematuria might be a sign of glomerular damage, interstitial nephritis, or infection of the kidney; or it may be seen with a lower urinary tract infection such as cystitis, an infection of the bladder. Hematuria may also accompany generalized bleeding disorders or be seen with anticoagulant therapy. Although detection of blood in urine is a serious finding, the presence of a few red blood cells in urine is normal, and hematuria may be associated with benign conditions.

The chemical reagent strip tests for blood in the urine will react with red blood cells, hemoglobin, or myoglobin (muscle hemoglobin). Although most positive reactions are caused by the presence of red blood cells in the urine, the tests are actually more sensitive to the presence of either hemoglobin or myoglobin. A distinction of which form is present is clinically significant. Reagent strip tests will detect **occult** or hidden **blood.** This is blood that is not suspected from the physical appearance of the urine specimen. Nevertheless, the presence of blood in urine is associated with a change in the appearance (color and transparency) of the urine and the presence of red cells in the microscopic examination of the urine sediment. Urine containing blood may appear normal, smoky, pink, amber, red to red-brown, brown, or bloody. In general, if the urine appears pink to red or brown in color, the presence of red blood cells, hemoglobin, or myoglobin should be suspected.

Differentiation between the presence of red blood cells and hemoglobin in the urine is clinically significant. Both will result in a positive reagent strip test for blood. Theoretically, hematuria is accompanied by the presence of red blood cells in the urine sediment, whereas the absence of red cells indicates hemoglobinuria. Unfortunately, red cells rapidly lyse in the urine, especially when the specific gravity is low (<1.010 by reagent strip) and/or the pH is alkaline. Therefore the absence of red cells in the urine sediment does not rule out hematuria or confirm hemoglobinuria. In difficult cases, tests for serum creatine kinase (CK), serum haptoglobin, and serum lactate dehydrogenase (LD) may be necessary to differentiate red cells, hemoglobin, and myoglobin (Table 4-3).

Red Blood Cells. Hematuria is the presence of red blood cells in the urine. It may result from bleeding at any point in the urinary system because of renal disease or dysfunction, infection, tumor or lesions, stone formation, generalized bleeding disorders, or anticoagulant usage. It is a sensitive early indicator of renal disease that should not be missed. Although there may be little correlation between the amount of blood and the severity of the disorder, hematuria may be the only indication of renal disease. It is associated with glomerular damage and is a typical finding in glomerular nephritis. Other findings in the routine urinalysis

Table 4-3

DIFFERENTIATION OF RED BLOOD CELLS, HEMOGLOBIN, AND MYOGLOBIN IN URINE

Finding	Red Cells	Hemoglobin	Myoglobin
Reagent strip blood test	Positive	Positive	Positive
Red blood cells in sediment	Present	Absent (few)	Absent (few)
Urine appearance	Cloudy red	Clear red	Clear red-brown
Plasma appearance	Normal	Pink to red (hemolysis)	Normal
Total serum creatine kinase (CK)	Normal	Slight elevation (10 times normal upper limit)	Marked elevation (40 times normal upper limit)
Total serum lactate dehydrogenase (LD)	Normal	Elevated	Elevated
LD isoenzymes 1 and 2	Normal	Elevated	Normal
LD isoenzymes 4 and 5	Normal	Normal	Elevated

associated with hematuria are the presence and degree of proteinuria and the presence and morphology of red cells (especially dysmorphic forms) and casts (especially red cell casts) in the urine sediment.

Hemoglobin. Hemoglobinuria is the presence of free hemoglobin in the urine. It may indicate significant intravascular hemolysis or hemolysis within the kidney or the lower urinary tract, or in the voided urine specimen itself. Hemoglobin in the bloodstream is carried by haptoglobin. When this plasma carrier is saturated, hemoglobin is excreted in the urine. Some of the excreted hemoglobin is absorbed into tubular cells, converted to ferritin and hemosiderin, and subsequently excreted several days after an acute hemolytic episode. These hemosiderin-containing cells and granules may be observed in the urinary sediment, especially when stained with Prussian blue.

Myoglobin. Myoglobinuria is the presence of myoglobin in urine. It is a rare but important finding. Myoglobin is released after acute destruction of muscle fibers (rhabdomyolysis) and is rapidly cleared from the bloodstream and excreted in urine as a red-brown pigment. Large amounts of myoglobin in the urine damages the kidneys. However, renal failure from myoglobinuria may not be recognized until a week or more after the clinical event, at which time the myoglobinuria is usually absent. Following rhabdomyolysis such as from strenuous exercise in an untrained person or traumatic injury, red-brown urine is voided within 1 or 2 days. In addition to a strongly positive test for blood, urinalysis findings include the presence of protein, few to no red cells, and casts—especially brown myoglobin casts. Other findings include normal colored serum (hemoglobinuria serum is pink), markedly elevated serum creatine kinase (CK), normal serum haptoglobin, and elevated serum lactate dehydrogenase (LD) with predominant LD isoenzymes 4 and 5 (see Table 4-3).

Principle and Specificity

Reagent strip tests for blood (hemoglobin, myoglobin) in urine are based on the **peroxidase** activity of the heme portion of the hemoglobin molecule. Reagent strip tests for blood contain an organic peroxide and the reduced form of a chromogen. The heme portion of the hemoglobin molecule has peroxidase activity. This catalyzes the release of oxygen from the organic peroxide contained in the reagent strip. The released oxygen reacts with the reduced form of the chromogen, producing an oxidized chromogen. The reaction is seen as a color change that is compared with the color chart provided by the manufacturer. The reaction is summarized as:

Peroxide + reduced chromogen $\xrightarrow{\text{(peroxidase activity)}}$ heme → water + oxidized chromogen

Reagent strips are equally sensitive to hemoglobin and myoglobin. Red blood cells are hemolyzed by contact with the reagent strip and the released hemoglobin reacts as described. Intact red cells must come in contact with the reagent strip and lyse in order to react. Thus urine must be well-mixed when tested for blood since false-negative results will occur if only a few intact red blood cells are present and allowed to settle before testing.

Sensitivity (Minimum Detectable Level)

Reagent Strip Test	Sensitivity (manufacturer's value)
Multistix/Hemastix	0.015-0.062 mg/dL hemoglobin (equivalent to 5 to 20 Ery/μL)
Chemstrip	5 Ery/μL or hemoglobin corresponding to 10 Ery/μL in 90% urines tested
Rapignost	0.015-0.03 mg free hemoglobin/dL urine (equivalent to 5 to 10 Ery/μL)

Interferences

False-Positive Results
- Strong oxidizing cleaning agents such as chlorine bleach cause false-positive results because of oxidation of the chromogen in the absence of peroxide.
- Microbial peroxidase activity associated with urinary tract infection may result in a positive reaction.
- Blood as a contaminant from menstruation will give positive results of no clinical significance.

False-Negative Results
- **Ascorbic acid** (generally more than 25 mg/dL) may cause false negative or delayed results—seen after ingestion of large doses of vitamin C or when included as a reducing agent in certain parenteral antibiotics such as tetracycline. Both Multistix and Chemstrip reagent strips claim no interference at reasonable or normally encountered levels. Chemstrip products include a blood-iodate scavenger to reduce false-negative results. Multistix products containing diisopropylbenzene dihydroperoxide as the organic peroxide are less subject to interference with ascorbic acid. Falsely low results may be seen with Rapignost products;

however, these multiple reagent strips include a test for ascorbic acid to rule out unsuspected false-negative results.

- Testing the supernatant urine from centrifugation or settling when only a few intact red cells are present will result in false-negative results.
- Elevated specific gravity (high salt concentration) and elevated protein levels may reduce the lysis of red cells.
- Other causes of false-negative results include formalin used as a preservative, large amounts of nitrite (more than 10 mg/dL), and treatment with captopril (an antihypertensive).

Additional Comments

Ascorbic acid remains a potential problem in a practical sense in reagent strip tests for blood. Any of the reagent strip tests that depend on the release of oxygen and subsequent oxidation of a chromogen are subject to false-negative or delayed results caused by the presence of ascorbic acid. When present in sufficient quantity, the ascorbic acid, which is a strong reducing agent, reacts with the released hydrogen peroxide rather than chromogen, causing inhibited (negative) results or delayed color reaction.

Interference by ascorbic acid is suspected when the reagent strip test for blood is negative, yet red blood cells are observed in the microscopic analysis of the urine sediment. The presence of ascorbic acid may be confirmed by testing the urine with a reagent strip for ascorbic acid or by the patient's clinical history.

Confirmatory Tests

- Microscopic examination of the urine sediment.
- Reagent strip test for ascorbic acid if the test for blood is negative and red cells are seen in the microscopic examination, or if blood is suspected on the basis of the appearance of the urine specimen.

■ NITRITE

Clinical Importance

Reagent strip tests for nitrite are used as a rapid method for detecting asymptomatic urinary tract infection. This test is most useful when combined with reagent strip tests for leukocyte esterase, another indicator of urinary tract infection. When certain (not all) bacteria are present in the urinary tract, they will convert nitrate (a normal urine constituent) to nitrite. Nitrite converters are generally gram-negative bacteria, and gram-positive organisms may not be

detected. In addition, there must be sufficient nitrate, a constituent derived from vegetables in the diet, for the reaction to occur. A significant disadvantage of this test is that urine must remain in the bladder for a sufficient period (generally 4 hours) for the conversion reaction to take place. Thus a first-morning specimen or a specimen collected at least 4 hours after the last voiding is preferred. This is difficult to obtain from a patient with a urinary tract infection; a common complaint with this condition is frequent urination.

To prevent kidney damage, infection must be detected as soon as possible. Most infections begin in the lower urinary tract as a result of fecal contamination from organisms normally present in the feces, such as *Escherichia coli*. The urinary tract is normally sterile. Infection is introduced via the urethra and ascends to the bladder, ureters, and finally the kidney. Early detection and treatment is important to prevent this ascending infection and subsequent renal involvement. Urinary tract infection is typically a disease of women. Exceptions are just after birth and, because of incontinance, old age.

Other indicators of urinary tract infection that may be used with tests for nitrite include reagent strip tests for leukocyte esterase, protein, and pH. Urinary sediment findings include bacteria and white blood cells. The presence of casts, especially white cell or bacteria casts, locate the infection within the kidney. Final diagnosis requires quantitative urine culture.

Principle

Reagent strip tests are based on the **Griess test**, which involves a **diazo reaction**. In an acid medium, nitrite will react with an aromatic amine (arsanilic or sulfanilic acid) to produce a diazonium salt. The diazonium salt is then coupled with another aromatic ring (quinolin) to form an azo dye, which is a pink or red color.

Specificity

The reaction is specific for nitrite.

Results

Results are reported as positive or negative. Any degree of uniform pink coloration is reported as positive. However, pink spots or pink edges are a negative reaction. The intensity of color formation does not indicate the degree of bacterial infection. Any pink coloration suggests a significant infection, equivalent to 100,000 or more microorganisms per mL.

Sensitivity (Minimum Detectable Level)

Reagent Strip Test for urine nitrite	Sensitivity manufacturer's value
Multistix	0.06 to 0.1 mg/dL nitrite ion
Chemstrip	as low as 0.05 mg/dL nitrite
Rapignost	0.05 to 0.1 mg/dL nitrite

Interferences

False-Positive Results

- In vitro conversion of nitrate to nitrite because of bacterial contamination in an improperly collected or stored urine specimen may give false-positive results.
- Medication such as phenazopyridine or other azo-containing compounds or other dyes that color urine red or that turn red in an acidic medium may mask color development or cause false-positive results.

False-Negative Results

- Insufficient incubation time in the bladder (in vivo) for conversion of nitrate to nitrite may result in false-negative results.
- Insufficient dietary nitrate present in urine for bacteria to reduce nitrate to nitrite (such as with starvation, fasting, or intravenous feeding) may yield negative results, even with a significant bacterial infection.
- Negative or delayed results may be seen with ascorbic acid in concentrations of 25 mg/dL or greater in specimens with small amounts of nitrite, because of reduction of the diazonium salt by ascorbic acid.
- Degradation of nitrite to nitrogen will give false-negative results.
- Reduced sensitivity is seen in concentrated urine with low pH (less than 6). These conditions are not typical of urinary tract infection, however.

Additional Comments

The test is primarily useful, if positive. If the reagent strip shows a negative reaction, urinary infection cannot be ruled out, and there are many causes of false-negative reaction. Organisms must contain the reductase enzyme necessary to reduce nitrate to nitrite. This is true of most of the gram-negative enteric pathogens that cause urinary tract infection. However, the gram-positive enterococci and yeast do not contain the reductase enzyme. The 4-hour incubation time in the bladder is necessary for conversion of nitrate to nitrite and is probably the main obstacle to positive reagent strip results with significant infection.

◼ LEUKOCYTE ESTERASE

Clinical Importance

Reagent strip tests for leukocyte esterase are used as another means of detecting urinary tract infection. Measurement of leukocyte esterase is an indirect measure of leukocytes (white blood cells) in the urine. Leukocyte esterase is present in azurophilic or primary granules of granulocytic leukocytes, including polymorphonuclear neutrophils (PMNs or neutrophils), monocytes (histiocytes), eosinophils, and basophils. Positive leukocyte esterase reactions in urine occur most often with increased neutrophils, which are present in response to bacterial infection. Conditions associated with sufficient quantities of other granulocytes to give a positive reaction are extremely rare. The lymphocytes and epithelial cells do not contain leukocyte esterase and are not measured in this test.

When the urinary tract is infected at any point from the urethra to the kidney, increased numbers of leukocytes, especially neutrophils, are typical. These cells are also seen in the urinary sediment. However, neutrophils are rapidly lysed or destroyed in urine, possibly a result of their phagocytic activity. Once lysed, they are undetectable in the microscopic examination of the sediment. However, the reagent strip test for leukocyte esterase remains positive whether lysed or intact cells are present in the urine.

Normal urine contains about 0 to 2 leukocytes per high power field in a 12:1 or 10:1 concentrated urine sediment. The sensitivity of the reagent strip tests for leukocyte esterase is about 5 to 15 leukocytes per high power field. Therefore normal urine will give a negative reagent strip reaction, yet the absence of leukocyte esterase does not rule out a urinary tract infection. Test results for leukocyte esterase are useful in combination with tests for nitrite, pH, and protein. The presence of bacteria and leukocytes in the urine sediment also are typical of infection.

Increased leukocyte esterase also may be seen in the absence of bacteria in the sediment or on routine urine culture. Inflammatory conditions may result in increased numbers of leukocytes without bacterial infection. Increased leukocytes may remain after treatment with antibiotics, without bacteria. Infections by organisms such as trichomonads and chlamydia may show increased leukocytes in the urine sediment with a positive reagent strip test for leukocyte esterase while routine urine culture results are negative. Immunosuppressed patients with urinary tract infection are unable to produce adequate quantities of leukocytes in response to their infection. Therefore the leukocyte esterase reaction is low or negative in the presence of significant infection in immunosupressed patients.

Principle

Reagent strip tests for leukocyte esterase use a diazo reaction, much like the reagent strip tests for nitrite. Reactive ingredients include an ester and a diazonium salt. The ester is hydrolyzed by leukocyte esterase to form its alcohol (which contains an aromatic ring) and acid. The aromatic ring is then coupled with the diazonium salt to form an azo dye. Positive reactions produce a purple color.

Specificity

The reaction is specific for esterase that is present in granulocytic leukocytes and histiocytes.

Sensitivity (Minimum Detectable Level)

Reagent Strip Test for urine leukocyte esterase	Sensitivity (manufacturer's value)
Multistix	5-15 cells/hpf in clinical urine
Chemstrip	10-25 cells/μL in first positive color block
Rapignost	10-25 cells/μL urine

Interferences

Substances that color urine, such as nitrofurantoin or bilirubin, may make color interpretation difficult.

False-Positive Results
- Strong oxidizing agents such as chlorine bleach and formalin (formaldehyde) preservative may cause positive reactions.

False-Negative Results
- Decreased results may be seen with elevated glucose (more than 3 g/dL), high specific gravity, oxalic acid, and high levels of albumin (more than 500 mg/dL).
- Drugs (antibiotics) causing decreased or false-negative results include cephalexin, cephalothin, tetracycline, and gentamicin.
- Large amounts of ascorbic acid may inhibit the reaction because of the reduction of the diazonium salt.

Additional Comments

The presence of repeated trace and positive values are clinically significant and indicate the need for further testing to determine the cause of leukocytes in the urine. Follow-up tests may include microscopic analysis of the urinary sediment, Gram stain, and quantitative urine culture.

The test is not affected by the presence of blood, bacteria, or epithelial cells. Reagent strips are available with tests for leukocyte esterase and nitrite, a clinically useful combination.

■ GLUCOSE (SUGAR)

Clinical Importance

Unlike the reagent strips previously described, tests for urine glucose are used to diagnose and monitor a metabolic rather than renal or urinary tract condition. The presence of measurable glucose (also called *dextrose*) in the urine is termed glycosuria (or glucosuria). This is not a normal finding. Although there are other causes of glycosuria, suspect the metabolic disorder diabetes mellitus when glucose is present in the urine. Tests for urine and blood glucose are used to diagnose and monitor this condition.

As mentioned, the presence of glucose in urine is not a normal finding. The blood glucose concentration normally varies between about 60 and 110 mg/dL. This may increase to 120 to 160 mg/dL after a meal. In normal individuals, all of the glucose in the blood is filtered through the glomerulus and reabsorbed into the bloodstream by an active transport mechanism at the proximal renal tubules. If the renal threshold (the lowest blood glucose concentration that will result in glycosuria) is exceeded (usually greater than 180 to 200 mg/dL), the excess glucose will not be reabsorbed into the blood and will be eliminated from the body by way of the urine. The most common condition in which the renal threshold for glucose is exceeded is diabetes mellitus, a condition characterized by the passage of a large quantity of urine (diabetes) containing sugar (mellitus). This condition results from a deficiency in the production of, or an inhibition in the action of the hormone insulin. Insulin is a hormone that has the effect of lowering the blood glucose concentration. If deficient, the blood glucose concentration exceeds the renal threshold and glucose is spilled over into the urine. Other factors that might result in glycosuria are reduced glomerular blood flow, reduced tubular reabsorption, and reduced urine flow.

Tests for urine glucose are among the oldest of laboratory tests. The "taste test" was used to distinguish sweet (caused by sugar) from the normal salty taste of urine. Hindu physicians noticed that ants were attracted to "honey urine." In 1956 the first reagent strip test appeared, namely, Clinistix (Miles Inc.), an enzymatic test for urine glucose, as did a similar paper tear strip test for glucose, Tes-Tape (Eli Lily & Co., Indianapolis, Ind.)[2] Together with Clinitest (Miles, Inc.), a tablet copper reduction test developed in 1945, urine glucose tests were routinely used by diabetic patients to self-monitor the adequacy of insulin control. These urine tests have been replaced by home blood glucose testing; however, urine glucose tests are less expensive and non-invasive, and still have a place in diabetes monitoring.

The presence of glycosuria is not diagnostic of diabetes mellitus. For example, glycosuria may be observed after large amounts of sugar or foods containing sugar are ingested. It may also occur in cases of acute emotional stress in which glucose is liberated by the liver for energy, and after heavy exercise. Glycosuria may also be associated with pregnancy, certain types of meningitis, hypothyroidism, certain tumors of the adrenal medulla, and some brain injuries.

■ REAGENT STRIP TESTS FOR GLUCOSE

Principle

Reagent strip tests for urine glucose are double sequential enzyme reactions based on use of the enzyme **glucose oxidase**. Glucose oxidase will oxidize glucose to gluconic acid and at the same time reduce atmospheric oxygen to hydrogen peroxide. In the presence of the enzyme peroxidase, the hydrogen peroxide formed will oxidize the reduced form of a dye (chromogen) to the oxidized form. This is seen as a color change. This reaction is diagrammed:

Step 1:

$$\text{Glucose (in urine)} + \text{O}_2 \text{ (from air)} \xrightarrow{\text{glucose oxidase}} \text{Gluconic acid} + \text{H}_2\text{O}_2$$

Step 2:

$$\text{H}_2\text{O}_2 + \text{reduced chromogen} \xrightarrow{\text{peroxidase}} \text{oxidized chromogen} + \text{H}_2\text{O}$$

Test products vary in the chromogen used as the oxidation-reduction indicator. They all contain glucose oxidase and peroxidase.

Specificity

All reagent strip tests are specific for glucose. They will not detect other sugars such as galactose, lactose, fructose, pentose, and sucrose, which might be clinically significant if present in urine. Detection of these sugars (with the exception of sucrose) may be done with a copper reduction test for reducing substances (sugars) such as the Clinitest Tablet Test (Miles, Inc.).

Sensitivity (Minimum Detectable Level)

Tests for urine glucose and sugar	Sensitivity (manufacturer's values)
Multistix/Diastix	75-125 mg/dL glucose (as low as 40 mg/dL in dilute urine containing less than 5 mg/dL ascorbic acid)
Chemstrip	40 mg/dL in 90% of urines tested
Rapignost	30 mg/dL maximum sensitivity 20 mg/dL
Clinitest Tablet Test	250 mg/dL reducing sugars (including glucose)

Table 4-4

RANGE OF VALUES IN TESTS FOR URINE GLUCOSE AND SUGAR

Test	Neg	50	100	150	250	500	750	1000	2000	3000	5000
Multistix/Diastix	Neg		100		250	500		1000	2000 or more		
Chemstrip (Multiple)	Neg	50	100		250	500		1000			
Rapignost	Norm	50		150	≥500						
Chemstrip uG & uGK	Neg		100		250	500		1000	2000	3000	5000
Clinitest 5 drop	Neg				250	500	750	1000	2000		
Clinitest 2 drop	Neg				Trace	500		1000	2000	3000	5000

Color blocks in mg/dL

*Units stated by manufacturers differ. All have been converted to mg/dL glucose.

Range of Values

The Multistix multiple reagent strips and Diastix contain color blocks allowing semiquantitation to 2000 mg/dL (2 g/dL). Chemstrip multiple reagent strips contain color blocks to 1000 mg/dL (1 gm/dL). Chemstrip uG (urine glucose) and Chemstrip uGK (urine glucose and ketone) allow for semiquantitation to 5000 mg/dL (5 g/dL); however, the reaction time is increased to 2 minutes. Rapignost strips allow for semiquantitation to 500 mg/dL. The range of values seen with various tests for urine glucose and reducing sugars (substances) is in Table 4-4.

Interferences

Because reagent strip tests are specific for glucose, most interferences cause reduced or false-negative results for glucose.

False-Positive Results
- Chlorine bleach or other strong oxidizing agents may oxidize the reduced form of dye, causing a color change in the absence of glucose.
- Sensitivity is increased with low specific gravity; trace values may be seen in very dilute urine.
- Reagent strips exposed to air by improper storage have been shown to give false-positive results.[1]

False-Negative Results
- Large urinary concentrations of ascorbic acid—from therapeutic doses of vitamin C or from drugs such as tetracyclines in which ascorbic acid is used as a reducing agent—may inhibit or delay color development. Ascorbic acid blocks or delays the reaction by acting as a reducing agent and reacting with hydrogen peroxide released by the presence of glucose in the urine.

  Multistix products may show inhibition with more than 50 mg/dL ascorbic acid in specimens containing small amounts (75-125 mg/dL) of glucose. Chemstrip is unaffected by ascorbic acid concentrations less than 100 mg/dL. Rapignost products may show false-negative results from the presence of ascorbic acid in specimens containing less than 100 mg/dL glucose.
- Moderate levels of ketones (40 mg/dL or higher) in specimens with small amounts of glucose (75-125 mg/dL) may show decreased values for glucose. However, this combination of high ketone and low glucose is unlikely in a diabetic patient.
- Use of sodium fluoride inhibits the enzyme.
- Cold, refrigerated urine specimens inhibit the enzyme reaction and yield decreased values.

Confirmatory and Follow-up Tests

If semiquantitation beyond the color blocks on usual multiple reagent strips is desired, urine may be tested with a test such as Chemstrip uG or uGK, or with the 2-drop Clinitest tablet test method for reducing sugars (see Table 4-4). The presence of ketones with glucose implies inadequate control of diabetes.

■ CLINITEST COPPER REDUCTION TEST FOR REDUCING SUGARS

Principle

The Clinitest Tablet Test (Miles, Inc.) is a nonspecific test for urine sugar and is based on the ability of glucose (or any other reducing substance) to reduce copper(II) *cupric ions*, to copper(I) *cuprous ions*, in the presence of heat and alkali. A positive reaction is seen as a change in color ranging from blue to green, yellow, and orange depending on the amount of sugar present. The reaction is:

$$2CuSO_4 + \text{reducing substance} \xrightarrow[\text{heat}]{\text{alkali}}$$
(copper II)   (e.g., glucose)

$$Cu_2O + \text{oxidized form of reducing substance}$$
(copper I)   (e.g., gluconic acid)

The reaction is essentially **Benedict's qualitative test** for urine sugar. Copper sulfate reagent is combined with anhydrous sodium hydroxide in an effervescent tablet containing citric acid and sodium carbonate. The interaction of sodium hydroxide with citric acid and water results in moderate boiling, making an external boiling water bath unnecessary.

Clinitest tests may be performed as either a 5-drop or a 2-drop method (Procedure 4-3). The 2-drop method was developed to avoid the so-called "pass-through" phenomenon. This may occur if very large amounts of sugar are present in urine, a possibility in certain diabetic patients. With the pass-through phenomenon, the color reaction goes through the entire range of colors back to a dark greenish brown because of the caramelization (burning) of the very large amount of sugar in the urine by heat. The final color does not compare with any of the color blocks; however, it most closely resembles a block representing a significantly lower result. To avoid falsely low results, it is extremely important to observe the entire Clinitest reaction from the addition of the tablet to the end point. A pass-through reaction is indicated by a bright orange color before caramelization occurs. Such reactions are minimized by use of the 2-drop method, since less sugar is present in the urine/reagent mixture. The 2-drop method is also useful to semiquantitate values greater than 2000 mg/dL (2 g/dL)—up to 5 g/dL are reportable.

Specificity

Copper reduction tests are nonspecific tests for reducing substances (sugars). They will react with any reducing sugar (including glucose) and other nonglucose-reducing substances.

Other nonglucose-reducing substances (NGRS) that may be found in urine include the reducing sugars galactose, fructose, lactose, and pentose, plus uric acid, creatinine, homogentisic acid, ascorbic acid, chloroform, and formaldehyde. The presence of certain sugars such as galactose and lactose is clinically significant, and their presence would not be detected with common reagent strip tests for glucose.

Sensitivity

Clinitest will detect 250 mg/dL sugar. This is significantly less than all of the reagent strip tests for glucose. Therefore with the presence of small amounts of glucose in urine, the reagent strip test may be positive whereas the copper reduction test is negative.

Interferences

Tablets must be protected from moisture. If not stored properly, they will change from a spotted bluish-white color to dark blue or blackish. These discolored tablets should not be used because they will not give reliable results. Tablets are available individually packaged in aluminum foil to prevent absorption of moisture. Although more expensive in this form, they may be cost effective when a limited number of tests are performed.

False-Positive Results

- The presence of extremely large amounts of ascorbic acid (more than 200 mg/dL) may cause low level positive results (equivalent to 500 mg/dL glucose or less).
- Specimens that have a low specific gravity and contain glucose may give a slightly elevated result with Clinitest.
- Large quantities of nalidixic acid, cephalosporins, and probenecid may give false-positive reactions.

Procedure 4-3

CLINITEST TABLET TEST FOR REDUCING SUGARS

5-drop Method

Follow the directions supplied with the Clinitest tablets.

1. Place 5 drops of urine in a 15 × 85 mm test tube and add 10 drops of water.
2. Add one Clinitest tablet.
3. Watch while boiling takes place, but do not shake.
4. Wait 15 seconds after boiling stops, then shake the tube gently, and compare the color of the solution with the color scale supplied for the 5-drop method.
5. Report results with the same units as used for reagent strip glucose results.
6. Watch the solution carefully while it is boiling. If it passes through orange to a dark shade of greenish brown, the sugar concentration is more than 2.0 g/dL, and the result should be recorded as greater than 2.0 g/dL without reference to the color scale. Urines showing this pass-through phenomenon should be retested with the 2-drop method.

2-drop Method

Follow the directions supplied with the Clinitest tablets.

1. Place 2 drops of urine in a 15 × 85 mm test tube and add 10 drops of water.
2. Add one Clinitest tablet.
3. Watch while boiling takes place, but do not shake.
4. Wait 15 seconds after boiling stops, then shake the tube gently, and compare the color of the solution with the color scale supplied for the 2-drop method.
5. Watch the test throughout the entire reaction and waiting period, since the pass-through phenomenon may also occur with the 2-drop test.
6. Report the results with the same units as used for other methods.

Modified from Linne JJ, Ringsrud KM: *Basic techniques in clinical laboratory science*, ed 3, St. Louis, 1992, Mosby, page 357.

False-Negative Results
- Mixing the Clinitest tube before the 15-second waiting period after boiling may cause falsely low values because of reoxidation of the cuprous ions to cupric ions by atmospheric oxygen.
- The presence of radiographic contrast media may result in reduced or false-negative reactions.

Additional Comments

The bottom of the test tube becomes very hot during the Clinitest reaction. Hold the tube at the lip (not the bottom) or place it in a test tube rack to avoid burns.

The urine from very young (less than 2 years of age) pediatric patients may be screened with the Clinitest test to detect the presence of **galactosuria**. The presence of galactose in the urine results from a metabolic error in which the enzyme galactose-1-phosphate uridyltransferase is lacking. This results in a failure to metabolize galactose, with increased levels in the blood (galactosemia) and urine. Galactosemia will result in permanent physical and mental deterioration, which may be controlled by early detection and dietary restriction of galactose.

Other reducing sugars such as lactose may be seen in the urine late in pregnancy or early lactation. Lactose intolerance in infancy and failure to gain weight may be because of intestinal lactase deficiency. Lactosuria may be seen.

Additional Tests

In cases in which nonglucose-reducing sugars are present in the urine, the reagent strip test for glucose is negative, whereas the copper reduction test (Clinitest) is positive. The specific sugar may be identified by thin layer chromatography.

■ KETONE BODIES

Clinical Importance

Like glucose, the presence of ketone bodies in the urine is a measure of metabolic, rather than renal, function. The ketone bodies are a group of three related compounds: acetoacetic (diacetic) acid, ß-hydroxybutyric acid, and acetone (Fig. 4-2).

When fat is used as a source of energy (fat catabolism), acetoacetic acid is produced first; this is converted either reversibly to ß-hydroxybutyric acid or irreversibly to acetone. Ketones are normal products of **fat metabolism**, which are eventually converted to carbon dioxide and water. They are not normally detectable in the urine, although some concentrated urine specimens may give reactions up to and includ-

Figure 4-2

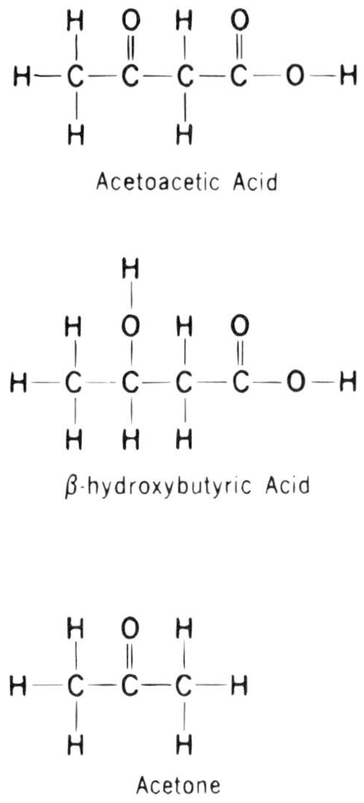

The ketone bodies. (From Linne JJ, Ringsrud KM: *Basic techniques in clinical laboratory science*, ed 3, St. Louis, 1992, Mosby.)

ing trace results. When increased quantities of fat are metabolized, the entire ketone production cannot be utilized as a source of energy. This is seen clinically as increased ketones in the blood (**ketonemia**) with increased ketones in the urine (**ketonuria**). This is **ketosis**, the combined increased concentration of ketones in the blood and the urine.

Two conditions associated with ketosis are diabetes mellitus and starvation. With diabetes mellitus, because of lack of insulin, the body is unable to use carbohydrate (glucose) as a source of energy and compensates by resorting to fat catabolism, a form of **glyconeogenesis**. This results in an accumulation of ketones in the blood and urine (ketosis). With starvation, the body is depleted of stored carbohydrate and must resort to fat as an energy source, with resulting ketosis. This is the mechanism for ketosis in dehydration and conditions associated with fever, vomiting, and diarrhea. With liver damage, the body lacks liver glycogen, the primary source of stored carbohydrate, and resorts to fat for its energy source. A ketogenic diet will also result in ketosis. This is a diet high in fat and low in carbohydrates; specifically, a diet containing more than 1.5 g of fat per 1.0 g of carbohydrate.

Since ketonuria is associated with the presence of glucose in urine in insulin-dependent diabetes mellitus, reagent strips that combine tests for glucose and ketones are available and useful for home or laboratory monitoring of diabetic control. Ketosis is an important finding, since acetoacetic acid and ß-hydroxybutyric acid contribute excess hydrogen ions to the blood. This can result in acidosis, which can lead to coma and even death. The body compensates for excess acid in the blood by eliminating hydrogen ions through the urine. The kidney is capable of producing urine with a pH as low as 4.5; thus uncontrolled diabetes is associated with a urine of an acid (low) pH. In the treatment of diabetes mellitus, it is important to control the dosage of insulin so that ketosis and acidosis do not occur. Reagent strip tests for ketonuria are an early indicator of inadequate control by insulin. A typical urine specimen from a patient with uncontrolled diabetes is very pale in color because of increased urine volume, contains a large amount of glucose, has a high specific gravity by refractometer or urinometer (because of the presence of glucose), a low urinary pH, and contains ketone bodies.

When ketonuria exists, the ketone bodies are not present in equal concentration. Of the ketones, 78% are present as ß-hydroxybutyric acid, 10% as acetoacetic acid, and only 2% as acetone. However, most laboratory tests for ketones are most sensitive to acetoacetic acid and there is no simple test for ß-hydroxybutyric acid.

Principle

Reagent strip tests for ketone bodies are based on Legal's test, a color reaction with sodium nitroprusside (nitroferricyanide). In an alkaline medium, acetoacetic acid will react with sodium nitroprusside to form a purple color. The test may be slightly sensitive to acetone if glycine is added. Tests for ketones are most sensitive to acetoacetic acid (AAA).

Specificity and Sensitivity

Tests for urine ketones	Specificity	Sensitivity (manufacturer's value)
Multistix/ Ketostix	acetoacetic acid	5-10 mg/dL
Chemstrip	acetoacetic acid acetone	9 mg/dL 70 mg/dL
Rapignost	acetoacetic acid acetone	>5 mg/dL 50 mg/dL
Acetest	acetoacetic acid acetone	5-10 mg/dL 20-25 mg/dL

Interferences

The presence of various pigments, drugs, or substances causing abnormally highly colored urine specimens presents problems when reading ketone results.

These may be falsely interpreted as positive results, or color may mask true positive reactions and therefore be interpreted as negative.

False-Positive Results

- Color reactions similar to those produced by ketones may be seen in urines containing phthaleins (Bromsulphalein, phenosulfonphthalein), very large amounts of phenylketones, or the preservative 8-hydroxyquinoline.
- Low-level false-positive reactions may be seen in highly concentrated urine specimens (high specific gravity) or in specimens containing large amounts of levodopa metabolites.
- Compounds containing sulfhydryl groups such as 2-mercaptoethanesulfonic acid (Mesna®) or acetylcysteine (Mucomyst®) may give an intense red or atypical color that forms immediately but fades to normal on standing. This interference is especially problematic when automatic reagent strip readers are used because reactions are read in a shorter time frame than with visual readings. If this interference is suspected, reagent strips should be checked visually, and the visual result reported. If the color persists and interference is still suspected, a drop of glacial acetic acid may be added to the test area on the reagent strip. Color caused by a sulfhydryl group will fade, whereas color caused by diacetic acid will remain.

False-Negative Results

- Negative or reduced reactions might be seen in improperly stored specimens because of the conversion of acetoacetic acid to acetone, with subsequent evaporation from the specimen.

Additional Comments

A tablet test (Acetest, Miles, Inc.) is also available that tests for acetoacetic acid and acetone based on a color reaction with sodium nitroprusside, like the reagent strip tests. It differs in that whole blood, serum, or plasma may be tested, in addition to urine.

In cases where large values for ketones are obtained, it is sometimes desirable to dilute subsequent specimens with water to monitor and observe a decrease in ketone excretion. The urine specimen is diluted 1:2, 1:4, and so on, until a large value is no longer seen. The report in such cases should state at what dilution a large value is no longer obtained (e.g., large, 1:4 dilution moderate).

■ BILIRUBIN

Clinical Importance

Tests for the presence of bilirubin in urine provide information concerning metabolic or systemic disorders, especially liver function. Bilirubin is a normal product of red cell breakdown. Normal red blood cells have a life span of about 120 days. The heme portion of the hemoglobin molecule is converted to the pigment bilirubin, which is normally eliminated from the body by way of the bile. A total of about 6 grams of hemoglobin is released each day. The heme portion of the hemoglobin molecule is converted to bilirubin by reticuloendothelial cells, primarily in the liver, spleen, and bone marrow. Bilirubin is insoluble in water when formed, and must be carried through the bloodstream as a bilirubin-albumin complex, referred to as **free bilirubin** or **unconjugated bilirubin.**

Once formed, free or unconjugated bilirubin circulates to the liver where it is made water soluble by **conjugation** with glucuronic acid and other hydrophilic substances to form **bilirubin glucuronide.** Bilirubin is conjugated by the Kupffer's cells of the liver. Once conjugated, bilirubin is normally excreted by the liver into the bile, transported to the common bile duct and then to the gallbladder, where it is concentrated and emptied into the small intestine. Here bilirubin is converted to urobilinogen, which is colorless, and eventually eliminated from the body in the feces as a colored oxidation product (**stercobilin**). Of the urobilinogen formed, about half is normally reabsorbed into the portal circulation and subsequently excreted again by the liver into the intestine. Therefore bilirubin is normally excreted from the body by the liver and eliminated by way of the intestine.

Because free or unconjugated bilirubin is insoluble in water and carried through the bloodstream linked to albumin, free bilirubin cannot pass through the glomerular membrane of the kidney and is not found in urine. Once conjugated, it is water soluble, and the molecule is small enough to be filtered through the kidney. Therefore conjugated bilirubin can be eliminated from the body by way of the urine. This is not a normal situation since once conjugated bilirubin is usually eliminated through the intestine. However, if, for a variety of reasons, conjugated bilirubin is present in increased concentration in the blood, conjugated bilirubin will be excreted by the kidney and detectable in the urine.

Bilirubin is a vivid yellow pigment. An increase in the concentration of free or conjugated bilirubin in the blood with accumulation of bilirubin in the body tissues is known as **jaundice.** The accumulation of this vivid yellow pigment in the tissues results in yellow pigmentation of the skin, the sclera (white of the eyes), and the mucous membranes. Urine containing bilirubin will typically show a vivid yellow, yellow-brown, or amber color. When shaken, it will show a large quantity of yellow foam.

Tests for urinary bilirubin (along with tests for urobilinogen) are important in detecting liver disease and in determining the cause of clinical jaundice. The causes of jaundice are numerous and must be discovered to initiate proper treatment. Detection of the presence of even very small amounts of bilirubin in the urine is important. The presence or absence of both bilirubin and urobilinogen in the urine and blood is used in determining the actual cause of jaundice and liver disease.

Among ways to explain and classify jaundice are prehepatic (hemolytic), hepatic (hepatocellular), and posthepatic (obstructive). Findings are summarized in Table 4-5.

Hemolytic (Prehepatic) Jaundice. Hemolytic jaundice occurs when there is increased destruction of red cells, such as in hemolytic anemia and hemolytic disease of the newborn. The liver functions normally, but since destruction of red cells increases, there is increased production of bilirubin, which must be conjugated by the liver and passed on to the intestine to be converted to urobilinogen, a colorless compound.

Table 4-5

LABORATORY FINDINGS IN VARIOUS TYPES OF JAUNDICE

Type of jaundice	Clinical examples	Unconjugated (free) bilirubin (blood)	Conjugated bilirubin (urine)	Urobilinogen (urine)	Feces color
Normal		0-1.3 mg/dL	Negative	≤ 1 mg/dL	Normal, brown
Hemolytic	Hemolytic anemia; hemolytic disease of the newborn	Increased	Negative	Increased	Increased (dark brown)
Hepatic	Hepatitis (viral, toxic, neonatal); cirrhosis	Increased (varies)	Increased (varies)	Increased or absent	Normal or pale
Obstructive	Gallstones; tumor	Normal	Increased	None (decreased)	Pale chalky-white "acholic"

Urobilinogen is oxidized to urobilin, a colored compound that gives the feces its normal color. Normally one half of the urobilinogen formed is reabsorbed into the portal circulation and returned to the liver, where it is reexcreted into the intestine. In the case of hemolytic jaundice, the liver is overwhelmed by the increased production of bilirubin and unable to excrete the increased portal concentration of urobilinogen back into the intestine. Thus increased quantities of urobilinogen are seen in the urine. Hemolytic or prehepatic jaundice is characterized by increased free or unconjugated bilirubin in the blood and increased urobilinogen in the feces and urine. However, bilirubin is not found in the urine because bilirubin conjugated by the liver goes into the intestine, where it is converted to urobilinogen.

Hepatic (Hepatocellular) Jaundice. This type of jaundice results from conditions that involve the liver cells directly and prevent normal excretion. Findings vary depending on the disease or condition and the stage of disease. There may be failure to conjugate bilirubin with increased concentration of free bilirubin in the blood. There also may be failure to transport conjugated bilirubin into the bile canaliculi with increased conjugated bilirubin backing up into the blood and urine. Or there may be failure to reexcrete urobilinogen with increased concentration in the blood and urine.

With conditions such as viral hepatitis, or toxic hepatitis caused by heavy metal or drug poisoning, and with cirrhosis, there is diffuse or overall hepatic cell involvement. The ability of the liver cells to remove and conjugate free bilirubin is decreased, with increased unconjugated bilirubin in the blood. The bilirubin conjugated by the liver may not be excreted into the bile, resulting in increased conjugated bilirubin in the blood and urine. From the conjugated bilirubin that reaches the gut, urobilinogen is formed and half is returned to the liver for reexcretion. However, the ability to remove urobilinogen from the blood is impaired early in liver disease so that urobilinogen remains and is eliminated by way of the urine. Eventually, when the liver is unable to pass conjugated bilirubin into the bile, the bilirubin regurgitates (backs up) into the blood and is eliminated from the body by way of the urine.

Obstructive (Posthepatic) Jaundice. Obstructive jaundice occurs when the common bile duct is obstructed and bile is unable to enter the intestine. This may be the result of stones (gallstones), tumors (cancer of the head of the pancreas), spasms, or stricture. As a result of this blockage to the normal outflow, conjugated bilirubin is regurgitated into the liver sinusoids and the blood and eliminated through the urine. Since conjugated bilirubin is unable to reach the intestine, no urobilinogen is formed, and urobilin is absent from the feces, resulting in a characteristic chalky white to light brown feces color, sometimes referred to as "acholic."

■ REAGENT STRIP TESTS FOR BILIRUBIN

Principle

Reagent strip tests for bilirubin are based on a diazo reaction. Bilirubin is coupled with a diazonium salt in an acid medium to form azobilirubin, a colored compound. Tests differ in the diazonium salt used and the color produced.

Specificity

Tests are specific for bilirubin. However, other highly colored pigments in the urine, such as azo or azo-containing compounds such as phenazopyridine, give the urine a characteristic vivid red-orange color that might be mistaken for, mask, or give atypical color reactions.

Sensitivity (Minimum Detectable Level)

Test for Urine Bilirubin	Sensitivity (manufacturer's values)
Multistix	0.4 - 0.8 mg/dL
Chemstrip	0.5 mg/dL in 90% of urines tested
Rapignost	0.5 mg/dL in 90% of urines tested
Ictotest Tablet Test	0.05 - 0.1 mg/dL

Interferences

The reagent strip tests for bilirubin are difficult to read, but interpretation improves with experience. Atypical colors may indicate that other bile pigments derived from bilirubin are present in the urine and mask the presence of bilirubin. Testing the urine with a more sensitive test such as the Ictotest Tablet Test (Miles, Inc.) may be indicated. Substances that color the urine red or that turn red in an acid medium may result in false-positive reactions. These same pigmented compounds may be mistaken for bilirubin in the gross urine specimen and may mask the reaction of small amounts of bilirubin.

False-Positive Results
- Drugs causing atypical colors and false-positive results include large doses of phenothiazine or chlorpromazine, metabolites of phenazopyridine (Pyridium) or ethoxazene (Serenium).
- Indican (indoxyl sulfate) can produce a yellow-orange to red color, which may interfere with interpretation of the color. Indoles form from bac-

terial overgrowth in the gut or in artificial urinary bladders made from the intestine.

False-Negative Results

- Exposure to light (especially ultraviolet) results in oxidation of bilirubin to biliverdin and low or negative results. Specimens must be absolutely fresh and protected from light.
- Results will be decreased if the bilirubin diglucuronide is hydrolyzed to free bilirubin in vitro because tests are most sensitive to the conjugated form of bilirubin.
- Ascorbic acid in concentrations of 25 mg/dL or more may interfere with the diazo reaction.
- Elevated nitrite concentration as seen in urinary tract infection may decrease sensitivity.

Additional Comments

Historically, several methods have been used to test for the presence of bilirubin in urine. One of the oldest is the foam test in which urine is shaken and observed for the presence of a yellow foam. Other early chemical tests used tincture of iodine, fuming nitric acid, and precipitation with barium chloride, then oxidation to biliverdin with trichloracetic acid and ferric chloride. These have all been replaced by the diazo methods used in reagent strip and tablet tests.

Confirmatory and Related Tests

Since the reagent strip tests are significantly less sensitive for bilirubin than the Ictotest tablet test, it may be necessary to routinely test all urine specimens suspected of containing bilirubin because of color or clinical history with a more sensitive method, even when reagent strip tests show negative reactions. Since colors are difficult to interpret and subject to masked and false-positive reactions, it has been recommended that all positive reactions with reagent strips be confirmed with another method, such as the Ictotest tablet test.

As described previously, the presence of bilirubin and urobilinogen in urine are related, and the presence or absence of both constituents is used in determining the cause of jaundice. However, specific serum tests for liver function, such as serum bilirubin, aspartate transaminase (AST), alkaline phosphatase, and γ-glutamyl transpeptidase are more useful than these urine tests.

ICTOTEST TABLET TEST

Principle

The Ictotest Tablet Test (Miles, Inc.) is based on a diazo reaction, in which bilirubin is coupled with a diazonium salt in an acid medium.

The tablets are supplied with a special absorbent mat. Urine is placed on the mat, the liquid portion of the urine is absorbed, and bilirubin remains on the outer surface. The tablet is placed over the urine on the mat, and water is added to the tablet. When bilirubin is present, it reacts with the diazonium salt present in the tablet to form azobilirubin. A positive reaction is indicated by a blue or purple color on the mat (Procedure 4-4).

Procedure 4-4

ICOTEST TABLET TEST FOR BILIRUBIN

Observe the precautions and follow the instructions supplied by the manufacturer.

1. Place 10 drops of urine on the center of either side of the special test mat supplied with the reagent tablets.

2. Place the Ictotest tablet in the center of the moistened area. Do not touch the tablet with your hands.

3. Place 1 drop of water onto the tablet. Wait 5 seconds, then place a second drop of water onto the tablet so that the water runs off the tablet onto the mat.

4. Observe the mat around or under the tablet for the appearance of a blue to purple color at 60 seconds.

5. Report the result as positive or negative according to the following criteria:

Negative: The mat shows no blue or purple within 60 seconds. Ignore any color that forms after 60 seconds, or a slight pink or red that may appear.
Positive: The mat around or under the tablet turns blue or purple within 60 seconds. Ignore any color change on the tablet itself.

Modified from Linne JJ, Ringsrud KM: *Basic techniques in clinical laboratory science,* ed 3, St. Louis, 1992, Mosby, p. 366.

Specificity

The test is specific for conjugated bilirubin. Use of the absorbent mat concentrates bilirubin on the surface and minimizes interfering pigments.

Sensitivity

Ictotest will detect as little as 0.05 to 0.1 mg/dL bilirubin. This is more sensitive than any of the reagent strip tests. For this reason, it has been recommended that urine be tested with Ictotest in any condition in which bilirubin is suspected.

Interferences

Interferences are generally the same as with reagent strip tests for bilirubin. Suppression of results by large amounts of ascorbic acid and interference by vivid pigments are especially troublesome.

Additional Comments

The special absorbent mat provided must be used to minimize interferences and increase sensitivity due to concentration of bilirubin. Either side may be used. The reagent tablet must begin to dissolve, and water flow from the tablet onto the mat that contains the possible bilirubin for the reaction to occur. However, it may be necessary to remove the tablet from the mat when reading the results, which must be read at the stated time interval. After that, a confusing pink color may appear. Finally, the tablets should be inspected for possible deterioration, seen as a tan to brown discoloration of the tablet. Improper storage with exposure to light, heat, and ambient moisture, will cause deterioration.

UROBILINOGEN AND PROPHOBILINOGEN

Clinical Importance of Urobilinogen

As described in the section on bilirubin, urobilinogens are normal by-products of red blood cell degradation, formed from bilirubin by bacterial action in the intestine and excreted in the feces as stercobilinogen. Urobilinogens are closely related tetrapyrroles; they are colorless, labile, and oxidize to colored urobilins in normal urine.

Increased urobilinogen may be seen in the urine in any condition with increased destruction of red blood cells, such as hemolytic anemias and megaloblastic anemia because of red cell precursor destruction in the bone marrow. It also may be seen in concentrated urine in fever and dehydration.

Urobilinogen in urine is associated with liver disease and dysfunction. One of the first functions lost in liver damage is the ability to remove urobilinogen from the blood and reexcrete it into the intestine. If this occurs, urobilinogen will be excreted in the urine. Urobilinogen is found in the urine in conditions such as infectious (viral) hepatitis, toxic hepatitis, cirrhosis, congestive heart failure, and infectious mononucleosis with liver involvement.

Normally, a small amount of urobilinogen is excreted into the urine, equal or less than 1 mg/dL urobilinogen (1 mg/dL ≈ 1 EU), and reagent strip results are reported as normal rather than negative. This represents about 1% of the urobilinogens produced. However, there are certain situations when urobilinogen is absent from the feces and the urine. Urobilinogen is produced from the actions of bacteria on bilirubin in the intestine. Therefore if the normal intestinal bacterial flora is altered or destroyed, such as from antibiotic therapy, urobilinogen is not produced. Or, if the liver is unable to conjugate bilirubin, or if there is obstruction to the flow of bile from the liver into the intestine, such as with gallstones or cancer of the head of the pancreas, urobilinogen cannot be formed in the intestine and will be absent in the urine and feces.

Clinical Importance of Porphobilinogen

Porphobilinogen is a normal, colorless precursor of the porphyrins. Porphyrins are a group of compounds used in the synthesis of hemoglobin. Ferroprotoporphyrin 9, a porphyrin, is the heme portion of hemoglobin. Porphyrins are normally eliminated from the body in the urine and feces primarily as coproporphyrin I with a small amount of coproporphyrin III. However, with certain inherited enzyme deficiencies such as lack of porphobilinogen deaminase, there is blockage in the normal pathway with increased excretion of other porphyrins in the urine. Porphobilinogen is seen in the urine in acute attacks of acute intermittent porphyria, variegate porphyria, and hereditary coproporphyria. An acute attack may be precipitated by drugs affecting the liver, such as certain anesthetics or barbituates. The discovery of porphobilinogen in urine is a critical value that can eliminate or reduce adverse effects from drugs or anesthetics.

Porphobilinogen is included is this section because tests for urobilinogen that use the Ehrlich's aldehyde reaction will detect urobilinogen and porphobilinogen, in addition to other Ehrlich-reactive compounds.

Principle of Reagent Strip Tests

Unlike most reagent strip tests, the principle of the various reagent strip tests for urobilinogen varies with the different manufacturers. Tests for urobilinogen traditionally employed **Ehrlich's aldehyde reaction**. In this reaction, urobilinogen, together with porphobilinogen and other Ehrlich-reactive compounds, react with p-dimethylaminobenzaldehyde in concentrated hydrochloric acid to form a colored (characteristically cherry-red) aldehyde. This is the basis for the Multistix reagent strip test and the Watson-Schwartz test. An inverse Ehrlich's aldeyhyde reaction is the basis of the Hoesch test for porphobilinogen.

The Multistix and Urobilistix (Miles, Inc.) reagent strips for urobilinogen use the Ehrlich's aldehyde reaction and will also react with porphobilinogen and various intermediate Ehrlich-reactive substances such as sulfonamides, p-aminosalicylic acid, procaine, and 5-hydroyxyindoleacetic acid.

The Chemstrip and Rapignost reagent strips employ a different principle for the measurement of urobilinogen. They use a diazo reaction in which a diazonium salt reacts with urobilinogen in an acid medium to form a red azo dye. The strips react with both urobilinogen and stercobilinogen. Differentiation between these two substances is not diagnostically significant since stercobilinogen is found in feces, not urine. Porphobilinogen and other Ehrlich-reactive substances are not detected with these reagent strips, which helps in ruling out interfering substances with Multistix. However, because porphobilinogen is not detected, the presence of unsuspected or undiagnosed porphyria would be completely missed with the Chemstrip and Rapignost strips.

Specificity and Sensitivity

Reagent strip tests and additional or confirmatory tests are included.

Test for urine urobilinogen	Specificity	Sensitivity (manufacturer's value—reagent strips)
Multistix/ Urobilistix	Urobilinogen Porphobilinogen Intermediate	As low as 0.2 mg/dL
Chemstrip	Urobilinogen	Approximately 0.4 mg/dL
Rapignost	Urobilinogen	1 mg/dL
Watson- Schwartz Test	Urobilinogen Porphobilinogen Intermediate	2.0 to 10 mg/dL (somewhat more sensitive to porphobilinogen than Hoesch test)*
Hoesch Test	Porphobilinogen	2.0 to 10 mg/dL

*Pietrach CA et al: Comparison of the Hoesch and Watson-Schwartz tests for urinary porphobilinogen, *Clin Chem* 23:1666 1977.

Interferences

The presence of Ehrlich-reacting substances other than urobilinogen is a problem in tests based on the Ehrlich aldehyde reaction (Multistix/Urobilistix). All strips are affected by highly colored pigments such as azo dyes or their metabolites in the urine specimen. Strips based on the diazo reaction show interferences similar to reagent strip tests for bilirubin.

False-Positive Results
- Intermediate Ehrlich-reactive substances such as sulfonamides, and p-aminosalicylic acid (PAS) metabolites, procaine, and 5-hydroxyindolacetic acid will react with the Multistix reagent strips.
- Methyldopa (Aldomet) will give a strong color reaction with Ehrlich's reagent.
- Highly colored pigments and their metabolites including ethoxazene (Serenium), drugs containing azo dyes (phenazopyridium), nitrofurantoin, and riboflavin and p-aminobenzoic acid may cause atypical or positive reactions with all reagent strips.
- Multistix strip reactivity increases with temperature and may give a false-positive warm aldehyde reaction if urine is tested at body temperature. The optimum temperature for testing is 22° to 26° C or room temperature.

False-Negative Results
- Specimens exposed to light or left at room temperature for more than 1 hour will show low or negative reactions because of conversion of urobilinogen to urobilin with all reagent strips.
- Formalin used as a preservative will cause false-negative reactions with all reagent strips.
- Tests based on the diazo reaction are affected by the presence of ascorbic acid and nitrite and will give decreased or negative results.
- Although porphobilinogen may be detected with the Miles reagent strips, the method is not reliable.
- Chemstrip and Rapignost strips based on a diazo reaction will not detect porphobilinogen in the urine.

Additional Comments

With all reagent strip tests, the absence of urobilinogen is not detectable.

It is particularly necessary to test a fresh urine specimen for urobilinogen. Urobilinogen (which is colorless) is unusually unstable and rapidly oxidizes to urobilin (an orange-red pigment). If urine is not tested within an hour of voiding, it should be refrigerated and protected from light. Urine preservatives generally interfere and should not be added. None of the tests described react with urobilin. However, the oxidation takes place so readily that most urine specimens containing urobilinogen show an abnormal orange-red or orange-brown color because of partial oxidation to urobilin. The color is similar to that seen when bilirubin is present in urine, and urine should generally be tested for both when testing is indicated on the basis of urine color.

Porphobilinogen is also a colorless compound that polymerizes (oxidizes) to a colored compound, porphobilin. Porphobilin gives a characteristic dark red or red-purple color, referred to as port wine red. Fresh urine containing porphobilinogen is not usually colored, but some patients may have a dark red urine, or it may darken on standing as porphobilinogen polymerizes. Therefore it is important that the urine specimen be fresh and properly stored when testing for porphobilinogen. To extend reactivity, adjust pH to 7 with sodium bicarbonate.

Confirmatory and Additional Tests

The normal urobilinogen concentration in urine is approximately 0.2 to 1.0 mg/dL. A reagent strip result of 2 mg/dL may or may not be abnormal and requires further evaluation.

The presence of intermediate Ehrlich-reactive substances is a problem in any test based on the Ehrlich reaction. Thus a combination of reagent strip tests that use different methodology with confirmation by the Hoesch test and Watson-Schwartz test is helpful in establishing the presence of abnormal concentrations of urobilinogen and porphobilinogen.

Generally, if tests based on both the Ehrlich aldehyde reaction and the diazo reaction show a similar reaction, results may be reported as urobilinogen from the reagent strip. If the Ehrlich reaction value is increased and the diazo reaction is normal, the presence of porphobilinogen or intermediate Ehrlich-reactive substances is suspected. This may be confirmed with the Hoesch test, which is specific for porphobilinogen. Positive results may be further confirmed with the Watson-Schwartz test. If the Hoesch test is negative, the substance showing increased results with Multistix is probably an intermediate Ehrlich-reactive substance. This may be confirmed with the Watson-Schwartz test if results are uncertain.

WATSON-SCHWARTZ QUALITATIVE TEST FOR UROBILINOGEN AND PORPHOBILINOGEN

Principle

The Watson-Schwartz test is a qualitative test that uses Ehrlich's aldehyde reaction for urobilinogen, porphobilinogen, and other Ehrlich-reactive compounds. These substances will react with Ehrlich's reagent and form a characteristic red (pink to deep cherry red) aldehyde. The color formed is enhanced by the presence of saturated sodium acetate, which also inhibits color formation by skatoles and indoles. If urobilinogen is present, the color development is characteristically delayed until the sodium acetate is added. If porphobilinogen is present, the aldehyde color characteristically develops as soon as the Ehrlich's reagent is added.

To differentiate color formed by urobilinogen, porphobilinogen, and intermediate compounds, the colored solution is extracted with the organic solvents chloroform and butanol. Color formed by urobilinogen is soluble in chloroform and butanol, porphobilinogen is not soluble in either organic solvent, whereas intermediate Ehrlich-reactive compounds are soluble in butanol, but not in chloroform (Table 4-6).

When performing the procedure, it is not necessary to continue on to a butanol extraction if the color goes into the chloroform layer. Urobilinogen is the only compound soluble in chloroform, porphobilinogen is the only compound insoluble in both organic solvents (soluble in aqueous solutions only), whereas intermediate compounds are soluble in butanol, but not chloroform.

Table 4-6

RESULTS OF WATSON-SCHWARTZ TEST			
Result	Urine Ehrlich's reagent Sodium acetate	Chloroform extract	Butanol extract
Negative	No pink color		
Urobilinogen	Pink	Pink	Pink
Porphobilinogen	Pink	Colorless	Colorless
Intermediate Ehrlich-Reactive Compounds	Pink	Colorless	Pink

Modified from Linne JJ, Ringsrud KM: *Basic techniques in clinical laboratory science*, ed 3, 1992, St. Louis, Mosby, p 368.

Reagents

1. **Ehrlich's reagent.** Dissolve 0.7 g of *p*-dimethyl-benzaldehyde in 200 mL of deionized or distilled water. Carefully add 150 mL of concentrated hydrochloric acid.
2. **Saturated sodium acetate.** Add deionized or distilled water directly to bottle of reagent grade sodium acetate. Shake daily for about 1 week. There should be a layer of undissolved crystals on the bottom of the stock and working reagent bottles.
3. **Chloroform.** Reagent grade.
4. **Butanol.** Reagent grade.

Interferences

Several compounds such as methyldopa, methyl red, and azo dyes give a confusing red color with Ehrlich's reagent. To rule out false-positive reactions because of reaction with acid alone rather than Ehrlich's reagent, include a control reaction using 6 mol/L hydrochloric acid in place of the Ehrlich's reagent.

False-Positive Results

- If urine is tested immediately after it is voided, the "warm aldehyde" reaction may be seen. This is a weak Ehrlich reaction that takes place at body temperature with a chromogen (probably indoxyl) present in normal urine. To avoid the interference, ensure urine is at room temperature before testing.
- The presence of intermediate Ehrlich-reactive compounds such as sulfonamides, procaine, 5-hydroxyindoleacetic acid, and others makes interpretation of results difficult.
- A strong color reaction is often seen in the urine of patients receiving methyldopa (Aldomet), with approximately equal color distribution in the aqueous and butanol layers.
- Indican will give an orange color in chloroform that should not be confused with urobilinogen.

Procedure 4-5

WATSON-SCHWARTZ TEST FOR UROBILINOGEN AND PORPHOBILINOGEN

1. Place 2.5 mL of urine in a test tube. Add 2.5 mL of Ehrlich's reagent. Mix well by inversion.

2. Add 5.0 mL of saturated sodium acetate and mix. Observe for the development of a pink to deep cherry-red color, indicating the presence of urobilinogen, porphobilinogen, or other Ehrlich-reactive compounds.

3. If color develops, add 5 mL of chloroform to the test tube, stopper, and shake vigorously to extract the color.
   - If color is caused by urobilinogen, it will be extracted into the lower chloroform layer. If all color is extracted into the chloroform layer, the test is positive for urobilinogen and further extraction is not necessary.
   - If color is caused by porphobilinogen or intermediate Ehrlich-reactive compounds, it will remain in the upper aqueous layer.

4. If color remains in the upper aqueous layer, remove one half of it to another test tube and add about 5 mL of butanol. Stopper and shake vigorously to extract the color.
   - If the color is caused by porphobilinogen, it will remain in the lower aqueous layer; porphobilinogen is not soluble in butanol.

- If the color is caused by intermediate Ehrlich-reactive compounds, it will be extracted into the upper butanol layer.
- If, in the first chloroform extraction, the color was caused by urobilinogen but was not completely extracted into chloroform, the color remaining in the aqueous layer will be extracted into butanol in the second extraction.
- If both urobilinogen and porphobilinogen are present (an extremely rare situation), color caused by urobilinogen will be extracted into the chloroform layer. Color due to porphobilinogen will remain in the aqueous layer. The butanol layer will remain colorless in this extraction.
- It is possible to have situations where the specimen contains intermediate Ehrlich-reactive compounds in addition to either urobilinogen or porphobilinogen. Interpretation is difficult and may require re-extraction with both chloroform and butanol.

5. Report the results as:
- Positive or negative for urobilinogen
- Positive for porphobilinogen
- Positive for both urobilinogen and porphobilinogen (very rare).

Do not report the finding of intermediate Ehrlich-reactive compounds. These are considered false-positive reactions.

- Pale peach and light orange colors should not be interpreted as positive reactions.
  False-Negative Results
- Specimens exposed to light or left at room temperature for more than 1 hour will show low or negative reactions because of conversion of urobilinogen to urobilin or porphobilinogen to porphobilin.

Additional Comments

The sodium acetate solution must be saturated for complete color enhancement. A layer of undissolved crystals on the bottom of the stock and working reagent bottles indicates saturation.

Chloroform is a known carcinogen, and exposure should be avoided. It should only be used if there is an adequate fume hood available. To avoid exposure to chloroform, screen specimens suspected of containing porphobilinogen with the Hoesch test and confirm positive reactions with the Watson-Schwartz test. In most cases, the presence of intermediate Ehrlich-reactive compounds can be established and false-positive reactions ruled out by comparing the results for urobilinogen on products based on the Ehrlich reaction with products based on a diazo reaction.

■ HOESCH TEST FOR PORPHOBILINOGEN

Principle

The Hoesch test is a confirmatory test for porphobilinogen based on an inverse Ehrlich's aldehyde reaction. In this test, an acid solution is maintained by adding a small volume of urine to a relatively large volume of Ehrlich's reagent (Procedure 4-6).

The Hoesch test may be used to confirm results with the Watson-Schwartz test or to confirm results for porphobilinogen when a positive reaction is seen with the Multistix reagent strip test together with a negative diazo reaction for urobilinogen with Chemstrip or Rapignost strips.

Reagents

1. Hydrochloric acid 6 mol/L. Dilute concentrated hydrochloric acid (reagent grade) 1:2 with deionized or distilled water by slowly adding acid to water.
2. Hoesch reagent. Dissolve 2.0 g *p*-dimethylaminobenzaldehyde in 6 mol/L HCl and dilute to 100 mL with 6 mol/L HCl.

Interferences

These are similar to those seen with the Watson-Schwartz Test.
False-Positive Results
- Large doses of methyldopa, the presence of indoles in some patients with intestinal ileus, and the presence of phenazopyridine have been reported to yield false-positive results.
- A rose color, which might be confused with the color caused by porphobilinogen, may be seen from urosein, a pigment related to indoleacetic acid, in response to strong HCl. To rule out this interference, test the specimen separately with 6 mol/L HCl and compare color with that formed with the Hoesch reagent.
- The presence of urobilinogen is not a practical problem since very large quantities (>20 mg/dL) are needed to give a positive reaction with Hoesch reagent.

Procedure 4-6

HOESCH TEST FOR PORPHOBILINOGEN

1. Pour approximately 2 mL of Hoesch reagent into a test tube.
2. Add 2 drops of well-mixed urine.
3. Observe for the appearance of an instantaneous cherry-red or bright red color that appears on top of the solution. Agitate briefly, and look for a light to bright pink color throughout the test tube.
4. Report results as positive or negative for porphobilinogen.

Modified from Linne JJ, Ringsrud KM: *Basic techniques in clinical laboratory science*, ed 3, 1992, St. Louis, Mosby p 370.

CHEMICAL EXAMINATION OF URINE

Additional Comments

A quantitative test for porphobilinogen is necessary when either the Watson-Schwartz or Hoesch test is questionable.

■ ASCORBIC ACID

Clinical Importance

Ascorbic acid or **vitamin C** is neither a normal nor pathologic constituent of urine. However, the presence of ascorbic acid may interfere with the measurement of other chemical tests. This is especially important in the reagent strip tests for blood and glucose that depend on the release of hydrogen peroxide by peroxidase and subsequent oxidation of a chromogen to indicate a reaction. Ascorbic acid may also react with the diazonium salt formed in reagent strip tests based on the diazo reaction, causing reduced or false-negative reactions.

The urine of persons who have ingested large quantities of vitamin C or who are receiving medications, such as intravenous antibiotics that contain vitamin C, may contain inhibiting quantities of ascorbic acid. It has been reported that up to 500 mg/dL ascorbic acid may be found in urine from the ingestion of large quantities of fruit.[3] Excess vitamin C is rapidly eliminated from the body through the urine. With large amounts of ascorbic acid, generally more than 25 mg/dL, inhibition is usually seen with low levels of the analyte in question in dilute urine.

Urine is not routinely tested for the presence of ascorbic acid, although the Rapignost multiple reagent strips contain a test area for ascorbic acid. The presence of ascorbic acid in the urine may be suspected when a reagent strip test for blood is negative, yet red blood cells are seen in the microscopic analysis of the urinary sediment. Or, it may be suspected when reagent strip tests for glucose from diabetic patients give inconsistent results, showing negative or reduced reactions, even though tests for ketones and copper reduction tests for sugar are positive. If suspected, the urine may be tested with a reagent strip test specific for ascorbic acid. If inhibiting quantities of ascorbic acid are found to be present or suspected on the basis of clinical his-

tory, or if discrepant test results are observed, a urine specimen voided at least 10 hours after the last administration of vitamin C should be retested.

Reagent Strip Tests

At present, neither Miles, Inc., nor Boehringer Mannheim Corp. offer a reagent strip test for ascorbic acid. Many of the Rapignost reagent strips (Behring Diagnostics Inc.) contain a test area for ascorbic acid. The Merckoquant ascorbic acid test (available from EM Science Div., EM Industries, Gibbstown, NJ, a division of E. Merck, Darmstadt, Federal Republic of Germany) is intended for the semiquantitative determination of ascorbic acid in foodstuffs such as fruit and vegetable juices and wine. It has been used to test urine for ascorbic acid by default, without the availability of reagent strips intended specifically for urine.

Principle

Both tests are based on the strong reducing properties of ascorbic acid. The Rapignost ascorbic test is based on Tillmann's reaction. Positive results are seen as the orange-colored background dye in Tillmann's reagent (2,6-dichlorophenolindophenol) becomes visible because of decolorization of the blue indophenol dye by ascorbic acid. The Merckoquant test for ascorbic acid is based on the reduction of the yellow-colored phosphomolybdate complex by ascorbic acid to give molybdenum blue.

Specificity

Tests are based on the reducing ability of ascorbic acid and will react with other reducing substances with similar redox-potential.

Additional Comments

The color chart for the Merckoquant reagent strips gives values in mg/L. Values for ascorbic acid throughout this chapter have been given in mg/dL; thus values with the Merckoquant reagent strips should be converted to mg/dL.

REVIEW QUESTIONS

1 Match the following test principles and constituents detected. Some test principles have more than one constituent.

    A. bilirubin
    B. blood
    C. glucose
    D. ketones
    E. leukocyte esterase
    F. nitrite
    G. pH
    H. protein
    I. reducing sugars
    J. specific gravity
    K. urobilinogen

    __I__ copper reduction test.
    __K__ diazo reaction. *(A,E,F, written to left)*
    __G__ double pH indicator system.
    __C__ double sequential enzyme reaction based on glucose oxidase.
    __K__ Ehrlich's aldehyde reaction.
    __B__ peroxidase activity of heme resulting in oxidation of chromogen on reagent strip.
    __J__ pK_a change of polyelectrolytes in relation to ionic concentration.
    __H__ protein error of pH indicators.
    __D__ reaction with sodium nitroprusside (Legal's test).

2 Which of the following is **not** a reason for measurement of urine pH:
    a. assessment of specimen acceptability for examination
    b. indication of urinary tract infection
    c. crystal identification
    d. indication of proteinuria

3 Measurement of urine specific gravity is useful in assessing what two general areas?
    a. Kidney status
    b. State of hydration

4 The presence and concentration of which of the following is **most** significant in the detection and diagnosis of renal disease:
    a. blood
    b. leukocyte esterase
    c. nitrite
    d. protein
    e. specific gravity

5 Which of the following is associated with proteinuria due to glomerular damage:
    a. albumin
    b. gamma globulin
    c. hemoglobin
    d. Tamm-Horsfall protein

6 The presence of light-chain immunoglobulins in the urine are associated with which of the following forms of proteinuria?
    a. asymptomatic disorders
    b. glomerular damage
    c. lower urinary tract infection
    d. prerenal disorders
    e. tubular damage

7 Which of the following is **not** detected by reagent strip tests for blood?
    a. hemosiderin
    b. hemoglobin
    c. myoglobin
    d. red blood cells

8 Why is it important to test the uncentrifuged, well-mixed urine specimen when testing with reagent strips for blood?

9 Reagent strip tests that depend on the release of oxygen and subsequent oxidation of a chromogen are all subject to false-negative reactions because of the presence of:
    a. ascorbic acid
    b. chlorine bleach
    c. low specific gravity
    d. phenazopyridine
    e. vitamin D

10 Detection of the presence of nitrite in the urine is useful:
    a. in the detection of asymptomatic urinary tract infection
    b. in the detection of infection by gram-positive organisms
    c. in the prevention of kidney damage by treatment of early infection
    d. more than one of the above
    e. all of the above

11 Finding leukocyte esterase in the urine is most useful in the detection of:
    a. early renal transplant rejection
    b. immunosuppression
    c. malignancy
    d. urinary tract infection

12 The most common cause of glucosuria is
diabetes mellitus. .

13 Explain the difference between reagent strip and copper reduction tests for urine sugar in terms of specificity and sensitivity.

14 Children less than 2 years of age are tested with a copper reduction test for sugar in addition to reagent strip tests to detect:
a. nonglucose-reducing sugars
b. smaller amounts of glucose than is detectable with reagent strips
c. sucrose overdose
d. the presence of ascorbic acid

15 Which of the following is not a cause of false-negative reagent strip tests for urine glucose?
a. ascorbic acid
b. dilute urine (low specific gravity)
c. moderate ketones with low glucose levels
d. sodium fluoride used as a preservative
e. urine specimen tested at refrigerator temperature

16 Name the three ketone bodies:
a. _acetoacetic_
b. _aceto butyric acid_
c. _β-hydroxybutyric acid_

17 Two conditions associated with ketosis are:
a. _diabetes mellitus_
b. _starvation._

18 Compounds containing sulfhydryl groups will give an atypical (false-positive) color reaction that fades on standing with reagent strips for:
a. bilirubin
b. glucose
c. ketones
d. urobilinogen

19 In order to be present in the urine, bilirubin must be:
a. bilirubin glucuronide
b. conjugated bilirubin
c. unconjugated bilirubin
d. more than one of the above
e. all of the above

20 Tests for urine bilirubin may be used to assess:
a. hormone production
b. kidney function
c. liver function
d. red cell destruction

21 False-positive reagent strip tests for bilirubin are seen with:
a. ascorbic acid
b. azo-containing compounds
c. elevated nitrite concentration
d. unconjugated (free) bilirubin
e. more than one of the above

22 Tests for urine urobilinogen may be used to assess:
a. hormone production
b. kidney function
c. liver function
d. red cell destruction
e. more than one of the above

23 Porphobilinogen in the urine may be detected by which of the following tests?
a. Hoesch test
b. reagent strip using a diazo reaction
c. reagent strips using Ehrlich's aldehyde reaction
d. Watson-Schwartz test
e. more than one of the above
f. all of the above

24 The presence of sufficient quantities of ascorbic acid in urine has the potential of causing false-positive reactions with which of the following?
a. copper reduction tests
b. tests based on a diazo reaction
c. tests based on release of oxygen from a peroxide and oxidation of a chromogen
d. protein precipitation tests
e. more than one of the above

25 The most common cause of false-negative reagent strip tests is probably:
a. ascorbic acid
b. azo dyes
c. chlorine bleach
d. dilute urine (low specific gravity)

CASE #1

As part of a routine physical examination, a urinalysis is performed on a midstream voided urine collection from an apparently healthy (asymptomatic), 8-year-old girl. The following results are obtained:

Urinalysis Results:

Physical Appearance:

color:	yellow
transparency:	hazy

Chemical Screening:

pH	6		
specific gravity	1.010		
protein (strip)	30 mg/dL	protein (SSA)	1+
blood	negative		
nitrite	negative		
leukocyte esterase	positive		
glucose	negative		
ketones	negative		
bilirubin	negative		
urobilinogen	normal		

Because of the results of the protein test by reagent strip, the urine was tested with the sulfosalicylic acid test for protein. A microscopic examination of the urine sediment was performed.

Microscopic Examination of Urinary Sediment:

red blood cells	0-2/hpf
white blood cells	10-25/hpf
casts	none seen
epithelial cells	few squamous
bacteria	moderate

After reviewing the results of the urinalysis, the physician requests a Gram stain and urine culture.

Microbiology Results:

Gram stain	Gram-positive cocci
Urine culture	Greater than 100,000 CFU/mL *Enterococcus* sp.

1. What urinalysis findings are abnormal?
2. This laboratory does not perform microscopics on all routine urinalysis tests. Why was a microscopic examination of the urine sediment performed in this case?
3. Can the urine collection already tested be Gram stained and cultured? _____ (yes or no)
   Explain:
4. Explain the negative nitrite result and presence of bacteria in the urine sediment.
5. Would these results be more likely to represent an upper or a lower urinary tract infection? _____
   Explain:

CASE #2

A 60-year-old female complains of low back pain. She is pale and tires easily. An x-ray examination shows a compression fracture of the spine. Blood is drawn for hematology, an erythrocyte sedimentation rate (ESR), and chemistries. Urine is collected for a routine urinalysis. Some results follow:

Urinalysis Results:

Physical Appearance:

color:	yellow
transparency:	clear

Chemical Screening:

pH	6		
specific gravity	1.015	(reagent strip)	
	1.018	(refractometer)	
protein (strip)	negative	protein (SSA)	2+
blood	negative		
nitrite	negative		
leukocyte esterase	negative		
glucose	negative		
ketones	negative		
bilirubin	negative		
urobilinogen	normal		

Hematology Results:

hemoglobin	10.0 g/dL
Blood film showed marked rouleaux	
ESR	100 mm/hour

Because this is a small clinic, the same person performed the urinalysis and hematology tests. Based on the laboratory findings, a SSA protein test and specific gravity by refractometer were performed (at no extra charge to the patient). The SSA protein result was 2+, representing about 100 mg protein/dL. A drop of the precipitate in the protein tube was placed on a microscope slide, coverslipped, and viewed microscopically with brightfield and polarizing microscopy.

1. What laboratory result(s) led to the decision to perform the SSA?
2. Explain the discrepancy between the urine reagent strip test for protein and the sulfosalicylic acid protein test results.
3. Why was the specific gravity repeated by refractometer?
4. Why was the precipitate from the SSA protein test viewed microscopically?
5. What follow-up test can be done to identify the urinary protein in this case?

CASE #3

An unconscious young man is taken to the hospital emergency room. His temperature is elevated; pulse rate increased; respiration rate increased; skin warm and dry, with poor turgor. His breath is noted to have an aromatic odor, and alcohol ingestion is suspected.

Venous blood is drawn for stat chemistry tests and hematology. A catheterized specimen of urine is tested with multiple reagent strips and refractometer in the emergency room. A drop of finger puncture blood is used to screen for glucose with a reflectance meter.

Urinalysis Results

(performed in emergency room)

Physical Appearance:
color:	pale
transparency:	clear

Chemical Screening (urine):
pH	5	
specific gravity	1.010	(reagent strip)
	1.031	(refractometer)
protein	negative	
blood	negative	
nitrite	negative	
leukocyte esterase	negative	
glucose	>2000 mg/dL	
ketones	moderate	
bilirubin	negative	
urobilinogen	normal	

Emergency room blood glucose: >500 mg/dL

1. What is the most likely cause of unconsciousness in this patient?
2. What is the cause of the aromatic odor noticed on the breath of this patient?
3. Explain the difference in the specific gravity values.
4. Why is it important to determine the cause of unconsciousness in this patient?

 CASE #4

A urine specimen is obtained from a 50-year-old woman who has had intermittent upper abdominal pain for the last 10 days. She is obese; her sclera appear yellow and she has right upper quadrant tenderness. She states that her stools have been paler than usual and her urine is a little darker. The following results are obtained:

Urinalysis Results:

Physical Appearance:
color:	brown (amber)
foam:	large quantity of yellow foam
transparency:	clear

Chemical Screening:
pH	6
specific gravity	1.015
protein (albumin)	negative

blood	negative		
nitrite	negative		
leukocyte esterase	negative		
glucose	negative		
ketones	negative		
bilirubin (strip)	large	tablet	positive
urobilinogen	normal		

1. What urinalysis findings are abnormal in this patient?
2. How does the color of the sclera and of the stool relate to the presence of bilirubin in the urine of this patient?
3. Why was an additional tablet test for bilirubin performed on the urine of this patient?
4. From the clinical history and urinalysis findings, classify the jaundice exhibited in this patient.
   a. hemolytic
   b. hepatic
   c. obstructive

CASE #5

A 23-year-old male comes to the emergency room of your hospital with acute abdominal pain. He has had a previous admission for psychiatric care. Laparotomy is planned to determine the cause of abdominal pain. Specimens are collected for hematology, chemistry, and urinalysis. The laboratory uses a reagent strip for urobilinogen, based on the Ehrlich aldehyde reaction.

Urinalysis Results:

Physical Appearance:
    color: red-purple (increasing on standing)
    transparency: hazy

Chemical Screening:
    pH   6
    specific gravity   1.010
    protein   negative
    blood   negative
    nitrite   negative
    leukocyte esterase   negative

glucose	negative
ketones	negative
bilirubin	negative
urobilinogen	8 EU (strip using Ehrlich's reaction)

Additional Tests:
    Urobilinogen   normal (strip using a diazo reaction)
    Hoesch test   positive
    Watson-Schwartz test positive for porphobilinogen

1. Why was the urine specimen tested with an additional reagent strip for urobilinogen based on a diazo reaction?
2. What is the significance of the positive Hoesch test?
3. Why was the Watson-Schwartz test performed?
4. What is causing the abnormal color in this urine specimen?
5. On the bases of these results, surgery (laparotomy) was canceled. Why?
6. What is the name of this patient's disease?

 CASE #6

A patient with known sickle cell disease is seen with symptoms of chronic anemia and jaundice.

Urinalysis Results:

Physical Appearance:
    color: amber (orange-red)
    transparency: clear

Chemical Screening:
    pH   6.5
    specific gravity   1.015
    protein   negative
    blood   negative
    nitrite   negative
    leukocyte esterase   negative
    glucose   negative
    ketones   negative
    bilirubin   negative
    urobilinogen   8 EU (Ehrlich aldehyde reaction)
                          8 EU (diazo based reaction)

1. What urinalysis findings are abnormal or discrepant in this patient?
2. Why was the urine tested with two different reagent strips for urobilinogen in this case?
3. If the patient has chronic hemolysis, why is the chemical test for blood (hemoglobin) negative in this patient?
4. Since the patient has jaundice (increased bilirubin in the blood), why is the reagent strip test for urine bilirubin negative?
5. Explain the presence of elevated levels of urine urobilinogen in this patient.
6. What is the cause of the abnormal color of the urine in this patient?
7. Classify the jaundice exhibited in this patient.
   a. hemolytic
   b. hepatic
   c. obstructive

REFERENCES

1. Cohen HT, Spiegel DM: Air-exposed urine dipsticks give false-positive results for glucose and false-negative results for blood. *Am J Clin Pathol* 96:398-400, 1991.

2. Free AH, Free HM: *Urinalysis in clinical laboratory practice*, Cleveland, 1975, CRC Press, p 5.

3. *Rapignost for more perspectives in urinalysis*, Somerville, NJ , Behring Diagnostics Inc., p 11.

BIBLIOGRAPHY

Bradley GM, Linne JJ: *The University of Minnesota hospital and clinic laboratory handbook*, ed 2, Hudson, Ohio, 1992, Lexi-Comp.

Factors affecting urine chemistry tests, Elkhart, Ind., 1982, Ames Div., Miles Laboratories.

Linne JJ, Ringsrud KM: *Basic techniques in clinical laboratory science*, ed 3, St. Louis, 1992, Mosby.

McNeely MDD, Brigden ML: *Urinalysis*. In Tilton RC et al: *Clinical laboratory medicine*, St. Louis, 1992, Mosby.

Modern urine chemistry application of urine chemistry and microscopic examination in health and disease, Elkhart, Ind., 1987, Ames Div., Miles Laboratories.

Physician's office laboratory guidelines, tentative guidelines, ed 2, Villanova, Pa., June 1992, National Committee for Clinical Laboratory Standards, 12(5) POL1-T2.

Rapignost for more perspectives in urinalysis, Somerville, NJ, Behring Diagnostics.

Routine urinalysis and collection, transportation, and preservation of urine specimens, Tentative guidelines, Villanova, Pa., Dec. 1992, National Committee for Clinical Laboratory Standards, 12(26) GP16-T.

Schumann GB, Schweitzer SC: *Examination of urine*. In Henry JB (ed): *Clinical diagnosis and management by laboratory methods*, ed 18, Philadelphia, 1991, WB Saunders.

Urinalysis today, Indianapolis, 1987, Boehringer Mannheim Diagnostics.

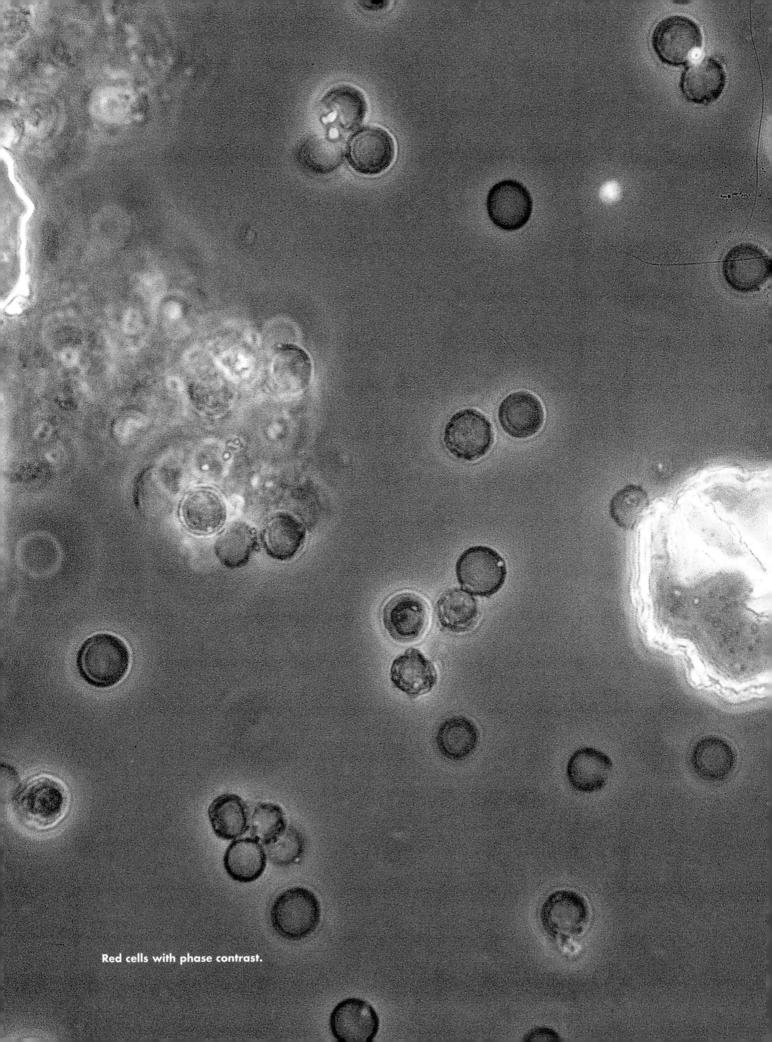

Red cells with phase contrast.

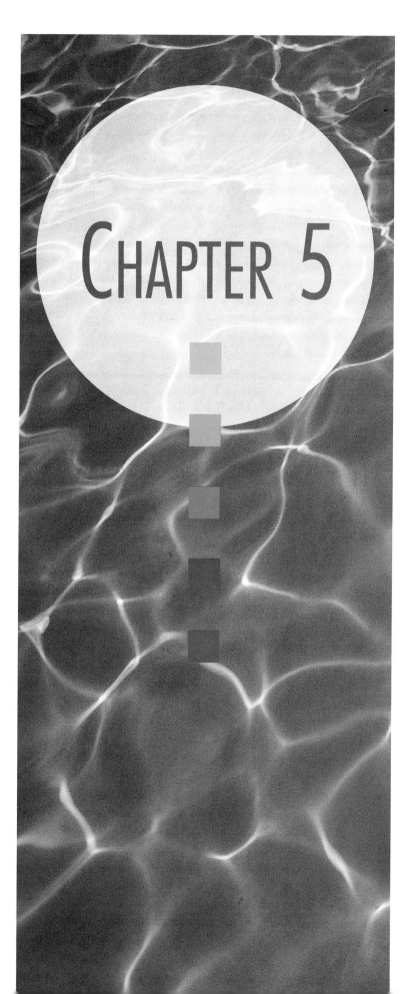

CHAPTER 5

MICROSCOPIC EXAMINATION OF THE URINE SEDIMENT

CHAPTER OUTLINE

● **Introduction**
Specimen Preparation
Standardization
Specimen Requirements
Normal Sediment

● **Microscopic Techniques**
Brightfield Microscopy
Phase Contrast Microscopy
Interference Contrast Microscopy
Polarizing Microscopy

● **Staining Techniques**
Supravital Stains
Fat Stains
Gram Stain
Acetic Acid

● **Cytocentrifugation**

● **Laboratory Procedure**

LEARNING OBJECTIVES

▶ Understand what is meant by standardized urinalysis systems and the advantages of such systems.

▶ List the factors that according to NCCLS must be standardized.

▶ Describe specimen preparation.

▶ Understand what constitutes a "normal" urine sediment.

▶ Describe and understand advantages and disadvantages of the following microscopic techniques:
brightfield
phase contrast
interference contrast
polarizing and compensated polarized
  microscopy

▶ Describe and understand the necessity, advantages, and disadvantages of various stains; namely, supravital stains (Sternheimer-Malbin and Toluidine blue), fat stains (Sudan stains and oil red O), Gram stain, Wright's stain, and Papanicolaou stain, as applied to urinalysis.

▶ Know what is meant by *birefringence*.

▶ Understand what is meant by cytocentrifugation and its usefulness.

▶ Follow the procedure for the microscopic analysis of the urine sediment, including the following:
centrifugation
concentration
staining as needed
preparing the microscope slide (mounting)
systematic microscopic examination
low power examination
high power examination
reporting results

◼ INTRODUCTION

The final portion of the urinalysis is the microscopic examination of the sediment. This is probably the most commonly used laboratory procedure for the detection of renal and/or urinary tract disease. The **urine sediment** consists of any solid material suspended in the urine. These solids may be cells, casts of precipitated protein (with or without inclusions), crystals and amorphous deposits of chemicals, or various miscellaneous and exogenous materials. Although they are indicated by lack of clarity in the urine specimen, the various elements that constitute the urine sediment can be identified only by microscopic examination. The sediment is sometimes referred to as **organized** (biologic) and **unorganized** (chemical).

Traditionally, a microscopic analysis of the urine sediment has been a part of every "routine urinalysis." However, several studies have shown that microscopic analysis may not be necessary or cost efficient on every urine specimen tested. Instead, the microscopic analysis of the sediment is performed when abnormal findings are seen in the physical and chemical analysis of the urine, or when indicated by the patient's condition or clinical history. As such, NCCLS states that, "The decision to perform microscopic examinations must be made by each individual laboratory based on its specific patient population."[1] They go on to suggest that the microscopic analysis should be performed when requested by the physician, when determined by laboratory protocol, or when any abnormal physiochemical result is obtained.

The examination of the urine sediment is neither simple nor inexpensive. It is time-consuming and requires well-trained, skilled, knowledgeable personnel. Although the visual chemical analysis of urine by reagent strip or tablets are "waived" tests according to CLIA '88, the microscopic analysis of the urine sediment is a "moderately complex" test. Personnel examining the urine sediment must follow a procedure that ensures consistency in all aspects of specimen preparation, examination, identification, and reporting. They must be skilled in the use of the microscope. They should be aware of various microscopic techniques such as brightfield, phase contrast, and polarizing microscopy, and know how to use the equipment available to them. They should be aware of various staining techniques and when and how to use them. They must be able to distinguish normal or contaminating entities from serious pathologic structures and know of resources such as atlases or textbooks (such as this publication) to aid in the identification of unusual findings. Finally, they must know the clinical correlation or significance of each of the elements that

may be encountered and the relationship of findings in the sediment to findings in the chemical and physical analysis of the urine specimen.

Specimen Preparation

To ensure detection of less abundant constituents, the urine specimen is usually concentrated before it is examined microscopically. This is accomplished by centrifuging a well-mixed and consistent volume of urine (usually 12, 15, or 10 mL). The clear supernatant is removed (decanted), and the solid material that settles to the bottom during centrifugation is examined under the microscope. A consistent volume of supernatant urine must be removed, leaving a uniform volume of sediment (usually 1 mL). This will result in a 12:1, 15:1, or 10:1 concentration of sediment, respectively. Other volumes may be used; however, it must be consistent within a given laboratory and the concentration of sediment included in the final report.

Standardization

To ensure consistency, various aids to the standardization and examination of the urine sediment are available. Complete systems or portions of systems may be used by a given laboratory. Complete standardized systems include specially designed graduated centrifuge tubes with devices or pipettes that allow for easy decanting of supernatant urine and retention of exactly the same volume of undisturbed, concentrated sediment. Systems differ in the final urine sediment volume, although they generally begin by centrifuging 12 mL of well-mixed urine. All standardized systems provide a capped centrifuge tube, transfer pipette, supravital stain, and choice of standardized slides. They also have various control solutions or preparations available. Systems include the KOVA system (ICL Scientific, Fountain Valley, Calif.), the UriSystem (Fisher Scientific, Pittsburgh, Pa.), and the Count-6 or Count-10 system (V-Tech, Inc., Palm Desert, Calif.).

Standardized systems employ specially designed slides of acrylic plastics with wells or applied cover glasses. They differ in the number of tests per slide, slide chamber volume (depth and surface area), availability of gridded slides, and type of coverglass material. People used to working with traditional slides and coverglasses may have trouble at first using standardized slides because of the greater depth of the chamber. **Compensated polarizing microscopy** may be more difficult, especially at the periphery of the examination area. Students who are new to microscopic examination of the urinary sediment prefer standardized slides to traditional slides and coverslips. NCCLS recommends the use of such standardized commercial systems so that abnormal sediment elements can be easily reported per unit volume rather than per low or high power field. If glass microscope slides and coverslips are used, a measured volume (20 µL) of uniformly concentrated sediment should be placed on the slide and covered with a standard coverslip (22 × 22 mm). NCCLS also recommends that results be calculated and reported in elements/mL of urine.

Whatever system is used, according to NCCLS, the following specific factors must be standardized.

1. **Urine volume.** Twelve mL is generally recommended and is the volume employed by standardized systems. If a different volume is used, the final concentration of urine examined must be applied to numerical counts.

2. **Time of centrifugation.** Five minutes is recommended.

3. **Speed of centrifugation.** NCCLS recommends a relative centrifugal force (RCF) of 400 g. Other standard textbooks recommend 450 or 400-450 g. Nomograms can be used to relate the revolutions per minute (RPM) to RCF by measuring the radius of the centrifuge head in centimeters from the center pin to the bottom of a horizontal cup or from the following formula:

$$RCF \text{ (g)} = 11.18 \times 10^{-6} \times \text{radius in cm} \times RPM^2$$

4. **Concentration factor of the sediment.** This is based on the volume of well-mixed urine centrifuged and the final volume of sediment remaining after the supernatant urine is removed.

5. **Volume of sediment examined.** Standardized slides hold a specific volume of urine sediment. The volume examined may be calculated for traditional slides and coverslips based on the volume of sediment placed on the slide, size (area) of coverslip, diameter of microscope objective, and concentration of urine sediment used.

6. **Reporting Format.** Every person in an institution who performs a microscopic examination of the urinary sediment should use the same terminology, reporting format, and reference ranges.

Specimen Requirements

Actual specimen requirements must be established by and for each laboratory. However, a first-morning, midstream, clean-catch urine specimen is generally the specimen of choice, although any freely voided urine collection is acceptable. The first specimen voided in the morning (an 8-hour concentration) is preferred, since it is most concentrated and therefore small amounts of abnormal constituents are more likely to be detected. Ideally, 25 to 50 mL of urine should be collected into a 100 mL screw-cap container. At least 12 mL is required for the normal concentration of the

sediment, although a 12:1 concentration can be done on 3 mL of specimen. Less than 3 mL of urine may be examined unconcentrated. All requests for microscopic examination of the urine must be accompanied by information about the type of specimen and time of collection. Physical and chemical results must be available and consulted at the time of examination.

Specimens should be centrifuged and examined as soon as possible after collection. They must be refrigerated if they cannot be examined within 2 hours of collection and should be refrigerated as soon as possible if they are not examined immediately. Specimens are unacceptable for microscopic examination if left unrefrigerated for more than 2 hours.

Red cells, white cells, and casts disintegrate rapidly in dilute (specific gravity <1.010) urine of an alkaline pH. Refrigeration serves to prevent the growth of bacteria, the growth of which increases urine pH because of ammonia production. As urine stands, red blood cells distort because of lack of isotonicity. They may swell and lyse, or shrink and crenate depending on the urine specific gravity (tonicity). Neutrophilic white blood cells disintegrate rapidly in hypotonic (low specific gravity) solutions. Casts also disintegrate, especially as dilute urine becomes alkaline.

Although refrigeration retards decomposition of these urinary sediment constituents, amorphous deposits of urates in acid urine and phosphates in alkaline urine tend to precipitate out of solution as the urine cools. These may obscure the presence of pathologic constituents in the urinary sediment. Although NCCLS does not recommend any chemical preservatives for routine urinalysis, they may be desirable in some cases. Formalin is a preservative that will fix the various formed elements, and formalin, or a formalin-containing formulation, is present in several commercially available urine preservatives. However, formalin interferes with several of the chemical tests on multiple reagent strips and cannot be used. If a chemical preservative is to be used to preserve the urinary sediment, the well-mixed urine specimen should be split so that an unaltered portion is available for chemical testing.

Normal Sediment

Normally urine contains little to no sediment. However, a few constituents may be seen in any urine specimen. These generally consist of very few red blood cells, white blood cells, hyaline casts, epithelial cells, and crystals. Each laboratory must establish its own reference values for normal urine based on its particular methodology and patient population. The reference values in Table 5-1 are those established for the University of Minnesota Hospital and Clinic and are included as an example of what may be "normally" encountered when the urine is examined microscopically.

Table 5-1

REFERENCE VALUES FOR URINARY SEDIMENT	
Sediment constituent	12:1 concentration
Red blood cells	0-2/hpf*
White blood cells (neutrophils)	0-5/hpf
Hyaline casts	0-2/lpf**
Renal epithelial cells	few/hpf
Transitional epithelial cells	few/hpf
Squamous epithelial cells	few/lpf
Bacteria	neg/hpf
Abnormal crystals	none/lpf

*hpf, high power (40x objective) field.
**lpf, low power (10x objective) field.

■ MICROSCOPIC TECHNIQUES

Traditionally the urine sediment has been examined as a wet mount of a preparation of concentrated unstained sediment using a regular brightfield microscope. Because it is a wet preparation, oil immersion cannot be used. The preparation is usually examined under low power with a 10× objective and high power using a 40× objective. The brightfield examination of such unstained sediment is difficult, and various microscopic techniques have been developed to aid in the identification of the various entities that might be encountered in urine sediment. Other useful techniques include staining and cytocentrifugation.

Brightfield Microscopy

This is the traditional microscopic method of observation of the urine sediment, and it is the most difficult. Correct light adjustment is essential. The light must be sufficiently reduced to give contrast to the various unstained structures and the background liquid. The light is adjusted by closing the aperture (condenser) iris diaphragm to increase contrast and by lowering the condenser slightly (only 1 or 2 mm). The condenser should not be "racked down"; instead, contrast is achieved by opening or closing the iris diaphragm. However, translucent elements that may occur in the urine sediment are easily overlooked with this technique. Especially difficult to visualize are hyaline casts, mucus, and various cells. Brightfield microscopy is enhanced by the use of stains, and if only a brightfield microscope is available, the use of a suitable stain is encouraged. Phase contrast microscopy is helpful, and a combination of phase contrast and brightfield microscopy is recommended. The hemoglobin pigment present in blood casts and red blood cell casts is more apparent with brightfield illumination as are certain cellular details and the presence of highly refractile fat (free and in cells or casts). Most crystals are more easily visualized with brightfield or brightfield and polarizing microscopy.

Phase Contrast Microscopy

The phase contrast microscope is especially useful in the examination of unstained urine sediment for the detection of translucent elements such as hyaline casts, mucus, cells, and bacteria that may be missed using brightfield microscopy. When available, phase contrast is an excellent microscope for the routine examination of the urine sediment. Phase contrast provides greater contrast between the urine sediment components and background fluid when the refractive indices are similar.

Some elements are better visualized with brightfield illumination, and the microscopist must be able to change from phase to brightfield with ease. For example, highly refractile structures such as fat or crystals are more easily identified with brightfield illumination. Although stained sediments may be examined with phase contrast, staining is not particularly helpful and represents an unnecessary step when phase contrast is used in the routine examination of the urine.

Interference Contrast Microscopy

Unlike phase contrast, interference contrast is not generally used in routine urinalysis because of the cost of the equipment. Like phase contrast it is useful for the examination of wet preparations, giving an apparent three-dimensional view of the object being observed. It allows for better visualization of inclusions such as granules or vacuoles within cells or casts by increasing contrast and showing geometric shape.

Polarizing Microscopy

Polarized light, with or without a full wave compensator, may be used to study structures that polarize light. Objects that polarize (bend or rotate) light are by definition **birefringent**. When viewed with crossed polarizing filters, they appear white against a black background. If a compensating filter is added, the birefringent body is seen against a magenta background, and certain crystals are identified by the pattern of their birefringence in relation to the direction of the slow wave of compensation.

Anything that is visualized with crossed polarizing filters is birefringent. Birefringent objects found in the urine sediment include various crystals, fat (as cholesterol ester droplets), starch (which may be confused with fat), and fibers (which might be confused with some casts). Both fat and starch show a characteristic Maltese cross pattern (a light cross against a black background) when polarized but appear different with brightfield illumination. Since protein material (i.e., casts, cells, bacteria) is not birefringent, polarizing microscopy may be used to differentiate certain amorphous crystals that polarize light from bacteria that do not, and an unusual ovoid form of calcium oxalate, which is strongly birefringent, from red blood cells that are not.

Both the College of American Pathologists and NCCLS recommend the use of polarizing microscopy in the examination of the urine sediment.

■ STAINING TECHNIQUES

Staining techniques have been used to help visualize various elements in the urine sediment that are difficult to see with brightfield illumination. NCCLS states, "Staining can be extremely helpful in the identification of cells and casts."[1] They go on to recommend the use of supravital stains such as a Sternheimer-Malbin Stain, which is commercially available, or 0.5% Toluidine blue, a nuclear stain.

Supravital Stains

Sternheimer-Malbin Stain. This crystal violet and safranin O stain may be used to aid in the identification of cellular elements. It is an easy-to-use, all-purpose stain available as Sedi-Stain (Clay Adams, division of Becton Dickinson and Co., Parsippany, NJ) and KOVA stain (ICL Scientific, Fountain Valley, Calif.). Staining reactions of the various cellular elements are listed on the package inserts. Very alkaline urines may cause the dyes to precipitate, forming fine brown stellate crystals or purple granules.

Toluidine Blue. A 0.5% solution of Toluidine blue is an easy-to-use nuclear stain that can be prepared in the laboratory. It also has the disadvantage of precipitating and causing clumping in some specimens.

Fat Stains

Sudan stains and oil red O are fat stains used to stain neutral fat or triglycerides. These fats do not polarize as a Maltese cross as cholesterol does, yet they have similar clinical significance. Both fat stains and polarizing microscopy should be used to help identify and confirm the presence of fat, either free, within renal epithelial cells or macrophages (oval fat bodies), or within casts (fatty casts).

Gram Stain

This is a routine stain used in microbiology to differentiate gram-negative (red) from gram-positive (purple) bacteria. It may be helpful in urinalysis but requires a dry preparation (smear or cytocentrifuged preparation), which is heat fixed and then stained.

Acetic Acid

Although not a stain, acetic acid has been used to differentiate white blood cells from red blood cells; however, phase contrast and supravital stains are preferable. A 2% solution of acetic acid may be added to a few drops of the concentrated sediment in a small test tube or flowed under the coverslip of a mounted specimen. The acetic acid will accentuate the nucleus of white cells and epithelial cells and lyse red cells. It will also dissolve certain crystals or convert them to other forms.

CYTOCENTRIFUGATION

A fairly recent but useful addition to microscopic examination of urine sediment is cytocentrifugation. This special slow centrifugation method is used to prepare permanent slides and gives excellent morphology. Specimens are traditionally stained with a Papanicolaou stain, the usual cytologic stain for tumor detection. This is a time-consuming method and not practical for routine urinalysis. However, either traditional or quick Wright's stains are relatively easy to prepare and adequate in most instances. Cytocentrifugation may be very helpful in difficult situations such as the differentiation of viral and nonviral inclusion cells, fungi, mononuclear cells, eosinophils, casts, and precancerous or malignant cells.

LABORATORY PROCEDURE

Procedure 5-1 is based on the procedure used by the University of Minnesota Hospital and Clinic, Minneapolis, Minn. It uses a 12:1 concentration of the urine specimen and employs parts of the KOVA system. Urine is measured and centrifuged in a special graduated centrifuge (KOVA) tube. It is decanted and exactly 1 mL retained for microscopic examination by using a special disposable pipette with a built-in plastic disk (KOVA petter). Results are reported according to the system in Table 5-2. Directions are included for both standardized slides and traditional glass microscope slides with coverglasses, using both unstained and stained sediment. If a phase contrast microscope is used, staining generally is unnecessary. However, if only a brightfield microscope is used, staining is recommended.

Table 5-2

REPORTING SYSTEM FOR URINE SEDIMENT

Average number per low power field (×100)

Casts	Negative	0-2	2-5	5-10	10-25	25-50	>50
Abnormal crystals	Negative	0-2	2-5	5-10	10-25	25-50	>50
Squamous epithelial cells		Few		Moderate		Many	
Mucus		Present					

Average number per high power field (×400)

Red blood cells	0-2	2-5	5-10	10-25	25-50	50-99	>100
White blood cells	0-2	2-5	5-10	10-25	25-50	50-99	>100
Normal crystals		Few		Moderate		Many	
Epithelial cells (renal tubular, oval fat bodies, transitional)		Few		Moderate		Many	
Miscellaneous (bacteria, yeast, *Trichomonas*, fat globules)		Few		Moderate		Many	
Sperm (males only)		Present					

Few means some are present; moderate means easily seen; many means prominent.

Modified from Linne JJ, Ringsrud KM: *Basic techniques in clinical laboratory science*, ed 3, St. Louis, 1992, Mosby, p 375.

MICROSCOPIC EXAMINATION OF THE URINE SEDIMENT

1. Pour exactly 12 mL of well-mixed urine into a labeled, graduated centrifuge (KOVA) tube.
   a. If less than 12 mL is available, use 3 mL.
   b. If less than 3 mL is available, examine the sediment without concentration. Include this information on the report form.

2. Centrifuge at a relative centrifugal force of 450 rpm for 5 minutes. Let the centrifuge come to a stop without using the brake. Use of the brake will cause resuspension of the sediment and falsely low results.

3. Decant 11 mL of clear supernatant urine into a test tube, leaving 1 mL of sediment in the KOVA tube.
   a. Insert the KOVA petter into the KOVA tube. Push it to the bottom of the tube until it is firmly seated. Holding the petter in place, decant the supernatant urine. This will leave exactly 1 mL of sediment in the bottom of the tube.
   b. If a 3 mL specimen was used, do not use a KOVA petter. Decant all liquid quickly, retaining a small drop in which to resuspend the sediment. This is approximately equivalent to a 12:1 concentration.
   c. If plain centrifuge tubes without a decanting device are used, pour off 11 mL of supernatant urine in one even motion so as not to resuspend the sediment. Use a disposable pipette to bring the volume of sediment to exactly 1 mL with the clear supernatant urine. Removal of more than 11 mL and readjustment to 1 mL is preferable to removal of less than 11 mL.

4. If using a brightfield microscope, use supravital staining. Add a drop or two of stain (e.g., Sedi-Stain) to the sediment and mix thoroughly. If the amount of original specimen is limited, or the urine is very alkaline, split the concentrated sediment and stain only one portion.

5. Thoroughly resuspend the sediment for examination by gently squeezing the KOVA petter.

6. Add the resuspended sediment to a standardized microscope slide following the manufacturer's directions. If traditional glass slides and coverglasses are used, place 20 µL of resuspended sediment on a microscope slide and cover with a 22 × 22 mm coverglass. The size of the drop is important. The fluid should completely fill the area under the coverglass without overflowing the area or causing the coverglass to float.

7. Place the prepared slide on the microscope stage and focus. Adjust the light using the low power objective by carefully positioning the condenser and iris diaphragm. The tendency is to have too much light, but the light must not be overly reduced. Be sure the sediment itself is brought into focus, rather than the coverglass. It is easier to achieve focus with specimens that are stained. Finally, vary the fine adjust continuously to maintain focus.

8. Be systematic in the examination. With standardized slides, scan the entire preparation. With traditional microscope slides and coverglasses, begin by looking around the four sides of the coverglass, then the center. First, look for the substances that are identified and graded under low power. Change to high power, refocus and readjust the light, and search for the substances that are graded and identified under high power. All gradings are based on the average number of structures seen in a minimum of 10 microscope fields. Describe separately each of the structures searched for under low and high power. Casts and cells are most important; look for these most carefully, observing the less important crystals and miscellaneous structures almost in retrospect.

9. Examine sediment preparations with the low and high power objectives as outlined below. Report results as indicated in Table 5-2. All entities encountered must be reported using the appropriate objective and within the grading scale established for the individual laboratory. For example, if a urinary sediment was examined and the microscopist found an average of 15 white blood cells, 3 hyaline casts, no red blood cells, and 2 squamous epithelial cells, the results would be reported as:

Concentration	12:1
Hyaline casts	2-5/lpf
Red cells	0-2/hpf
White blood cells	10-25/hpf
Squamous epithelial cells	Few

Low Power Examination

With the low power (10×) objective, search for the following:
a. **Casts.** With standardized slides, scan the entire area for the presence of casts. Since they tend to roll to the edges of the coverglass with traditional slides, look for casts around all four edges of the preparation, and then in the center.

MICROSCOPIC EXAMINATION OF THE URINE SEDIMENT, cont'd.

When a cast is discovered, change to high power to identify it. Grade and report casts on the basis of the average number seen per low power field as shown in Table 5-2. If more than one type of cast is found in a single specimen, identify and grade each type separately.

b. **Crystals and amorphous material.** Look for these structures in the same way as for casts.

   (1) **Normal crystals** are reported as few, moderate or many per high power field, but may be more apparent under low power.

   (2) Grade **abnormal crystals** as the average number seen per low power field using the criteria given in Table 5-2. Remember, abnormal crystals must be confirmed before they are reported.

   (3) Since crystals are generally identified by shape rather than size, a combination of low and high power observation is necessary in the detection and identification of these structures.

c. **Squamous epithelial cells.** Report as few, moderate, or many per low power field.

d. **Mucus.** This is reported as present when easily seen or prominent under low power. It is more apparent with phase contrast microscopy.

High Power Examination
With the high power (40×) objective, search for the following:

a. **Red blood cells.** Grade and report on the basis of the average number seen per high power field (see Table 5-2). Report the presence of unusual forms such as dysmorphic red cells, if encountered.

b. **White blood cells.** Grade and report on the basis of the average number seen per high power field (see Table 5-2). These are usually neutrophils (PMNs). If unusual cell types such as lymphocytes or eosinophils are morphologically identifiable, report this finding.

c. **Normal crystals.** Identify and report as few, moderate, or many per high power field for each type of crystal encountered.

d. **Identify casts,** which are graded under low power.

e. **Epithelial cells:** renal tubular, oval fat bodies (renal tubular cells with fat), and transitional. Specify type and report as few, moderate, or many per high power field.

f. **Miscellaneous.** This category includes various cell forms and other structures that may be encountered in the urine sediment: yeast, bacteria, trichomonads, fat globules. Identify the cell or structure and report as few, moderate, or many per high power field. Report the presence of sperm as present in males only. It is considered a contaminant in routine urinalysis specimens from females and is not reported.

URINALYSIS AND BODY FLUIDS: A COLORTEXT AND ATLAS

REVIEW QUESTIONS

1 List six factors that should be standardized in the microscopic examination of the urine sediment.
a.
b.
c.
d.
e.
f.

2 Which of the following changes is **not** associated with stored urine sediment?
a. growth of bacteria
b. loss of amorphous deposits and crystals
c. loss of casts
d. loss of red cells
e. loss of white cells

3 Translucent elements in the urinary sediment (hyaline casts, mucus, cells, and bacteria) are most easily visualized by use of:
a. brightfield microscopy
b. cytocentrifugation
c. phase contrast microscopy
d. polarized microscopy

4 The ability to polarize light is referred to as _____.

5 If a phase contrast microscope is not used for the microscopic analysis of the urine sediment, which of the following techniques is recommended for routine examination?
a. cytocentrifugation
b. polarizing microscopy
c. sudan staining
d. supravital staining

REFERENCES

1. *Routine urinalysis and collection, transportation, and preservation of urine specimens, tentative guidelines*, Villanova, Pa, Dec. 1992, National Committee for Clinical Laboratory Standards, 12(26) GP16-T, p 9.

BIBLIOGRAPHY

Benham L, O'Kell RT: Urinalysis: minimizing microscopy. (letter), *Clin Chem* 28(7):1722, 1982.

Ferris JA: Comparison and standardization of the urine microscopic examination, *Lab Med* 14:659-662, 1983.

Linne JJ, Ringsrud KM: *Basic techniques in clinical laboratory science*, ed 3, St. Louis, 1992, Mosby.

Physician's office laboratory guidelines, tentative guidelines, ed 2, Villanova, Pa, June 1992, National Committee for Clinical Laboratory Standards, 12(5) POL1-T2.

Schumann GB, Greenberg NF: Usefulness of macroscopic urinalysis as a screening procedure. A preliminary report, *Am J Clin Pathol* 71(4):452-456, 1979.

Schumann GB, Schumann JL, and Schweitzer S: The urine sediment examination. A coordinated approach, *Lab Management* 21:45, 1983.

Schumann GB, Schweitzer SC: Examination of urine. In Henry JB (ed): *Clinical diagnosis and management by laboratory methods*, ed 18, Philadelphia, 1991, WB Saunders.

Schumann GB, Tebbs RD: Comparison of slides used for standardized routine microscopic urinalysis, *J Med Tech* 3:54-58, 1986.

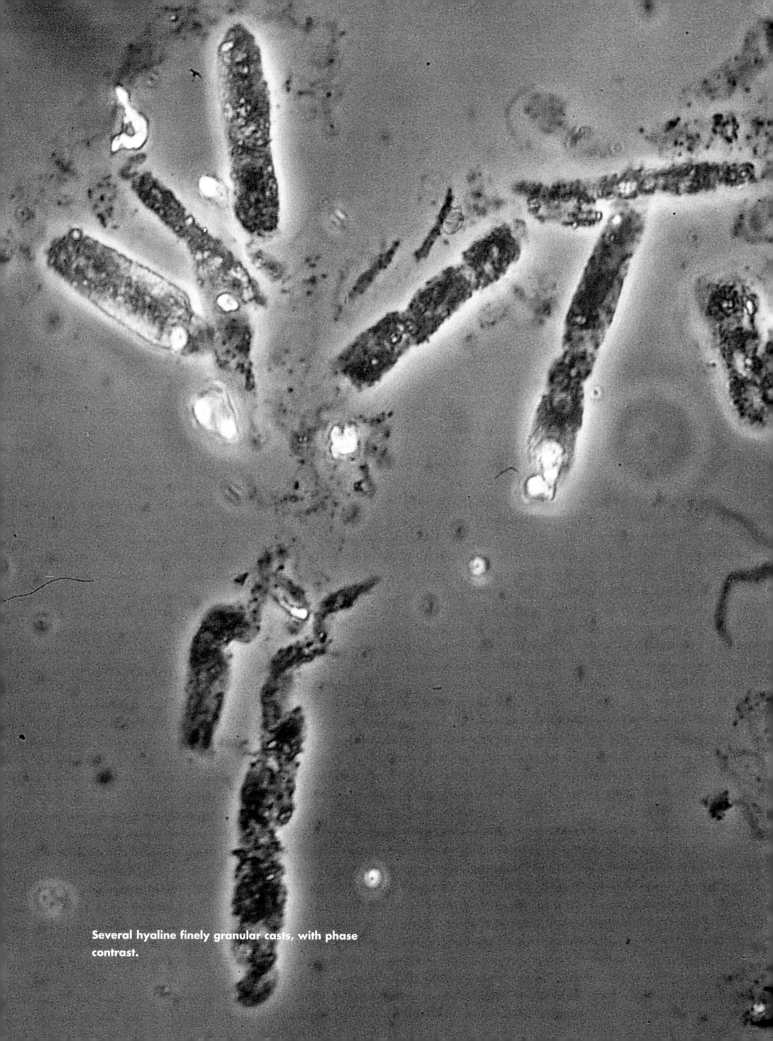

Several hyaline finely granular casts, with phase contrast.

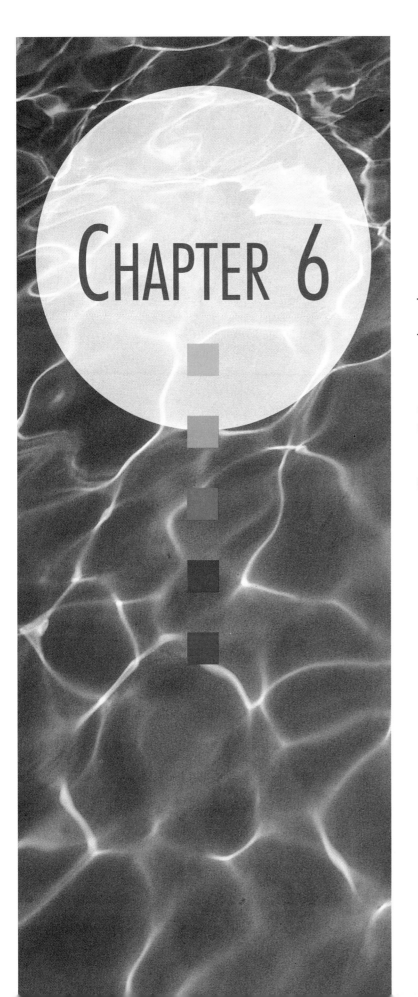

CHAPTER 6

ATLAS OF URINE SEDIMENT CONSTITUENTS

CHAPTER OUTLINE

● Introduction

● Hematopoietic Cells in the Urine Sediment
  Red Blood Cells (Erythrocytes)
  Clinical Importance
  Microscopic Appearance
  Structures Confused With Red Cells
  Other Considerations
  White Blood Cells (Leukocytes)
  Clinical Importance
  Microscopic Appearance
  Structures Confused With White Cells
  Glitter Cells
  Eosinophils
  Lymphocytes and Other Mononuclear Cells

● Epithelial Cells
  Squamous Epithelial Cells
  Transitional Epithelial (Urothelial) Cells
  Renal Epithelial Cells
  Tumor Cells

● Other Cellular Components
  Spermatozoa
  Bacteria
  Yeast
  Trichomonas
  Other Parasites

● Casts
  Formation and Significance
  Identification and Morphology of Casts
  Classification of Casts
  Hyaline Casts

Cellular Casts
Granular Casts
Waxy Casts
Fatty Casts
Pigmented Casts
Inclusion Casts
Pseudocasts and Structures Confused With Casts

● Crystals and Amorphous Material
  Clinical Significance
  Normal Acid Crystals
  Normal Alkaline Crystals
  Abnormal Urinary Crystals—Introduction
  Abnormal Crystals of Metabolic Origin
  Abnormal Crystals of Iatrogenic Origin (Drugs)

● Contaminants and Artifacts
  Starch
  Fibers (Including Disposable Diaper Fibers)
  Air Bubbles
  Oil Droplets
  Glass Fragments
  Stains
  Pollen Grains
  Fecal Contamination

● Review Questions
  Cells
  Casts
  Crystals

● References

● Bibliography

LEARNING OBJECTIVES

▶ Recognize the various constituents described and pictured when encountered including:
  Red cells
  White cells
  Epithelial cells
  Other cellular components
  Casts
  Crystals and amorphous material
  Contaminants and artifacts

▶ Understand microscopic and staining techniques used in the identification of various constituents.

▶ Understand the relative importance and pathophysiology of each of the constituents described.

▶ Define and understand the significance of:
  Dysmorphic red cells
  Glitter cells
  Clue cells
  Oval fat bodies (renal tubular fat)
  Hemosiderin

▶ Understand the terms *organized* and *unorganized* *sediment.*

▶ Understand the formation and significance of casts and how they are classified and reported.

▶ Understand what is meant by the terms acid, alkaline, normal and abnormal crystals, their significance, and how they are identified and reported.

▶ Know which are the most commonly encountered crystals in acid and alkaline urine specimens.

▶ Confirm the presence of the various abnormal crystals that might be encountered.

▶ Understand the relationship between findings in the urine sediment and physical and chemical findings in the urinalysis, including but not limited to:
    Appearance, blood, and red cells
    Appearance, leukocyte esterase, nitrite, and
        white cells
    Protein and casts
    pH and crystals.

INTRODUCTION

As mentioned in Chapter 5, the various constituents of urine sediment are either biologic or chemical in make-up. The biologic part is sometimes referred to as the **organized sediment** and consists of cells derived from blood or hematopoietic cells (red cells and white cells), epithelial cells (renal, transitional, squamous), casts (with or without inclusions), other cell forms (bacteria, yeast, fungi, parasites, and spermatozoa) and fat of biologic origin. The biologic portion of the urine sediment is generally more important than the chemical part.

The chemical part is sometimes referred to as the **unorganized sediment**. It consists of crystals and amorphous deposits of chemicals. Amorphous means without shape or form; amorphous deposits of urates may be seen in urine of an acid pH and phosphates in urine of an alkaline pH. There are certain "normal" crystal forms that occur in urine. These have limited clinical significance but may obscure the presence of important (pathologic) findings. In addition, there are certain abnormal crystals, which indicate serious pathology. These may be of metabolic or iatrogenic origin.

Finally, there are various contaminants or exogenous structures that may be present in the urine sediment of either biologic or chemical origin. These must be recognized so that they are not mistaken for clinically significant constituents.

All of these constituents will be described and illustrated with photomicrographs in the following section. As many techniques as possible (type of microscopic illumination, staining, and cytocentrifugation) will be used to illustrate the various characteristics and techniques used in the identification of each of the entities. Unless otherwise specified, the staining reactions are those of the Sternheimer-Malbin crystal violet safranin stain (Sedi-Stain, Clay Adams, division of Becton-Dickinson, Parsippany, NJ). Cytocentrifuged preparations in this Atlas were prepared using the Cytospin (Shandon, Inc., Pittsburgh, Pa.).

Photomicrographs are of unstained urine sediment using brightfield illumination unless stated otherwise.

Stated magnifications are as viewed through the microscope with consistent enlargement of the 35mm photomicrographs used throughout this text. Low-power magnifications are generally ×100 or ×160; high-power generally ×400 or ×450 and occasionally ×640 or ×512; and oil-immersion generally ×1000. These vary with the exact microscope and objectives used for the photomicrographs.

HEMATOPOIETIC CELLS IN THE URINE SEDIMENT

Any of the cells present in the blood (hematopoietic cells) may theoretically be found in the urine sediment. However, the most commonly encountered cells in the sediment are red blood cells or erythrocytes and white blood cells or leukocytes, usually as polymorphonuclear neutrophils (PMNs).

RED BLOOD CELLS (ERYTHROCYTES)

Clinical Importance

Reference values for red blood cells in the urine sediment are generally on the order of 0-2 red blood cells per high power field, or 3 to 12/µL.[6] According to the College of American Pathologists Glossary of Terms for Urine Sediment, there are normally less than five red blood cells per high power field in the urine sediment. Although the presence of a few red cells is normal and benign, **hematuria** (the presence of red blood cells in the urine) is a sensitive early indicator of renal disease that should not be missed. Hematuria may be the result of bleeding at any point in the urinary system caused by renal disease or dysfunction, infection, tumor or lesions, stone formation, generalized bleeding disorders, or anticoagulant usage. There may be little correlation between the amount of blood and the severity of the disorder, and the degree of hematuria may vary from a frankly bloody specimen to a specimen showing no alteration in appearance (microscopic hematuria).

Figure 6-1

Red cells, 5 intact, 1 crenated. Unstained, ×400.

Figure 6-2

Red cells (3) showing yellowish orange color from hemoglobin. One white cell also present. Unstained, ×400.

Determination of the cause of hematuria and site of bleeding requires a variety of information—both clinical and laboratory based. Results in other portions of the microscopic analysis, together with physical and chemical findings in the urinalysis, are taken into account. For example, the occurrence of **dysmorphic** (distorted, irregular, or misshapen) red cells, especially when accompanied by proteinuria and blood casts, indicates bleeding of glomerular origin. When hematuria is unaccompanied by proteinuria or casts, the site of bleeding is probably not within the kidney, but lower in the urogenital tract. It should also be remembered that contamination of the urine specimen with menstrual fluid is a common source of red blood cells in urine.

When blood is detected in the chemical screen, it is important to distinguish hematuria from hemoglobinuria and myoglobinuria. This is described in Chapter 4. In general, with hematuria, red blood cells are present in the microscopic analysis of the urine sediment but absent with hemoglobinuria and myoglobinuria.

Microscopic Appearance

Theoretically, the recognition of red blood cells in the urine sediment should be a simple matter. Red cells are intact biconcave disks, about 7 μm in diameter, have a characteristic bluish-green sheen and generally smooth appearance as shown in Fig. 6-1.

The hemoglobin pigment gives the intact red cell a pale yellowish-orange color when viewed with brightfield illumination in an unstained sediment. Such a classic appearance of red cells is seen in Fig. 6-2.

When stained with Sedi-Stain, red cells show a pink to purple color in urine of a neutral pH, purple color at an alkaline pH, and are either unstained or show a

Figure 6-3

Several red cells, intact and crenated, showing minimal staining. Sedi-Stain, ×400.

pink color at an acid pH. Therefore staining may or may not be helpful in recognition of red cells in urine. Fig. 6-3 shows a specimen with intact and crenated red blood cells stained with Sedi-Stain. In this case, staining is minimal, although cells are somewhat easier to visualize than when unstained.

Figs. 6-4 and 6-5 show a variety of staining within the same urine specimen.

Unfortunately red blood cells are not so easily recognized, and detection requires careful microscopic examination. They are searched for and enumerated with the high-power objective. Proper light adjustment is essential; light is reduced and contrast achieved by proper adjustment of the condenser and iris diaphragm. Most importantly, detection requires continual refocusing with the fine adjustment of the microscope as the preparation is scanned for the pres-

Figure 6-4

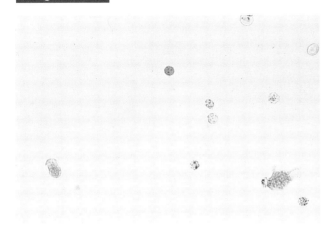

Stained red cells with variable staining. Two stained white cells also present for comparison. Sedi-Stain, ×400.

Figure 6-5

Red cells, two strongly stained, one unstained. Sedi-Stain, ×400.

Figure 6-6

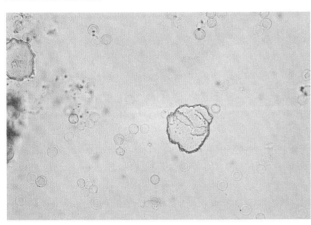

A

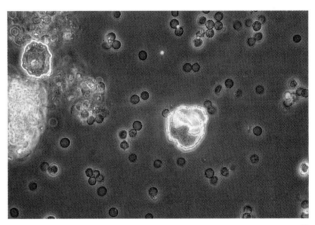

B

Red cells. Many ghost or shadow red cells, which are difficult to visualize with brightfield microscopy but are easily seen with phase contrast. Unusual uric acid crystal also present. A, Brightfield, ×400. B, Same field as A with phase contrast, ×400.

ence of cells. As mentioned, stain may be helpful in brightfield examination, but the use of phase contrast illumination is extremely helpful in the detection of red blood cells. Even after hemolysis, the remaining red cell membrane is clearly visible with phase contrast.

Intact red cells are seen in absolutely fresh urine which is approximately isotonic with blood (specific gravity about 1.010). They rapidly undergo morphologic changes both in the urinary tract and in the voided specimen, which is seldom isotonic with blood.

When urine is dilute or hypotonic (low specific gravity), the red cells appear **swollen** and **rounded** because of diffusion of fluid into the red cell. These will eventually burst, especially at an alkaline pH, leaving a **ghost** or **shadow** cell where only the red cell membrane

remains after the hemoglobin is released. Such ghost cells that have lost hemoglobin are extremely difficult to see with brightfield illumination; however, they are easily visualized with phase contrast, as shown in Fig. 6-6, *A* and *B*. Eventually, even the ghost cell membrane will disappear as the cell completely disintegrates.

In concentrated (high specific gravity) urine, hypertonicity causes the cell to lose fluid to the urine, and the red cells appear **crenated** and **shrunken**, as shown in Fig. 6-7.

These crenated cells have little spicules, or projections, and may be confused with white blood cells. However, crenated cells are significantly smaller than white blood cells and have a generally smooth, rather than granular, appearance (Fig. 6-8).

Figure 6-7

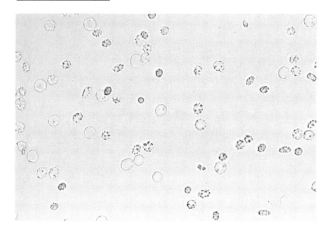

Crenated red cells, unstained, ×400.

Figure 6-8

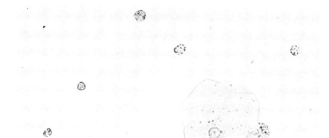

Stained crenated red cells, white cells, and one squamous epithelial cell. Sedi-Stain, ×400.

Figure 6-9

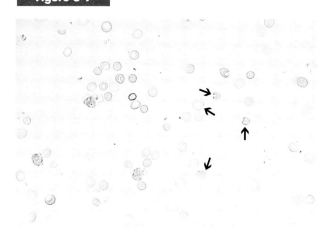

Dysmorphic red cells (*arrows*), with many other red cells and three white cells, Sedi-Stain, ×400.

Figure 6-10

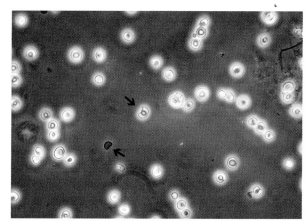

Dysmorphic red cells (*arrows*). Phase contrast, ×400.

    Dysmorphic, or distorted, red cells are an important finding that should be noted in the microscopic examination since they are indicative of renal (especially glomerular) hematuria. It is felt that the red cell becomes bent, twisted, or distorted and may even lose some cell membrane as it makes its way through the glomerulus (Fig. 6-9). Dysmorphic forms are best visualized with phase or interference contrast microscopy (Fig. 6-10).

    Nucleated red cells and even sickle cells may be seen in the urine on rare occasions (Figs. 6-11, 6-12, and 6-13).

Structures Confused With Red Cells

    In addition to being difficult to detect, red cells are often confused with other structures in the urine sedi-

ment. Aids to identification include the use of phase and polarizing microscopy, supravital stains, such as Sedi-Stain or 0.5% toluidine blue, acetic acid, cytocentrifugation, and chemical reagent strip tests.

    White cells (leukocytes). It may be difficult to distinguish red cells from white cells in the urine. This is especially true if the urine is very fresh and the white cells very intact, or if they are lymphocytes. Generally, the white cell is larger and has a generally granular appearance with a nucleus (which is lobed in fresh neutrophils). Before use of stains and phase microscopy became common, acetic acid was used to differentiate red and white blood cells. If acetic acid is added to a portion of the urine sediment, or introduced under the coverglass, red cells should lyse (disappear), whereas the white cell nucleus is accentuated (stained).

Figure 6-11

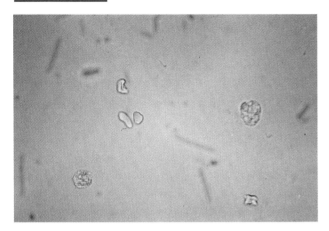

Dysmorphic red cells (sickle cells) from urine of patient with sickle cell anemia. Two white cells also present. Unstained, ×450.

Figure 6-12

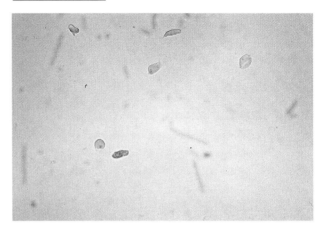

Dysmorphic and sickle cells in stained urine from a patient with sickle cell anemia. Sedi-Stain, ×450.

Figure 6-13

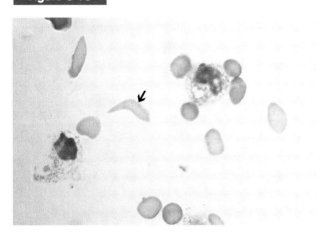

Sickle cell (*arrow*), red cells, and two white cells from cytocentrifuged urine sediment of a patient with sickle cell anemia. Cytospin, Wright's Stain, ×1000.

Figure 6-14

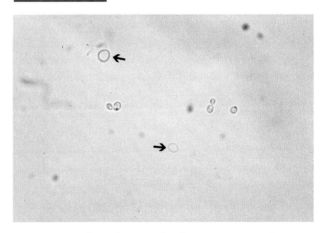

Yeast, several, and two red cells (*arrows*), ×400.

Yeast. Although they may be confused with red cells, yeast are generally smaller and rounder (spherical not flattened) and show considerable variation in size within a specimen. Their reproduction by budding is a valuable clue to their presence (Fig. 6-14).

Calcium Oxalate. A very rare ovoid form of calcium oxalate may be mistaken for red blood cells, especially with brightfield illumination. These birefringent crystals are readily recognized when viewed with polarized and compensated polarized microscopy as shown in Fig. 6-200.

Bubbles or Oil Droplets. Although air bubbles or oil droplets may be confused with red cells, their typical variation in size and highly refractive or reflective appearance is obvious with experience (see Figs. 6-239 and 6-241).

Other Considerations

Observation of a tiny red button on the bottom of the tube after centrifugation is a clue to the presence of red blood cells in the sediment. This finding, together with results of reagent strip tests for blood, is a useful tool in the identification of red cells in the urine sediment. Microscopic hematuria should be accompanied by a positive reagent strip test for blood. However, reagent strips are more sensitive to hemoglobin than red cells, and only a few very intact red blood cells may not react. Sensitivity is also reduced in concentrated (high specific gravity) urine. If all else fails, red cells may be demonstrated by adding distilled or deionized water to the sediment to lyse cells and then retesting with the reagent strip for blood.

More often, negative or delayed reagent strip results with microscopic hematuria are seen in urine specimens containing large amounts of ascorbic acid (Vitamin C). This may be confirmed by testing the specimen with a reagent strip for ascorbic acid. Vitamin C interference may be especially troublesome in outpatient situations where patients self-medicate.

■ WHITE BLOOD CELLS (LEUKOCYTES)

Clinical Importance

The concentrated urine sediment from a healthy person contains a few (as many as five) leukocytes per high power field. More than this is usually considered abnormal. They may enter the urine from any point along the urinary tract or from secretions of the male or female genital tract. Although results are often reported as white cells or leukocytes, the presence of such cells generally refers to a neutrophilic leukocyte (polymorphonuclear neutrophil or PMN) unless stated otherwise. Any leukocyte found in the blood may be found in the urine; the presence of lymphocytes and eosinophils is of diagnostic significance.

The presence of increased white cells in the urine is termed **pyuria**, and indicates inflammation at some point along the urogenital tract. Pyuria may result from bacterial infection or from other renal or urinary tract disease. With infection, bacteria and neutrophils are generally seen together, and clumps of leukocytes (neutrophils) are associated with acute infection. However, it is possible to see bacteria without leukocytes, or in certain infections such as from *Chlamydia* sp., leukocytes are seen without bacteria. It may be possible to see ingested bacteria within the neutrophil, although such cells are extremely labile and rapidly disappear from the urine specimen.

Infection within the kidney such as acute pyelonephritis is associated with the presence of casts, together with white cells (neutrophils), protein, and bacteria. The casts may be cellular (neutrophil), granular, or bacterial. When such casts are seen with bacteria and white cells, the infection is most likely located within the kidney and represents an upper rather than a lower urinary tract (bladder) infection. Upper urinary tract infections are generally associated with moderate proteinuria, whereas lower urinary tract infections tend to have minimal or small proteinuria.

Microscopic Appearance

Like red cells, white cells are searched for microscopically with the high-power objective. Since the urine sediment is examined as a wet preparation, the oil-immersion objective cannot be used. Proper light adjustment and continual readjustment of the fine

Figure 6-15

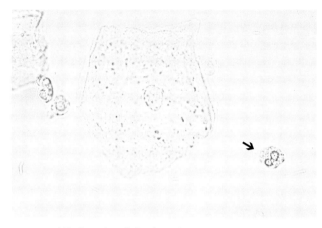

Neutrophil showing lobed nucleus (*arrow*). Squamous epithelial cell also present. Unstained ×640.

Figure 6-16

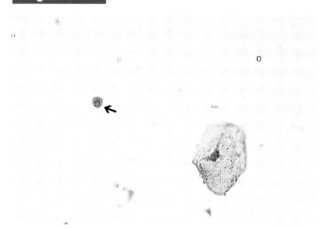

Stained neutrophil showing lobed nucleus (*arrow*) and folded squamous epithelial cell, which might be mistaken for a cast. Sedi-Stain, ×400.

Figure 6-17

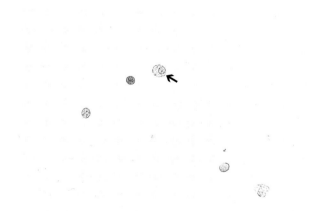

Probable neutrophil with lobes fused into single round nucleus, appearing like a mononuclear cell or renal tubular epithelial cell (*arrow*). Red cells also present. Sedi-Stain, ×400.

Figure 6-18

Clump of degenerating white cells. Unstained, ×400.

Figure 6-19

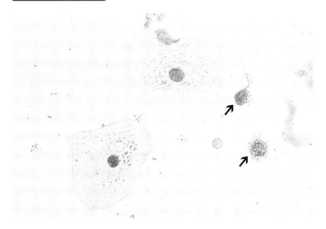

Degenerating (petaled) white cells at arrows, seen in a cytocentrifuged preparation. Red cell and two squamous epithelial cells also present. Cytospin, quick Wright's stain, ×400.

Figure 6-20

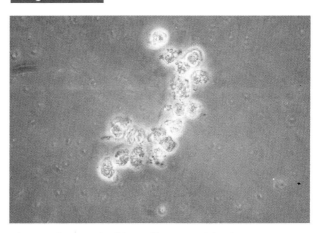

Clump of several white cells seen with phase contrast, ×400.

Figure 6-21

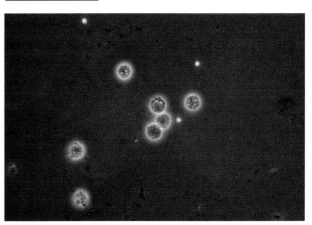

Several white cells with phase contrast illumination, ×400.

focus is essential. Typically, neutrophils are said to be about 10 to 12 μm in diameter, which is about twice the size of a red cell. However, this size difference may not be apparent, and the leukocyte may appear dense and granular, about the same size as—and difficult to distinguish from—a red cell. The cytoplasm may occasionally contain ingested bacteria or yeast, which crowds the nucleus and enlarges the cell two or three times its normal size.

Ideally, neutrophils have thin cytoplasmic granulation and a discrete lobed nucleus (Figs. 6-15 and 6-16).

This is true when cells are absolutely fresh; however, neutrophils rapidly degenerate, especially in dilute alkaline urine, and approximately 50% can be lost within 2 to 3 hours in unrefrigerated urine. As the cells degenerate, nuclear detail is lost, and the lobes fuse into a single round nucleus, losing cytoplasmic granulation. Such cells may be indistinguishable from mononuclear cell forms such as lymphocytes or renal tubular epithelial cells (Fig. 6-17). A small clump of disintegrating neutrophils is seen in Fig. 6-18.

Various stages of disintegration are often observed in a single urine specimen. In very dilute urine, the cell cytoplasm may expand into ungranulated petals before dissolution, as shown in Fig. 6-19.

Microscopic aids to identification of white cells are much the same as for red cells; namely, phase or interference contrast microscopy, use of supravital stains, acetic acid, and cytocentrifugation.

Phase or interference contrast microscopy is especially useful, allowing for better visualization of the nucleus and cytoplasmic granulation (Figs. 6-20 and 6-21).

Supravital staining is also helpful. A nuclear stain especially helpful with leukocyte identification is 0.5% Toluidine blue. Sternheimer-Malbin stain (Sedi-Stain, KOVA stain) is also helpful; however, precipitation of stain in the highly alkaline urine often associated with

Figure 6-22

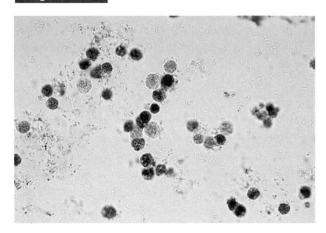

Many white cells showing varied staining. Many bacteria also present. Sedi-Stain, ×400.

Figure 6-23

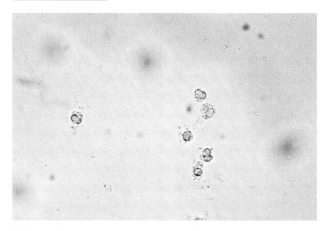

White cells treated with acetic acid to accentuate the nucleus and differentiate from red cells, ×400.

Figure 6-24

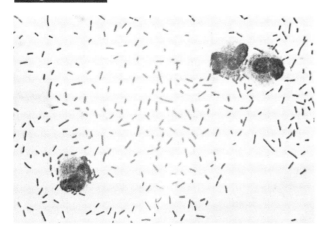

Neutrophils and blue staining rod-shaped bacteria in cytocentrifuged urine sediment stained with Wright's stain, ×1000.

Figure 6-25

White cells (*arrows*) and crenated red cells. Unstained sediment, ×400.

urinary tract infections may be confusing. The actual staining reactions with neutrophils vary somewhat, from a dark staining cell to a colorless or light blue cell, even within a given specimen (Fig. 6-22).

Generally the nucleus is purple with purple granulation, or the nucleus may be colorless to light blue with pale blue or gray cytoplasm in the so-called Sternheimer-Malbin positive, glitter cell.

Adding acetic acid may be useful in causing lysis of red cells with accentuation (staining) of the leukocyte nucleus (Fig. 6-23).

Cytocentrifugation and staining with Wright's (or Papanicolaou) stain may be particularly useful. In this case, identification of leukocytes is much the same as in peripheral blood films, unless the cells are too disintegrated for identification (Fig. 6-24).

Structures Confused With White Cells

Most often, white cells are confused with red cells or renal epithelial cells. White cells are usually described as larger than red cells and granular appearing with a nucleus. However, this distinction may be difficult, especially when the white cells are very fresh and intact, or the red cells are crenated (Figs. 6-25 and 6-26).

White cells difficult to distinguish from red cells may also be lymphocytes. These are about the same size as red cells but have a single rather than a lobulated nucleus.

Renal epithelial cells may be very difficult to distinguish from white cells, and the final decision is often based on the presence of other elements in the sediment. However, they are generally larger than white cells and have a proportionately smaller and more distinct nucle-

Figure 6-26

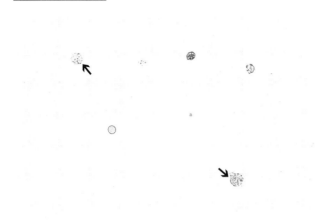

White cells (*arrows*) and crenated red cells appearing like white cells. Sedi-Stain, ×400.

Figure 6-28

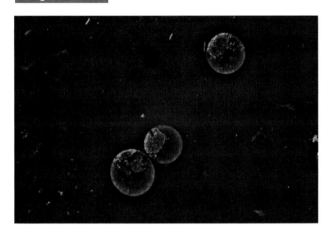

Glitter cells (swollen neutrophils showing Brownian motion in the wet preparation). Dark phase contrast, ×450.

us with more cytoplasm per cell. As the PMN degenerates, the nuclear lobes tend to fuse into one and granulation is lost from the cytoplasm, making distinction from renal epithelial cells extremely difficult (Fig. 6-27).

Glitter Cells

This is a type of neutrophil seen in dilute urine of specific gravity of 1.010 or less. The neutrophil swells because of hypotonicity, and the cytoplasmic granules exhibit constant, Brownian motion. This motion results in a shining or glittering appearance of the cell, hence "**glitter cell**." These cells are observed in wet preparations, and since the special appearance depends on motion, they are difficult to photograph. They are especially striking when viewed with phase contrast (Fig. 6-28).

Figure 6-27

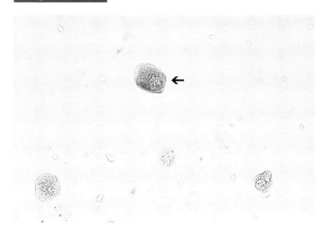

Probable white cell or cells and renal tubular epithelial cell (*arrow*) in stained sediment. Sedi-Stain, ×400.

When stained with Sedi-Stain, they have colorless or light blue nuclei and pale blue or gray cytoplasm. They are also referred to as Sternheimer-Malbin positive cells. Clinically, glitter cells are associated with dilute or hypotonic urine and may be seen in patients with lower urinary tract infections as well as chronic pyelonephritis, for which they were once thought to be diagnostic.

Eosinophils

Eosinophils may be seen in the urine sediment of patients with drug-induced interstitial nephritis, including hypersensitivity to drugs such as penicillin and its analogues, and with other acute genitourinary tract disorders. Detection is important, since treatment is effectively achieved by discontinuing of the drug.

Eosinophils are difficult to recognize in wet preparations, with either brightfield or phase contrast illumination. Supravital stains may be helpful. Eosinophils are generally larger than neutrophils and may be oval or elongated. The eosinophilic granules may not be visible on wet preparations, but the presence of a two- or three-lobed nucleus is helpful. Cytocentrifugation can help in detection. Slides may be stained with Wright's stain (Figs. 6-29 and 6-30). However, a special eosinophil stain such as Hansel's stain (methylene blue and eosin-Y in methanol, Lide Labs, Florissant, Mo.) is helpful since the eosinophils are more easily recognized than with Wright's stain (Fig. 6-31).

Lymphocytes and Other Mononuclear Cells

Normal urine contains a few small lymphocytes; however, they are rarely recognized. They are difficult to distinguish from red blood cells, especially on wet

Figure 6-29

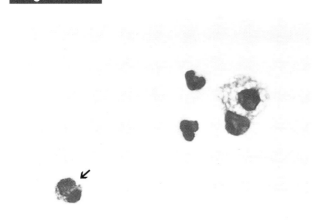

Eosinophil (*arrow*), two neutrophils, and macrophage. Cytospin, Wright's stain, ×1000.

Figure 6-30

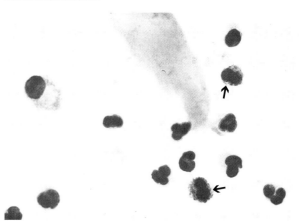

Eosinophils (*arrows*), several neutrophils, one renal cell, and part of a hyaline cast. Cytospin, Wright's stain, ×1000.

Figure 6-31

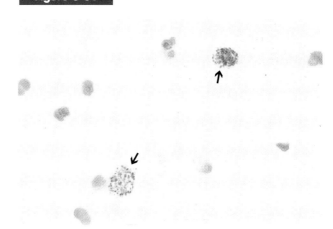

Eosinophils (*at arrows*) and neutrophils. Cytospin, Hansel's stain, ×1000.

preparations with both brightfield and phase contrast microscopy. They are about the same size as, or slightly larger than, red cells, have a single large nucleus that fills the cell, and show little to no cytoplasm. The presence of increased numbers of lymphocytes seen in the first few weeks after renal transplantation are an important early sign of rejection. Cytocentrifugation and staining with Wright's stain are helpful aids in identification (Fig. 6-32). Since lymphocytes are not granulocytes, they will not react with the reagent strip tests for leukocyte esterase.

Monocytes, macrophages, and histiocytes are all phagocytic cells that are related but vary in size and are difficult to recognize in wet preparations. Cytocentrifugation and staining with Wright or Papanicolaou stain help. These mononuclear cells resemble aging neutrophils and may be difficult to distinguish from renal epithelial cells. They are generally larger than neutrophils and have an indented, round, or oval nucleus and abundant (often vacuolated, sometimes foamy or frayed) cytoplasm.

Macrophages may be seen with ingested fat, hemosiderin, red cells, or crystals in the cytoplasm. Several macrophages are seen in Figs. 6-33 through 6-36 from a patient with mitral atresia. The urine contained a large quantity of protein (3+ SSA) and many casts.

Histiocytes may be multinucleated. These large cells are associated with chronic inflammation and with radiation therapy.

■ EPITHELIAL CELLS

Epithelial cells are the type of cells that line all of the urinary and genital tracts. Except for the tubules of the nephron, the structures of the urinary tract consist of multiple layers of epithelial cells. The layer of cells closest to the lumen throughout the urinary system,

but especially the urethra and bladder wall, are continually sloughed off (**exfoliated**) into the urine. They are replaced by cells that originate in deeper layers. A few of these cells are seen in most urine specimens. Although they consist of only a single layer of cells, epithelial cells from the nephron are also sloughed into the urine. However, only very few renal epithelial cells are normally seen in the sediment.

The epithelial cells seen in the urine sediment are of three different types: **squamous, transitional** (**urothelial**), and **renal**. Identification may be difficult but is clinically significant.

Squamous Epithelial Cells

Squamous epithelial cells line the female urethra and trigone and distal portion of the male urethra. They also line the vagina, and large numbers often rep-

Figure 6-32

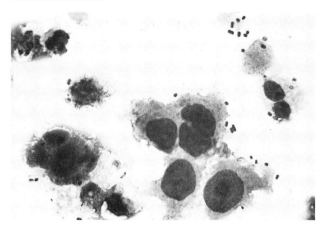

Mononuclear cells, possibly lymphocytes. Cytospin, Wright's stain, ×1000.

Figure 6-33

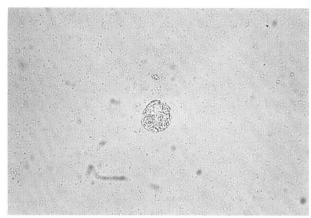

Macrophage. Unstained, ×400.

Figure 6-34

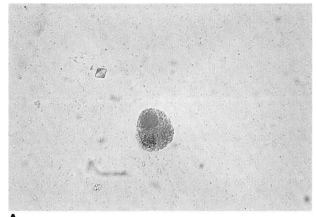

A

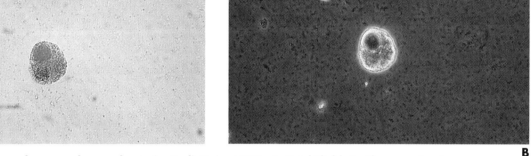

B

Macrophage, and many bacteria. Sedi-Stain, ×400. **A**, Brightfield. **B**, Phase contrast.

Figure 6-35

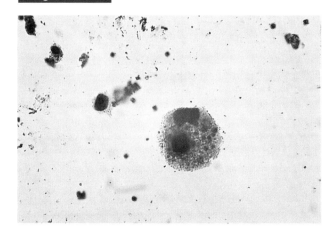

Macrophage. Cytospin, Wright's stain, ×400.

Figure 6-36

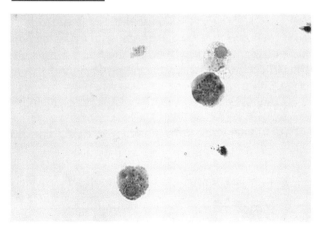

Macrophages. Cytospin, Papanicolaou stain, ×400.

Figure 6-37

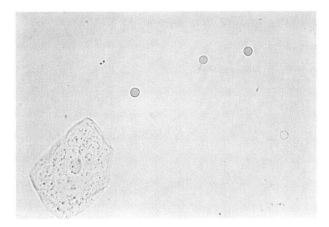

Squamous epithelial cell and red cells. Unstained, ×400.

Figure 6-38

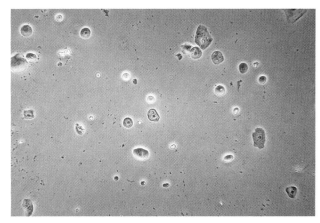

Several squamous epithelial cells under low-power magnification. Phase contrast, ×100.

Figure 6-39

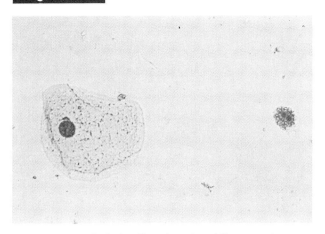

Squamous epithelial cell and eosinophil. Cytospin, Wright's stain, ×400.

Figure 6-40

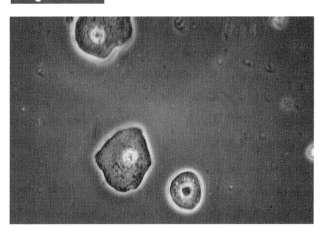

Two squamous epithelial cells and one transitional epithelial cell. Phase contrast, ×400.

resent vaginal or perineal contamination in urine collected from females or foreskin contamination in urine from males. A few squamous epithelial cells are seen in most urine specimens and are useful as a tool to obtain microscopic focus in a basically normal or negative urine sediment. Their presence has little clinical significance and usually represents contamination.

Squamous epithelial cells are large, flat cells about 30 to 50 μm in diameter, with a single distinct nucleus about the size of a lymphocyte or red cell (Fig. 6-37). The cell may be rectangular or round, and the edges may be curled. They are large enough to be seen easily under low-power (10× objective) magnification and are usually searched for and enumerated as few, moderate, or many at this magnification (Fig. 6-38). When stained with Sternheimer-Malbin stain, the cytoplasm is light purple or blue with a dark shade of orange-purple nucleus. They are easily recognized with brightfield (Fig. 6-39) and phase microscopy (Fig. 6-40), both unstained and

stained, but may eventually degenerate into an amorphous mass. They sometimes roll into a cigar shape, which should not be mistaken for casts (Fig. 6-41).

Clue Cell. This is a special type of squamous epithelial cell of vaginal origin that may be seen in the urine sediment. They are usually searched for in wet mounts of vaginal swabs. **Clue cells** are squamous epithelial cells covered (encrusted) with a coccobacilli, *Gardnerella vaginalis*, and indicate bacterial vaginitis caused by Gardnerella. The bacterium coating the cells gives the cytoplasm a characteristic refractile, stippled, or granular appearance with shaggy or bearded cell borders. To be reported as a clue cell, most (but not all) of the cell surface should be covered with bacteria, and the bacteria should be seen to extend past the cytoplasmic margins (Figs. 6-42-45). Squamous epithelial cells may have occasional irregular keratohyaline granules in the cytoplasm that should not be mistaken for adherent bacteria.

Figure 6-41

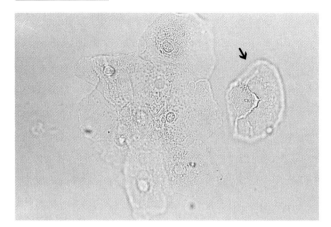

Several degenerating squamous epithelial cells with one folded cell (*arrow*) like a possible cast. Unstained, ×400.

Figure 6-42

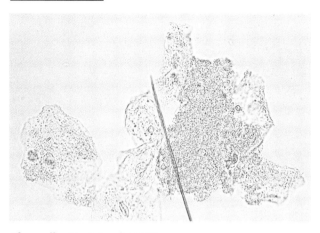

Clue cells. Unstained, ×400.

Figure 6-43

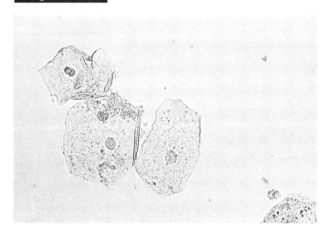

Squamous epithelial cells, with one beginning to appear as a clue cell. Sedi-Stain, ×400.

Figure 6-44

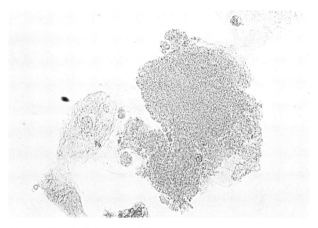

Clue cells. Sedi-Stain, ×400.

Transitional Epithelial (Urothelial) Cells

Transitional epithelial cells, also referred to as **urothelial** cells, form a stratified epithelial lining of the urinary tract from the pelvis of the kidney to the base of the bladder (trigone) in females and the proximal part of the urethra in males. Cells from the most superficial layer (especially of the bladder) resemble squamous epithelial cells. As the cell layers become deeper or cells originate in sites closer to the kidney, they become thicker and rounder, eventually becoming very difficult to distinguish from the renal epithelium of the kidney tubules or from white cells.

Transitional epithelial cells are generally about four to six times the size of a red blood cell (20 to 30 μm) and are spherical or polyhedral in shape with a relatively large, distinct round or oval nucleus located centrally or slightly off center. Since transitional epithelial cells readily take on water, these cells lining the lumen of the urinary tract are in direct contact with urine,

Figure 6-45

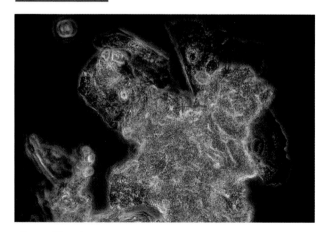

Clue cells. Phase contrast, ×400.

Figure 6-46

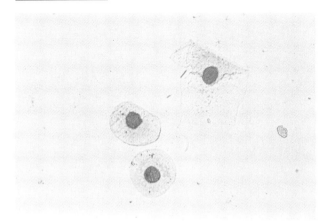

Two transitional epithelial cells, one folded squamous epithelial cell. Cytospin, Wright's stain, ×400.

Figure 6-47

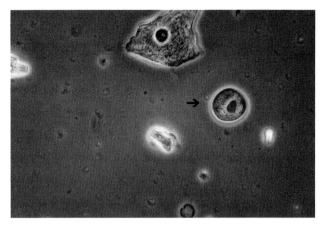

Transitional epithelial cell (*arrow*) and squamous epithelial cell. Phase contrast, ×400.

Figure 6-48

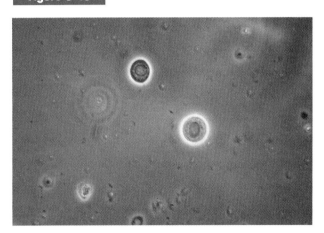

Two medium-sized transitional epithelial cells. Phase contrast, ×400.

Figure 6-49

Cluster of small unstained transitional epithelial cells, ×400.

and are observably spherical from swelling, like a balloon of water. The nucleus is about the same size as in a squamous epithelial cell, roughly the size of a lymphocyte or red cell. Binucleated cells also may be seen. When stained with a Sternheimer-Malbin stain, the nucleus is blue purple, and the cytoplasm light purple. The cytoplasm may be vacuolated and may have inclusions. Some transitional cells have tails of cytoplasm and are referred to as **caudate cells**. These originate from the renal pelvis or the bladder trigone and are not significantly diagnostic.

Transitional epithelial cells ranging from large round cells (almost squamous), to medium-sized cells, to smaller forms (almost renal) and caudate are seen in Figs. 6-46 through 6-50.

The urine of normal persons contains a few transitional epithelial cells. They may occur singly, in pairs, or in small groups. Numbers are increased in infections, where they are seen together with neutrophils.

Figure 6-50

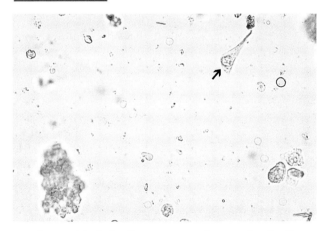

Caudate epithelial cell (*arrow*), and several red cells. Unstained ×400.

Figure 6-51

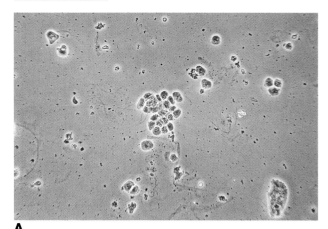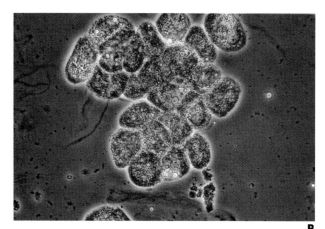

A   B

Cluster of transitional epithelial cells showing changes caused by virus or drugs.
A, Phase contrast, ×100. B, Same grouping of cells as in A at higher magnification.
Phase contrast, ×400.

Figure 6-52

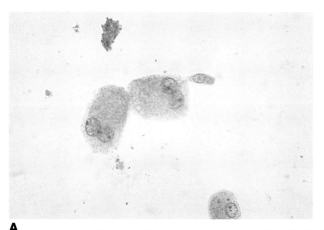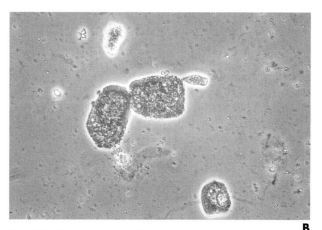

A   B

Unusual binucleated transitional epithelial cells with changes caused by virus or
drugs. Sedi-stain, ×400. A, Brightfield. B, Same field as A with phase contrast.

The cells shown in Figs. 6-51 and 6-52 show unusual multinucleated and vacuolated forms of transitional epithelial cells with changes caused by drugs or infection from a patient with viral associated hemophagocytic syndrome.

Clusters or sheets of transitional epithelial cells may be seen after catheterization or bladder washings (Fig. 6-53). The cells in this example are unusually small because the patient was a 1-month-old infant.

Urothelial cells may also be seen with neoplasms and should be referred for cytologic examination when large numbers with nuclear irregularities are observed. After radiation therapy, extremely large transitional cells with multiple nuclei and vacuoles may be seen (Fig. 6-54).

Renal Epithelial Cells

The nephron from the proximal to the distal convoluted tubules, plus the small and large collecting ducts, are lined with a layer of renal epithelial cells. Although a few **renal epithelial cells** (also called **renal tubular epithelium** or **RTE**) may be found in normal urine specimens, increased numbers are significant. According to Schumann, "The presence of more than 15 renal tubular epithelial cells per 10 high power fields (430×) provides strong evidence of active renal disease or tubular injury."[9] They are the most clinically important of the epithelial cells that may be found in urine and result from a variety of renal disorders, especially acute tubular necrosis, viral infections involving the kidney, and in renal transplant rejection.

Figure 6-53

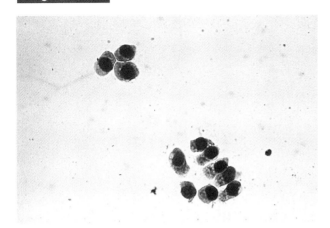

Many small transitional epithelial cells after catheterization of 1-month-old infant. Sedi-Stain, ×400.

Figure 6-54

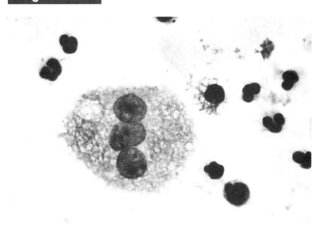

Multinucleated and vacuolated transitional epithelial cell as seen after radiation therapy. Cytospin, Wright's stain, ×1000.

The rate of renal exfoliation is increased with fever, chemical toxins, inflammation, infections, and neoplasms.

Renal epithelial cells are difficult to identify in wet preparations with both brightfield and phase microscopy. Supravital staining may be helpful, and cytocentrifugation and staining with Wright's stain and especially Papanicolaou stain is most useful. Renal epithelial cells resemble leukocytes (especially degenerating neutrophils with rounded nuclei), other mononuclear leukocytes such as histiocytes and monocytes, and small transitional epithelial cells. The presence of other findings in the urinalysis, such as protein, casts (epithelial, cellular, or granular), and dysmorphic red cells, is useful.

Morphology also depends on the actual site of origin within the kidney. Renal cells are typically polyhedral in shape and elongated or ovoid with granular cytoplasm. Size varies, but renal cells are generally from three to five times the size of a red cell or slightly larger to twice as large as a neutrophil—about the same size as smaller transitional epithelial cells. There is usually a single distinct round nucleus, which may be eccentric. Renal cells do not absorb water and swell as do transitional cells; therefore they tend to retain their polyhedral shape, unlike transitional cells, which tend to be round. The observation of at least one flattened side is helpful, if not diagnostic (Figs. 6-55 and 6-56). When stained with a Sternheimer Malbin stain, the nucleus stains a dark shade of blue-purple and cytoplasm a light shade of blue-purple.

Cells originating from the proximal and distal convoluted tubules are relatively large and elongated or oval with a granular cytoplasm and relatively small, dense nuclei. They are associated with acute tubular necrosis and drug or heavy metal toxicity. Proximal tubular cells contain a microvillus border that may be

Figure 6-55

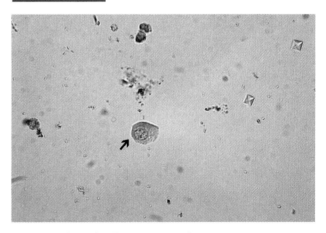

Renal epithelial cell (*arrow*). Sedi-Stain, ×400.

visible microscopically. The granularity makes the proximal tubular cells, in particular, appear as small or fragmented granular casts (Figs. 6-57 and 6-58).

Cytocentrifugation and staining with Wright's or Papanicoulaou stain is especially helpful in visualizing these structures as cells rather than casts, as shown in Figs. 6-59 and 6-60.

The most commonly seen renal epithelial cells probably originate from the small collecting ducts or tubules. These are seen as cuboidal or polyhedral-shaped cells as seen in Fig. 6-61, which are difficult to distinguish from small transitional epithelial cells originating in the bladder.

Columnar cell forms originating from the large collecting ducts also may be seen.

Polyhedral or columnar epithelial cells originating in glands that empty into the urethra such as the prostate gland, seminal vesicle, and paraurethral

Figure 6-56

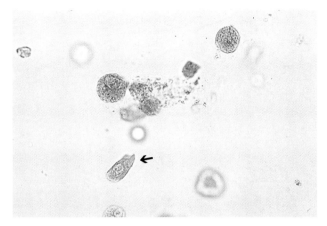

Renal epithelial cell (*arrow*). Sedi-Stain, ×400.

Figure 6-57

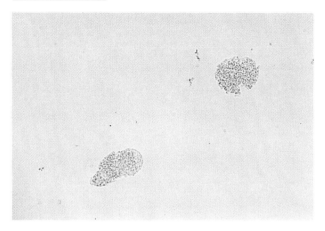

Two unstained proximal renal tubular epithelial cells appearing like granular casts. Unstained, ×400.

Figure 6-58

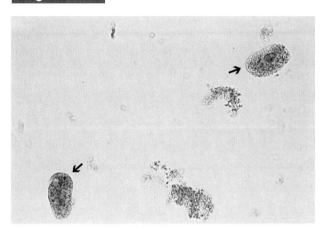

Stained proximal renal tubular epithelial cells (*arrows*) appearing like granular casts. Sedi-Stain, ×400.

Figure 6-59

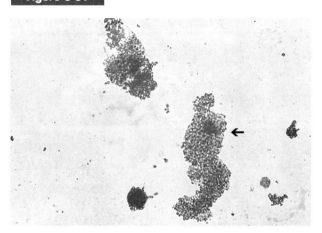

Cytocentrifuged preparation of proximal renal tubular epithelial cells appearing like granular casts (*arrow*). Cytospin, Wright's stain, ×400.

Figure 6-60

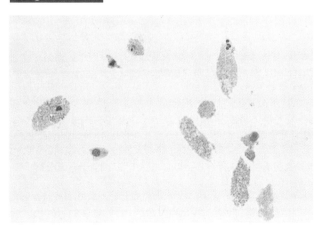

Cytocentrifuged preparation of proximal renal tubular epithelial cells appearing like granular casts. Cytospin, Papanicolaou stain, ×400.

Figure 6-61

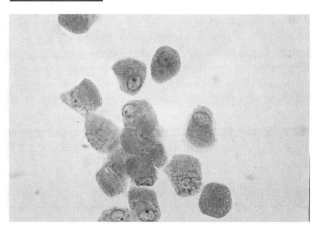

Cuboidal or polyhedral renal tubular epithelial cells probably from the small collecting ducts; very difficult to differentiate from transitional epithelial cells. Sedi-Stain, ×400.

Figure 6-62

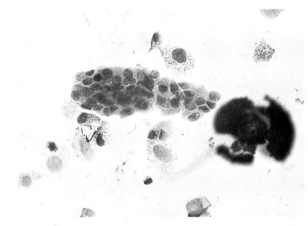

Renal epithelial fragment; much like a renal epithelial cell cast but without a visable protein matrix, in a cytocentrifuged urine sediment. Cytospin, Papanicolaou stain, ×400.

Figure 6-63

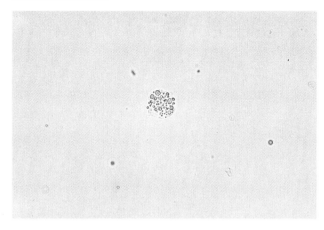

Oval fat body and free fat. Unstained, ×400.

Figure 6-64

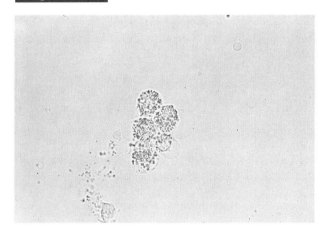

Oval fat bodies, small cluster. Unstained, ×400.

Figure 6-65

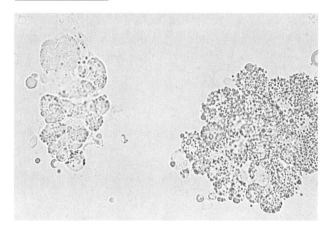

Many oval fat bodies, in clumps. Unstained, ×400.

glands may be present and difficult or impossible to distinguish from renal epithelial cells. Urine containing fecal material (such as from a fistula between the bowel and bladder) or from bladders surgically formed from the ileum (ileal bladder) may contain columnar epithelial cells.

Renal Epithelial Fragments. Fragments of renal epithelial cells originating from the collecting ducts (but not the proximal or distal tubules) have been described. A **renal epithelial fragment** may be defined as three or more renal cells of collecting duct origin[7] (Fig. 6-62). The presence of renal fragments is more serious than single renal epithelial cells and indicates renal tubular injury with disruption of the basement membrane.

Oval Fat Bodies and Fat Globules. The presence of fat of biologic origin in urine is called **lipiduria** and is an important pathologic finding indicating severe renal

dysfunction. It is associated with the nephrotic syndrome, advanced diabetes mellitus, lupus, and conditions that result in severe damage of renal tubular epithelial cells due to ethylene glycol or mercury poisoning. The **nephrotic syndrome** is a clinical syndrome that is generally the result of excessive permeability of the glomerulus to plasma protein and is seen as massive proteinuria and lipiduria. The loss of protein (albumin) into the urine results in hypoalbuminemia or decreased blood albumin, and hyperlipidemia or increased blood lipids (as cholesterol). The liver responds to low serum albumin resulting in low oncotic pressure with increased liver synthesis of albumin. This causes increased synthesis of lipoproteins. The overall clinical result is generalized edema (or swelling in all of the body tissues) resulting from the fall in oncotic pressure and low intravascular volume from loss of albumin

Figure 6-66

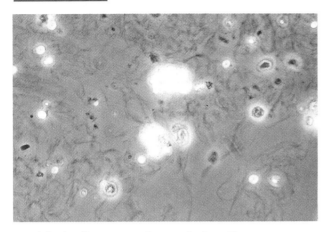

Oval fat bodies, somewhat confusing. Phase contrast, ×400.

Figure 6-67

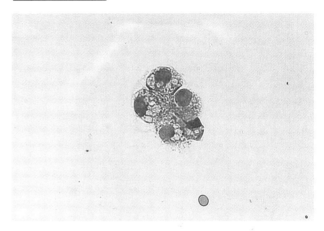

Oval fat bodies, cytocentrifuged and stained with a quick Wright's stain showing cell nucleus and vacuoles where fat was present, ×400.

Figure 6-68

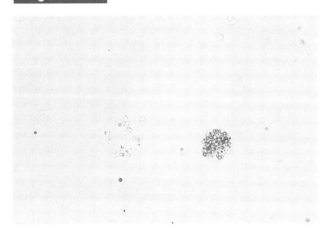

Oval fat body, and free fat. Sudan III stain, ×400.

Figure 6-69

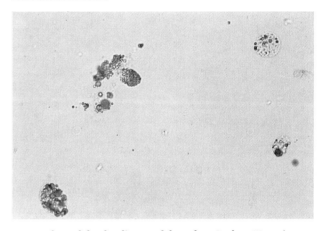

Several oval fat bodies and free fat. Sudan III stain, ×400,

and subsequent sodium retention. The lipiduria (urinary fat) may be in the form of cholesterol or triglyceride (neutral fat) and seen in the urine sediment as free fat globules, fat within cells, or fat within casts.

Oval fat bodies are renal epithelial cells filled with fat (lipid) droplets. They are also sometimes referred to as **renal tubular fat (RTF)** or **renal tubular fat bodies**. The fat droplets are probably contained within degenerating or necrotic renal epithelial cells, although the lipid-containing cells may be macrophages or histiocytes. The fat droplets within the oval fat body are very refractile droplets that vary in size (Figs. 6-63, 6-64, and 6-65). They are probably more easily recognized with brightfield rather than phase contrast microscopy (Fig. 6-66), and if suspected, the specimen should be viewed with brightfield illumination.

Although the oval fat body is considered to be a cell filled with fat, the cell nucleus is barely visible in wet

preparations. It is more likely to be visualized in cytocentrifuged stained preparations (Fig. 6-67).

When wet preparations are stained with a Sternheimer-Malbin stain, the fat globules do not become colored but appear highly refractile in a blue purple matrix.

Special fat stains such as Sudan stains (Sudan III) or oil red O are useful in the identification of triglycerides or neutral fat, which stain orange or red in wet preparations (Figs. 6-68, 6-69, and 6-70).

Failure to stain with fat stains does not rule out the presence of fat or lipid globules. If cholesterol esters are present in the fat globules, they may be visualized with polarized light. In the case of cholesterol, a typical Maltese cross pattern (white cross on a black background) is seen when the specimen is viewed with crossed polarizing filters. It may also be viewed with compensated polarized light by the addition of a

Figure 6-70

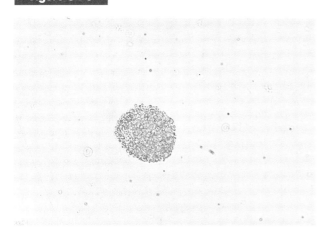

Large fat-filled oval fat body weakly stained with Sudan III, ×400.

Figure 6-71

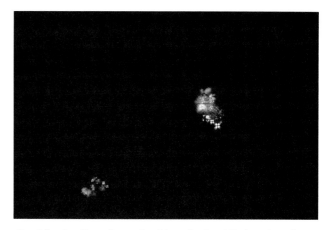

Oval fat bodies viewed with polarized light, showing Maltese cross formation, ×400.

Figure 6-72

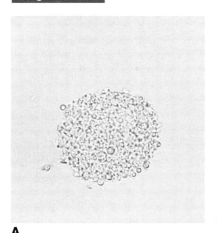
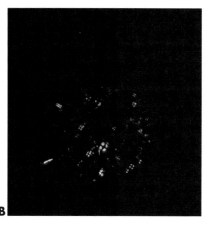
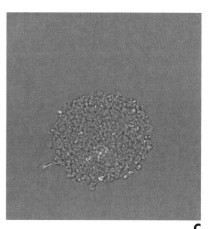

A   B   C

Large fat-filled oval fat body unstained and with polarized and compensated polarized light showing the presence of cholesterol esters that polarize as a Maltese cross, ×640. A, Brightfield. B, Polarized light. C, Compensated polarized light.

full-wave compensator (first order red filter) (Figs. 6-71, 6-72, A, B, and C).

Polarized light should not be used exclusively to determine the presence or absence of fat or oval fat bodies in urine. Many small crystals will also polarize light and may be confusing. Urine contaminated with starch will give the same Maltese cross pattern with polarized and compensated polarized light. These "beach balls" seen with compensated polarized light should not be confused with starch—a common, ubiquitous contaminant in laboratory specimens most easily appreciated with brightfield illumination (see Fig. 6-235, A, B, C).

When the urine sediment is cytocentrifuged and stained with Wright's stain, the fat is dissolved from the cells and/or casts within which it was contained. The remaining structures show holes or vacuoles where the fat was present.

Oval fat bodies are rarely seen by themselves in the urine sediment. They are associated with the presence of free globules or droplets of fat and fatty casts (further described under casts). As renal tubular epithelial cells undergo degeneration, lipid droplets may be seen in the cytoplasm. This fatty degeneration may take place in stored urine specimens, such as those retained for teaching students and staff.

Fat globules are clinically significant when of biologic origin, being equivalent to oval fat bodies and fatty casts. They are seen as highly refractile globules of various sizes (Figs. 6-73, 6-74, A, B, C).

Like fat contained within cells and casts, fat globules may be identified with fat stains such as Sudan III or oil red O, and polarized microscopy. The globules may be made up of cholesterol esters or triglycerides.

Unfortunately, fat globules may be seen in the urine because of contamination with extraneous sources

Figure 6-73

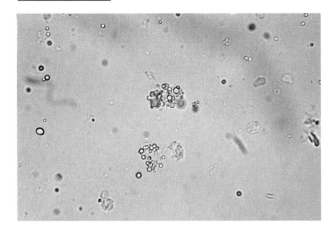

Free fat and oval fat bodies. Unstained, ×400.

Figure 6-74

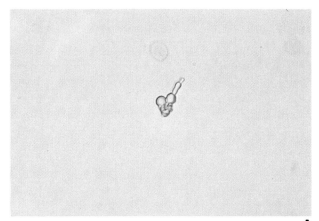

A

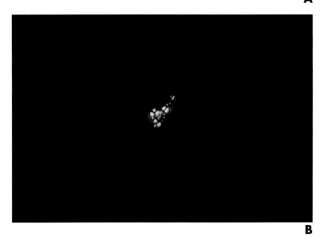

B

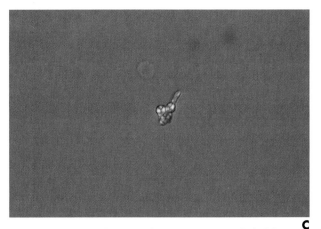

C

Large unstained fat globule, ×640. A, Brightfield.
B, Polarized light. C, Compensated polarized light.

such as unclean collection utensils, oiled catheters, and vaginal creams (see Fig. 6-241 and 6-242). These globules may be difficult to distinguish from fat globules of biologic origin; however, the presence of oval fat bodies and fatty casts, together with chemical findings such as large quantities of protein (albumin) in the urine, implies significant lipiduria. See also the section on Contaminants and Artifacts.

Fat globules may be identified microscopically from either the surface of a centrifuged urine or the concentrated sediment. Since the density of fat is less than water, the globules may float and be discovered by removing a drop from the surface of the centrifuged urine before it is decanted for the usual urinary sediment concentration. This should be examined microscopically, along with the usual sediment examination when the discovery of lipiduria is desired clinically.

Hemosiderin Inclusions. Renal epithelial cells containing granules of hemosiderin occasionally may be seen in the urinary sediment. Hemosiderin is a form of iron, formed by renal tubular epithelial cells from hemoglobin present in the renal tubules. The presence of hemosiderin in the urine sediment 2 to 3 days after an acute hemolytic episode indicates severe intravascular hemolysis. It is commonly seen in paroxysmal nocturnal hemoglobinuria and may be seen as the result of hemochromatosis.

Hemosiderin granules appear as coarse yellow-brown granules that are morphologically similar to **amorphous** urates in wet preparations. The color is similar to hemoglobin, to which it is related. Unlike urates, hemosiderin will stain blue with a Prussian blue stain for iron. This may be done as a wet staining procedure referred to as **Rous Test**[5] (Procedure 6-1). As an alternative, the specimen may be cytocentrifuged and stained for iron with a Prussian blue stain used for blood films.

ROUS TEST FOR HEMOSIDERIN IN URINE

Reagents:

Potassium ferrocyanide, 2% solution
> Dilute 10 g potassium ferrocyanide to 500 mL
> with deionized or distilled water.

Hydrochloric acid, 1% solution
> Add 5 mL of concentrated HCl to 500 mL
> deionized or distilled water.

Working Reagent
> Immediately before using, combine 5 mL of 2%
> potassium ferrocyanide and 5 mL of 1% HCl.

Procedure:

1. Centrifuge 12 mL of urine (preferably first-morning specimen) at 400 to 450 rpm for 5 minutes. Decant the supernatant. Examine a drop of the concentrated sediment microscopically for yellow brown granules, especially within renal tubular epithelial cells or casts.

2. Suspend the remaining sediment in the freshly prepared working reagent and allow to stand for 10 minutes.

3. Centrifuge and decant the supernatant. Examine the concentrated sediment microscopically for the presence of blue granules of hemosiderin. These may be free granules or granules seen within renal epithelial cells, macrophages, or casts.

4. If unstained granules are seen, reexamine after 30 minutes to rule out a delayed reaction.

5. Report as positive or negative for hemosiderin.

Figure 6-75

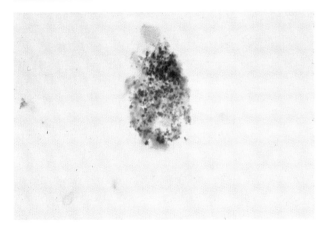

Hemosiderin containing cell, showing a positive Rous Test. Prussian blue stain for iron, ×400.

Figure 6-76

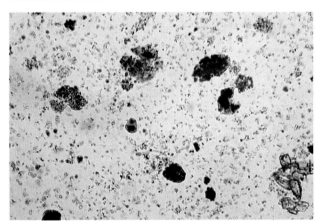

Many cells and granules showing a positive Rous Test for hemosiderin. Prussian blue stain, ×400.

Granules of hemosiderin may be seen within renal tubular epithelial cells, macrophages, casts, or as free amorphous granules in the urine (Figs. 6-75 and 6-76). (See also Figs. 6-171, 6-172, 6-173, under Hemosiderin Casts and 6-224 and 6-225 under Crystals.)

Inclusion Bodies. In cases of viral infections such as rubella and herpes, renal epithelial cells may contain **inclusion bodies**. With cytomegalovirus, especially large intranuclear inclusions may be seen. In cases of lead poisoning, cytoplasmic inclusions may be seen. All of these inclusions are difficult to visualize in wet preparations (Fig. 6-77), but cytocentrifugation and staining, especially with Papanicolaou stain, is helpful (Fig. 6-78).

Tumor Cells

A description of the various tumor or altered cell forms that may occur in urine is beyond this text although they may occur in urine specimens. Diagnosis requires special cytologic techniques of collection and preparation with examination by qualified cytologists. However, the microscopist examining the urinary sediment should be aware of possible irregularities and refer the specimen accordingly. The presence of red cells in the chemical examination of the urine is an early diagnostic clue.

Figure 6-77

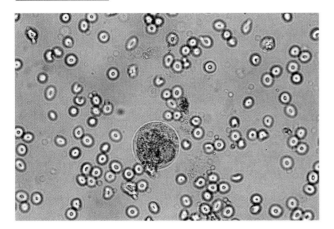

Inclusion bodies in macrophage or epithelial cell.
Sedi-Stain, ×400.

Figure 6-78

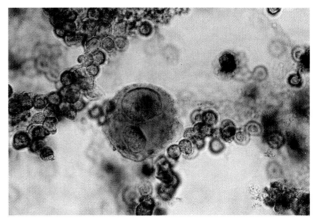

Inclusion bodies in cytocentrifuged urine sediment.
Papanicolaou stain, ×1000.

OTHER CELLULAR COMPONENTS

Spermatozoa

Spermatozoa may be present in the urine of both males and females. It should be recognized by the microscopist when present but is not routinely reported in some laboratories. The presence of spermatozoa may be an important finding in fertility studies and cases of possible sexual abuse. Individual laboratory protocol should be established and followed. See also the section on Semen Analysis.

Spermatozoa are fairly easily recognized by their oval body (head) and long delicate tail. The sperm head is about 4 to 6 μm long—smaller and narrower than a red cell—and the tail is about 40 to 60 μm long (Figs. 6-79 and 6-80).

Spermatozoa may be motile in wet preparations, an aid to identification. Phase contrast microscopy is especially helpful (Fig. 6-81). Identification is more difficult if the tail is separated from the head.

Bacteria

The urinary tract is normally sterile or free of bacteria. However, most urine specimens contain a few bacteria as a result of contamination from the vagina or urethra (**perineal contamination**) as the specimen is voided. If the specimen is allowed to stand for a period of time at room temperature before analysis, bacteria will rapidly multiply and be apparent in the urine sediment. If the specimen is collected in a manner suitable for urine culture, stored, and examined in a timely manner, the presence of bacteria may indicate a urinary tract infection. Other indicators of actual

Figure 6-79

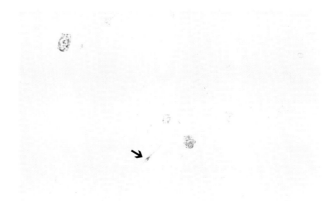

Sperm (*arrow*). Sedi-Stain, ×400.

Figure 6-80

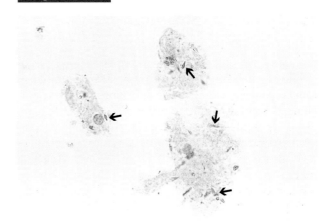

Sperm (*arrows*), trapped in mucus. Sedi-Stain, ×400.

Figure 6-81

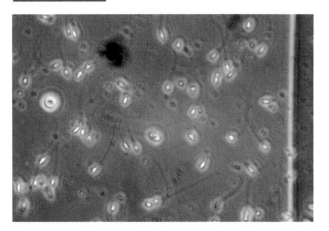

Sperm, many in counting chamber. Phase contrast, ×400.

Figure 6-82

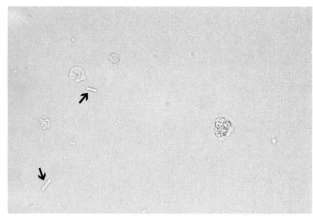

Rod-shaped bacteria (*arrows*), white cells and red cell also present. Unstained, ×640.

Figure 6-83

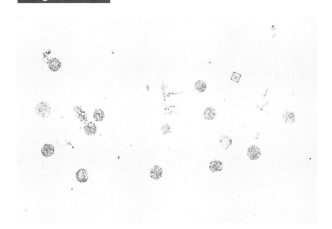

Several rod-shaped bacteria, some in clumps, white cells, and calcium oxalate crystal. Sedi-Stain, ×400.

Figure 6-84

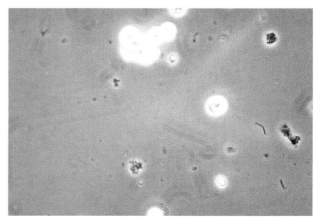

Rod-shaped bacteria and white cells. Phase contrast, ×400.

infections include the presence of white cells (neutrophils), leukocyte esterase, nitrite, and protein. Infection should be confirmed by quantitative urine culture.

Although extremely small (only a few millimeters long), bacteria are recognizable morphologically in wet preparations under high-power (Figs. 6-82 and 6-83). The use of phase contrast microscopy is extremely helpful (Fig. 6-84). They may occur as rods or cocci either singly or in chains—rods are more easily visualized, especially when motile. Most infections are from medium-sized gram negative enteric organisms of fecal origin such as *E. coli* or *Proteus* species.

Some infecting organisms are extremely small and difficult to distinguish from cocci in wet preparations (Fig. 6-85).

Occasionally, unusually long rod-shaped forms with central swelling are seen. These **protoplasts** are the result of damage to the cell wall by antibiotics (especially penicillins) used in therapy (Figs. 6-86, 6-87, and 6-88).

Gram-positive lactobacilli from vaginal or fecal contamination appear as large rods longer than the usual infecting organisms.

Cocci as infecting organisms may pose a problem in identification. Smaller forms such as *enterococci* may be difficult to visualize, or the short chains mistaken for rods (Fig. 6-89). Large, refractile coccal forms such as staphylococci may be mistaken for crystals (Fig. 6-90, A and B).

Although not normally part of urinalysis, Gram staining a drop of concentrated sediment is helpful in recognition of bacteria in difficult specimens. Fig. 6-91 shows

Figure 6-85

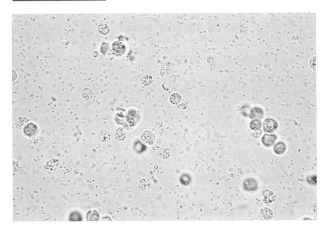

Many small rod-shaped bacteria appearing like possible cocci and white cells. Unstained ×400.

Figure 6-86

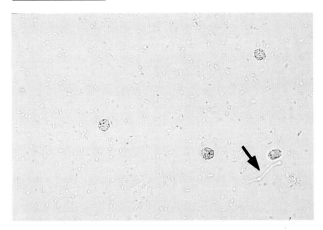

Proplast (*arrow*), many rod-shaped bacteria and four white cells. Unstained, ×400.

Figure 6-87

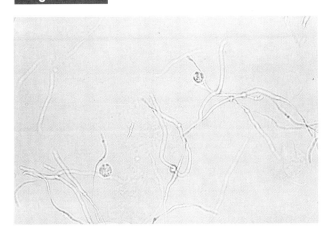

Protoplasts (many long thread-like forms), and white cells. Unstained, ×400.

Figure 6-88

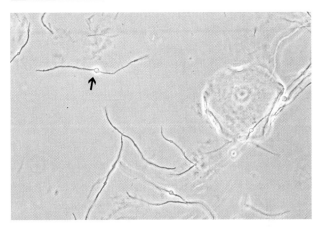

Many protophasts (*one at arrow*), and a squamous epithelial cell. Phase contrast, ×400.

a Gram stain of Gram-positive (purple) staphylococci from the same specimen as shown in Fig. 6-90. It should be remembered that all bacteria, both gram positive and gram negative, will appear purple in a Wright's stained cytocentrifuged specimen. This is illustrated by the Gram negative but purple-appearing rods in Fig. 6-92.

When a urinary tract infection (UTI) is present, it is important for the clinician to differentiate a lower (bladder) from an upper (kidney) infection. The presence of white cells (neutrophils), leukocyte esterase, and nitrite may be seen with both lower and upper urinary tract infections. The absence of any or all of these findings does not rule out infection. Proteinuria is associated with all infections; mild (trace to 1+) with lower UTIs and a larger degree (moderate) with upper UTIs. The presence of casts, which may be cellular, white cell, granular, or bacterial, places the infection within the kidney.

Figure 6-89

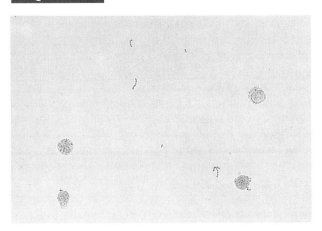

Bacteria, short chains of enterococci, and white cells. Sedi-Stain, ×400.

Figure 6-90

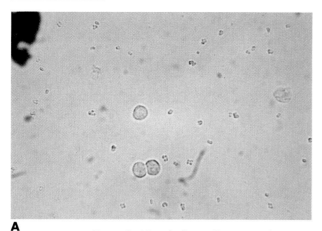
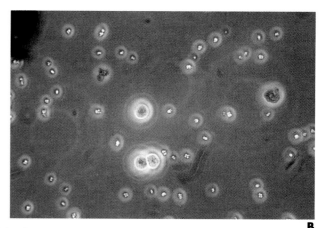

A

B

Bacteria (Staphylococci) seen as large cocci in clusters and tetrads appearing like small crystals with phase contrast. White cells also present. **A,** Brightfield, ×450. **B,** Same field as A with phase contrast, showing how these cocci might be mistaken for small crystals, ×400.

Figure 6-91

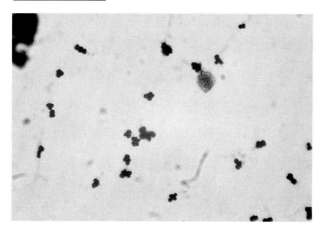

Gram-positive Staphylococci, on Gram stain of concentrated sediment, ×1000.

Figure 6-92

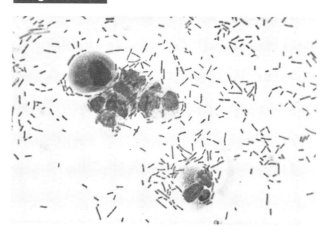

White cells and purple-staining gram-negative bacteria (rods) on cytocentrifuged preparation of urine sediment stained with Wright's stain, ×1000.

Yeast

Yeast are most often present in urine as *Candida* species. They may be the result of vaginal contamination with vaginal yeast infections and are often the result of contamination from skin and air. They are also associated with the presence of sugar in urine, and seen in specimens from diabetic patients with yeast infections, because sugar is utilized as an energy source for the growth of yeast cells. They may be seen in the urine of immunosuppressed patients who have true kidney infections caused by yeast, especially *Candida* species, and are associated with the presence of pseudohyphae in such cases.

Yeast have a typically ovoid shape, are colorless, and have a smooth, refractile appearance. They may

be mistaken for red cells, but are generally smaller (5 to 7 μm) and have a relatively thick cell wall and exhibit considerable variation in size. The presence of a single bud is especially helpful in differentiation from red cells. They are relatively easy to visualize with brightfield microscopy in wet preparations and phase contrast is helpful (Figs. 6-93 and 6-94).

Supravital staining is not always helpful as yeast may or may not stain as in the case of red cells (Figs. 6-95 and 6-96). They are strongly gram positive, and Gram staining of a drop of concentrated sediment helps in difficult cases. Wright's staining of a cytocentrifuged preparation clearly differentiates yeast from red blood cells, as shown in Fig. 6-97.

Figure 6-93

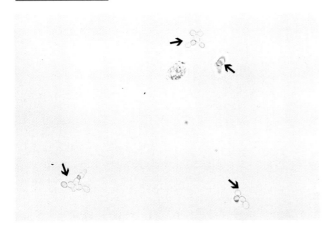

Typical budding yeast (*arrows*), and one white cell. Unstained, ×400.

Figure 6-94

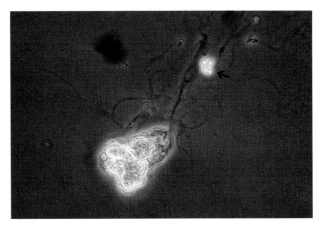

Budding yeast (*arrow*), white cells (in clumps), and mucus. Phase contrast, ×400.

Figure 6-95

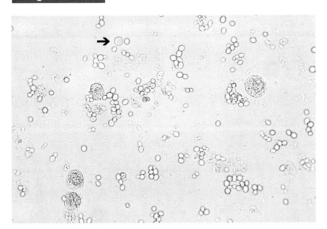

Many slightly stained yeast, white cells (4), and red cell (*arrow*). Sedi-Stain, ×400.

Figure 6-96

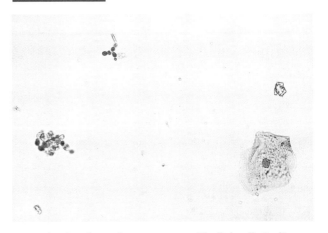

Yeast (stained), and squamous epithelial cell. Sedi-Stain, ×400.

Elongated cells, which may be up to 50 µm long and resemble mycelia, may be seen. These are **pseudohyphae** and may be branched and have terminal buds (Figs. 6-98 and 6-99). They are clinically significant in the urine from debilitated patients with severe *Candida* infections such as seen in immunosuppressed patients.

Other mycelial forms of yeast have been seen that should not be mistaken for casts (Figs. 6-100, *A* and *B*).

Trichomonas

The parasite most often seen in urine specimens is *Trichomonas vaginalis*. This protozoan is primarily responsible for vaginal infections; however, it also may infect the urethra, periurethral glands, bladder, and prostate. If present, it normally resides in the vagina in women and the prostate in men. It feeds on the mucos-

Figure 6-97

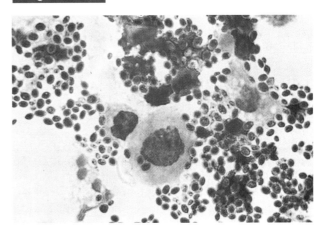

Yeast and white cells in cytocentrifuged preparation, of the same specimen as Fig. 6-95. Wright's stain, ×1000.

Figure 6-98

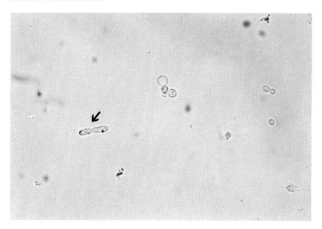

Yeast, normal budding and pseudohyphae (*arrow*). Unstained, ×400.

Figure 6-99

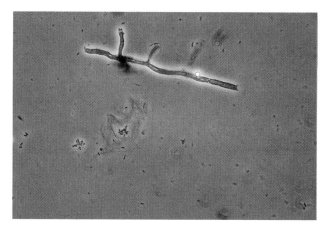

Large pseudohyphae (**Candida** sp.), and bacteria. Phase contrast, ×400.

Figure 6-100

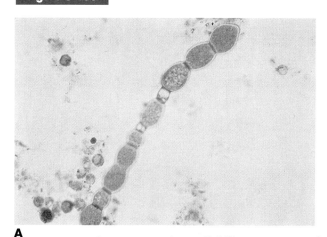

A

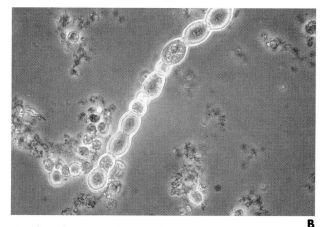

B

Large unusual mycelial-like yeast not to be mistaken for casts. Sedi-Stain, ×400.
A, Brightfield. B, Same field as A with phase contrast.

al surface and ingests bacteria and leukocytes that may be present. Wet preparations of direct swabs from the vagina or urethra are usually examined for *T. vaginalis* infections, although the organisms may be seen contaminating the urine sediment.

Trichomonads are usually searched for in wet preparations because their most distinguishing feature is motility. They show a rapid, jerky, rotating, nondirectional motion and are often first noticed by the microscopist when they move. *T. vaginalis* is a flagellated protozoan. It is usually pear-shaped and up to 30 µm long—about the size of large white cells or transitional epithelial cells, both of which it resembles, especially when no longer motile. The organism has a single nucleus, four anterior flagella, an anterior undulating membrane, and sharp protruding posterior axostyle (Figs. 6-101 and 6-102).

The flagella are most easily seen with phase contrast microscopy, and phase is most helpful in the discovery of these organisms (Fig. 6-103).

Dead cells are very difficult to identify. The addition of supravital stain tends to destroy motility and cause the cells to round-up and appear very similar to degenerating transitional epithelial cell forms (Fig. 6-104).

Observation of "rippling" of the undulating membrane is helpful and remains for several hours after the organism is no longer motile.

Other Parasites

The urine may contain a variety of parasites as the result of fecal or vaginal contamination. *Enterobius vermicularis*, or pinworm, a fairly common helminth

Figure 6-101

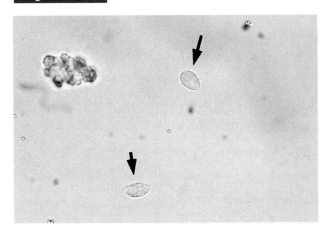

Trichomonas, pear shaped (*arrows*). Unstained, ×400.

Figure 6-102

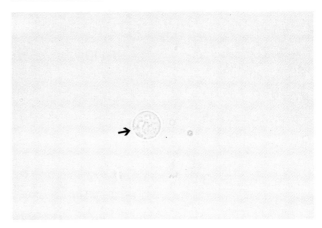

Trichomonas, rounded with very hard to see flagella (*arrow*). Unstained, ×640.

Figure 6-103

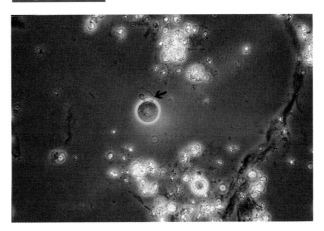

Trichomonas, rounded with flagella (*arrow*). Phase contrast, ×400.

Figure 6-104

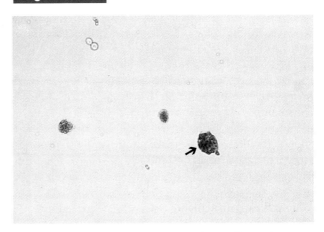

Presumed Trichomonas (*arrow*), white cells and yeast. Sedi-Stain, ×400.

infecting the intestinal tract, may occasionally be seen in the urine in larval or egg (ova) form.

Other parasites occasionally seen in urine include *Trichuris* or whipworm, *Schistosomes, Strongyloides,* and *Giardia* and various ameba. Various insects or "bugs" possibly seen in urine specimens include lice, fleas, bedbugs, mites, and ticks. All of these need special knowledge for identification; however, they may be noticed initially during urinalysis and then referred for identification. Infections also vary with different geographic regions and patient populations.

■ CASTS

Formation and Significance

The discovery of **casts** in the urine sediment is an extremely important finding. Casts are the result of solidification of protein within the lumen of the kidney tubules (nephron). As the name implies, this solidification results in a cast that was molded by the tubule. Cast formation may be the result of either precipitation of protein or conglutination (clumping together) of material within the tubular lumen. In either case, at the time of cast formation, any material present within the tubule (such as cells, fat, bacteria, or other inclusion) is trapped within the cast matrix and may be visualized in the urine sediment. In effect, this gives a biopsy of the renal tubule, and anything within the cast represents the condition within the nephron at the time the cast was formed.

The basic structure of any cast is a protein matrix. All casts have a matrix of Tamm-Horsfall mucoprotein; in addition, plasma proteins may or may not be present. Anything present within the renal tubule may adhere to or be enmeshed within the cast matrix as it forms. Although the high molecular weight Tamm-Horsfall glycoprotein is secreted by renal tubular cells, cast formation is associated with detectable proteinuria derived from plasma proteins, as described in Chapter 4. Other immunoproteins have been identified in certain casts, although they are not found in any given cast type or disease. Cast formation is enhanced by the presence of plasma proteins, an acid pH, and a sufficient concentration of solutes. For this reason, casts are not likely to be present in urine, which is dilute and alkaline and will disappear from a urine specimen improperly stored as the pH becomes alkaline.

Casts consisting of only precipitated Tamm-Horsfall protein are referred to as hyaline casts. A few hyaline casts may be seen in normal urine specimens, and increased numbers of hyaline casts may be seen with mild irritation of the kidney associated with dehydration or physical exercise. A few granular casts may also be seen in nonpathologic situations. However, the presence of other types of casts indicates a serious (pathologic) situation with renal involvement.

Identification and Morphology of Casts

The basic cast morphology is shown in Fig. 6-105.

As shown in this archetypal example, the cast is a cylindrical structure with rounded ends. Indeed, to be identified as a cast, the structure should have an even definite outline, parallel sides, and rounded ends. Size varies somewhat; however, the cast diameter should be uniform, and it should be several times longer than it is wide. This ideal shape is not always seen, since casts take on the shape of the tubule in which they are formed. Structures may be seen that are serpentine or convoluted and folded. One end may taper off into a tail or point. This has been referred to as a **cylindroid**, a term that has the same significance as a hyaline cast (cylindroids are generally hyaline). They are troublesome, since they may be mistaken for strands of mucus. Cylindroids should be enumerated and reported as a hyaline cast. Casts may also be fragmented or broken, a common finding with waxy casts that typically show blunt, not rounded, ends. Judgment is necessary when atypical forms are encountered; the whole specimen must be considered before a morphologic decision is made, including other sediment findings and results of the chemical screen. Casts are important pathologic structures that must be reported when present, but they should not be falsely identified or reported when they are absent.

Casts are difficult to visualize, especially with brightfield microscopy, because the refractive index of the protein matrix is nearly the same as that of glass. Correct light adjustment is essential. Casts are searched for and enumerated with the low-power

Figure 6-105

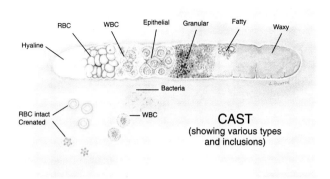

Archetypal cast (showing various types and inclusions). (From Linne JJ, Ringsrud KM: *Basic techniques in clinical laboratory science*, ed 3, St. Louis, 1992, Mosby.)

objective but identified with the high-power objective. Discovery and identification is greatly enhanced by phase or interference contrast microscopy. Phase contrast microscopy gives contrast between the cast and background fluid (urine), whereas interference contrast enhances the dimensionality of the cast so that shape and inclusions are better appreciated. The use of supravital stains such as a Sternheimer-Malbin stain (Sedi-Stain, KOVA stain) is also very useful, especially if only a brightfield microscope is available. Cells or other inclusions within the cast usually take on stain and enhance visualization. Cytocentrifugation may also be helpful in difficult cases.

Classification of Casts

Once it is determined that a cast is present, it must be named or classified so that it can be reported. This classification is not always easy, and many classification schemes exist. In the laboratory, classification is usually done on the basis of morphology, such as hyaline, granular, cellular, fatty, other inclusions, and waxy. A given urine specimen may contain more than one type of cast, and a particular cast may have mixed morphology, such as hyaline at one end, and red cell at the other. This mixed morphology is shown in the extreme in Fig. 6-105, where an all-inclusive cast showing a hyaline matrix, the various cellular cast types, granules, fatty inclusions, and waxy matrix are all shown in one cast.

As mentioned, casts may form as either the result of precipitation of protein or conglutination of material within the renal tubular lumen. In both cases, the cast may contain various inclusions. These may be seen as inclusions of red cells, leukocytes, exfoliated renal epithelial cells, fat, or granules within what appears to be a basic hyaline matrix, or the cast may appear to be made up of a grouping or conglutination of any of the various inclusions described previously.

In addition, once the cast is formed, it does not remain static, but changes when the cells or other inclusions degenerate as the cast makes its way through the kidney and into the urine. Degenerative changes within the cast are associated with renal stasis, where the cast is retained within the kidney for a period of time before it is flushed into the urine. Cellular degeneration is seen as increasing cytoplasmic granularity with a loss of cell membrane. Eventually the cellular origin is not visible and only large to small granules remain. These granules undergo further degredation and eventually lose structure. The cast matrix becomes a thick, refractile, opaque, waxlike-appearing substance in a cast referred to as **waxy**. Pathologically, the waxy cast is the most serious type seen, since its formation implies a greatly lengthened transit time or shutdown of the portion of the kidney where the structure evolved. For this reason, waxy casts are sometimes referred to as **renal failure casts**.

The width or diameter of the cast is also clinically significant. Most casts have a fairly consistent diameter as do the tubules in which they are formed, although casts from infants are narrower than those of adults. **Narrow** casts may be seen, probably formed in tubules that have swollen and the lumen narrowed because of an inflammatory process. They tend to be of the hyaline type. **Broad** casts indicate more serious pathology. Their diameter is several times greater than normal casts and are probably formed in dilated renal tubules or in the larger collecting tubules that serve several nephrons. Chronic renal disease or obstruction (stasis) may result in dilation and destruction of renal tubules and broad casts. Casts forming in the collecting tubules implies urinary stasis, since the hydrostatic

pressure within these tubules is normally too high for cast formation to take place. Broad casts can be of any type; however, since their presence implies stasis, they tend to be waxy, and waxy casts are most often broad.

A morphologic classification of casts is presented in Box 6-1.

More than one type of cast may be present in any given specimen. Each type of cast that is seen must be enumerated and identified.

The various casts that might be encountered as summarized in Box 6-1 will now be described. Staining reactions are for Sedi-Stain, a Sternheimer-Malbin crystal violet safranin stain, unless otherwise stated.

Hyaline Casts

Hyaline casts are both the most difficult to visualize and least important of casts in the urine sediment. A few hyaline casts (less than two per low-power field in the concentrated sediment) may be seen in the urine from normal healthy persons. They are the result of solidification of Tamm-Horsfall protein secreted by the renal tubular epithelium and may be seen without significant proteinuria. They may be seen in increased numbers after strenuous exercise; the sediment returns to normal after 24 to 48 hours. Hyaline casts may be seen in large numbers (20-30 per low-power field) in moderate or severe renal disease.

Hyaline casts are colorless, homogeneous, nonrefractive, semitransparent structures. Examination with brightfield microscopy is especially difficult and requires careful light adjustment. The light is adjusted to give contrast by lowering the condenser slightly (1-2 mm) and closing the iris diaphragm. As mentioned under Identification and Morphology of Casts, phase and interfering contrast microscopy are especially useful when searching for hyaline casts. The dif-

Box 6-1

MORPHOLOGIC CLASSIFICATION OF CASTS

Hyaline cast
Cellular cast
  White blood cell (leukocyte, neutrophil, pus) cast
  Epithelial (renal tubular) cell cast
  Red blood cell (blood and hemoglobin pigment) cast
  Bacteria cast
  Mixed cell cast
Granular cast
Waxy cast

Fatty (and oval fat body) cast
Pigmented cast
  Hemoglobin (and blood) cast
  Myoglobin cast
  Bilirubin and drug pigment cast
Inclusion cast
  (Granular cast)
  (Fatty cast)
  Hemosiderin cast
  Crystal cast

From Linne JJ, Ringsrud KM: *Basic techniques in clinical laboratory science*, ed 3, St. Louis, 1992, Mosby.

Figure 6-106

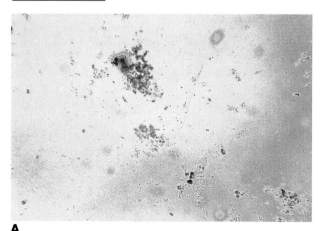

A

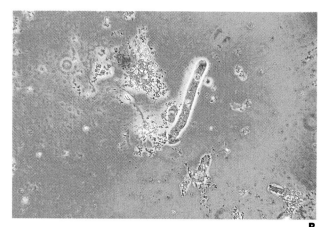

B

Hyaline casts. Unstained sediment, ×100. **A,** Brightfield, showing very difficult to visualize casts. **B,** Same field as A with phase contrast showing much more apparent hyaline casts, also mucus and amorphous material.

Figure 6-107

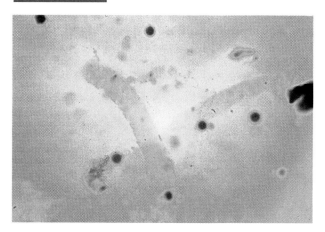

Hyaline casts, stained with Sedi-Stain, ×400.

Figure 6-108

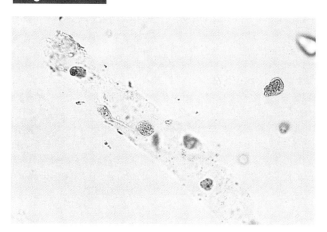

Hyaline cellular cast. Sedi-Stain, ×400.

ference in appearance between brightfield and phase contrast microscopy is seen in Fig. 6-106, *A* and *B*.

The use of supravital stains such as Sedi-Stain is also helpful. Hyaline casts stain pale pink or pale purple with a very uniform color (Fig. 6-107). They stain slightly darker than mucous threads. However, they may take up a minimum of stain and remain difficult to visualize. The presence of a few entrapped or adherent cells help visualization, as shown in Fig. 6-108.

Hyaline casts may be difficult to distinguish from mucous threads, which are often present under the same circumstances (see Figs. 6-179, 6-180, and 6-181). The use of phase contrast microscopy is especially helpful, and stain may also be useful as shown in Fig. 6-109, *A* and *B*.

Morphologically, hyaline casts usually are seen with the classic cast shape—parallel sides, uniform diameter, definite border, and rounded ends. However, narrower

diameters than usual may occur, and one end may taper off into a tail referred to as a cylindroid (Fig. 6-110). Cylindroids should be considered and reported the same as hyaline casts. Unusual convoluted, serpentine, folded, thin, and elongated forms may also be seen.

Hyaline casts are most likely to be found in concentrated, acidic urine. They are soluble in water and even more soluble in slightly alkaline solutions. They will dissolve as urine becomes alkaline because of improper storage and are difficult to maintain even when refrigerated for more than a few hours. They may not be able to form in advanced renal failure because of the loss of concentrating ability and failure to maintain the normal acid urine pH.

Since hyaline casts result from the solidification of protein within the renal tubule, they may contain inclusions of any structure that is present in the tubule at the time of formation. Therefore casts may be seen

Figure 6-109

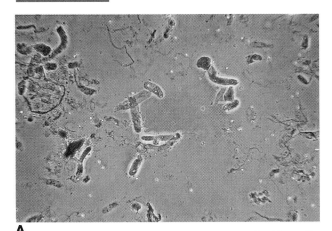
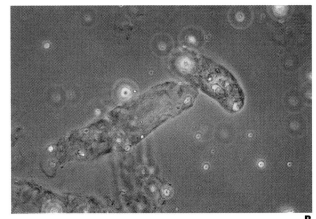

A   B

Several hyaline casts stained with Sedi-Stain and viewed with phase contrast at low-power and high-power magnification. **A,** ×100. **B,** Same field as A, ×400.

that are primarily hyaline but contain granules (proteinaceous or cellular debris), fat, or cells. Most hyaline casts will appear to contain fine granules when viewed with phase contrast microscopy but should be classified merely as hyaline casts.

Cellular Casts

Cellular casts are made up of any of the cells that might be present within the renal tubules. The cellular cast often appears to be the result of the clumping or conglutination of cells. Although it may be difficult or impossible to see microscopically, the cells are still embedded or enmeshed in a protein matrix. Cellular casts, basically hyaline casts with a few embedded cells, may be seen. Any of the cells present in the renal tubules may form a cellular cast. Most often they may be classified as white cell, red cell, or renal tubular epithelial casts. Bacteria casts have also been described. Often, the cells begin to degenerate, and the cell of origin is impossible to identify. It is especially difficult to differentiate a white cell from a renal epithelial cell cast. If in doubt, the cast is merely reported as cellular, as shown in Figs. 6-111, 6-112, 6-113, *A* and *B*, 6-114, *A* and *B*, and 6-115. Other findings in the urine specimen, both chemical and microscopic, will imply the cell type or source to the clinician.

The presence of cellular casts is an important finding that should not be missed. The casts indicate the presence of cells within the renal tubules. This is not normal; however, cells within the cast make them easier to visualize than plain hyaline casts. Care and proper microscopic technique, especially light adjustment, is still essential. Phase or interference contrast and supravital staining plus cytocentrifugation and appropriate staining are also useful tools in the identification of cellular casts.

Figure 6-110

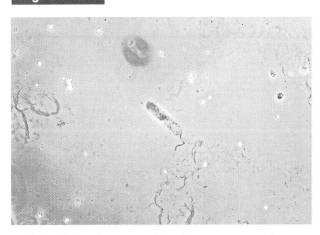

Cylindroid (hyaline cast with tail), and mucus. Phase contrast, ×100.

White Blood Cell Casts. White blood cell casts are also referred to as leukocyte casts or pus casts. They are not a normal finding. The white cells may be any of the white cell types that appear in blood; however, they are most often neutrophils (PMNs). When leukocytes are present in the urine sediment with leukocyte casts, the origin of the leukocytes may be placed within the kidney. Theoretically leukocytes may enter the kidney at any point of the nephron. They may originate in the blood and enter through the glomerulus in glomerular disease. However, they are most often the result of interstitial disease (inflammation or infection), in which the leukocytes (usually as phagocytic neutrophils) enter from the blood by squeezing through or between the renal tubular epithelial cells. This is most often in response to bacterial infection of the tubular interstitium called **pyelonephritis**. In such cases, white cells and bacteria would also be seen in

Figure 6-111

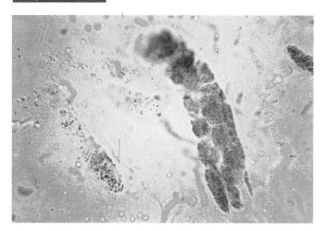

Cellular cast, (probably epithelial cell cast). Sedi-Stain, ×450.

Figure 6-112

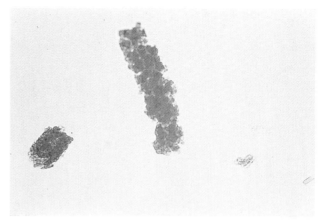

Cellular cast (probably red cell origin). Sedi-Stain, ×400.

Figure 6-113

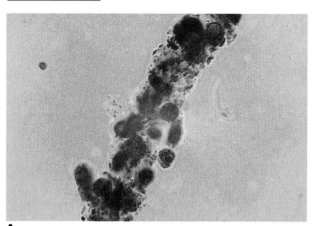

A

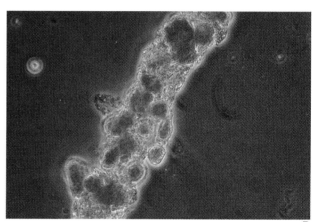

B

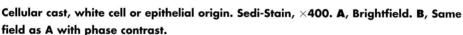

Cellular cast, white cell or epithelial origin. Sedi-Stain, ×400. A, Brightfield. B, Same field as A with phase contrast.

the urine sediment, and the presence of white cell casts differentiates an upper (kidney) from a lower (bladder) urinary tract infection.

White blood cell casts are relatively easy to see with brightfield microscopy (Fig. 6-116), especially when stained (Figs. 6-117, 6-118, and 6-119).

Phase and interference contrast microscopy is very helpful as shown in Fig. 6-120, *A* and *B*.

The characteristic multilobulated nucleus of the neutrophil identifies the white blood cell cast. Leukocytes within the cast will stain as they do in urine—purple to violet or pale blue. Neutrophils within casts degenerate rapidly, as they do in urine. This degeneration is seen as increased granulation of the cytoplasm, merging of cell borders, and loss of nuclear detail. Eventually the cast can be referred to only as cellular, and finally even cellular origin is uncertain and the cast must be referred to as granular.

The number of cells within a white blood cell cast varies from a cast packed with cells to only a few white blood cells in a hyaline matrix. Casts that appear to be entirely packed cells still have a protein matrix and should have parallel sides and rounded ends. It may be difficult to distinguish this sort of leukocyte cast from a **pseudocast** made up of a clump of white blood cells originating in the lower urinary tract. Such pseudocasts may be the result of white blood cells adhering to a strand or clump of mucus. The use of phase contrast microscopy and degree of proteinuria are helpful in distinguishing these pseudo-casts from true white blood cell casts (Fig. 6-121).

White cell casts may also be difficult or impossible to distinguish from epithelial cell casts, especially as the cells begin to degenerate. Once again, when the cell origin is uncertain, the cast should be referred to as a cellular cast. Other urinary findings will help the clin-

Figure 6-114

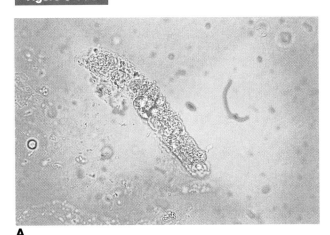
A

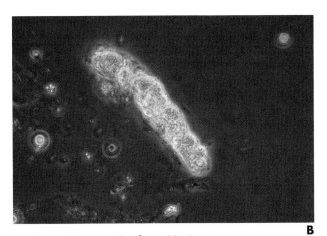
B

Cellular casts, with degenerating cells of uncertain origin. Unstained, ×400. **A,** Brightfield. **B,** Same field as A with phase contrast.

Figure 6-115

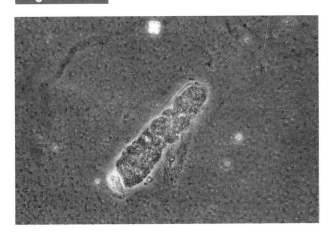

Cellular (almost granular) cast with cells barely visable. Phase contrast, ×400.

Figure 6-116

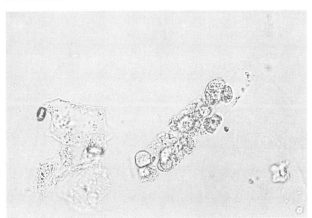

Probable white blood cell cast. Unstained, ×400.

ician decide the most likely cell type. The presence of leukocytes and bacteria implies white cell casts, whereas the presence of renal tubular epithelial cells implies epithelial cell casts with significant loss of renal tubular epithelium.

Renal Tubular Epithelial Cell Casts. At this point, it should be obvious that to be called an **epithelial cell** cast, the epithelial cell must be renal tubular in origin. Although relatively infrequent, epithelial cell casts are an important pathologic finding. They result from destruction or desquamation of the cells that line the renal tubules, and damage may be irreversible depending on the severity of the disease process. Epithelial cell casts may be seen after exposure to nephrotoxic substances such as mercury or ethylene glycol (antifreeze), or they may be associated with viral infections such as cytomegalovirus or hepatitis virus.

Figure 6-117

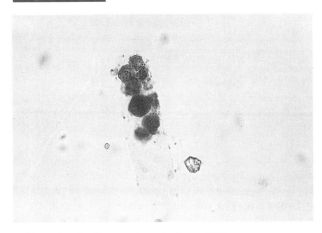

White blood cell cast. Sedi-Stain, ×400.

Figure 6-118

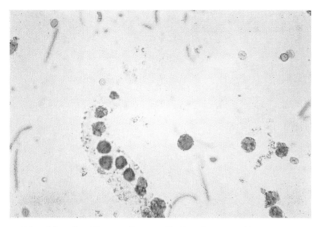

White blood cell cast, basically hyaline. Sedi-Stain, ×450.

Figure 6-119

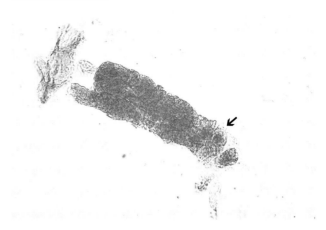

White blood cell cast with degenerating cells (*one lobed neutrophil at the arrow*). Sedi-Stain, ×400.

Figure 6-120

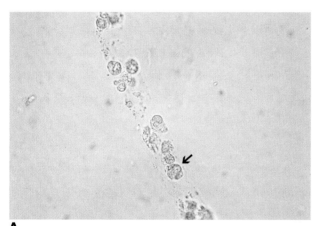
A

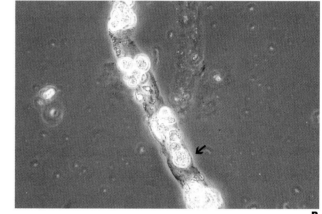
B

White blood cell cast (hyaline white cell cast). Unstained, ×400. **A**, Brightfield. **B**, Same cast, as in A with phase contrast showing lobed neutrophil at arrow.

Figure 6-121

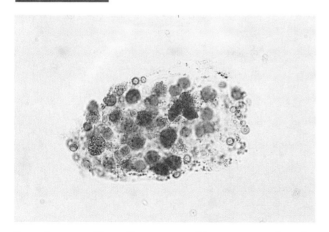

Pseudocast, white cells entrapped in mucus. Sedi-Stain, ×400.

An epithelial cell cast often appears to consist of one or two rows of renal epithelial cells. This implies tubular desquamation or destruction.

Supravital staining, phase or interference contrast, and cytocentrifugation are all helpful techniques in the identification of epithelial cell casts (Figs. 6-122, 6-123, 6-124, *A* and *B*, and 6-125).

Epithelial cell casts may also be seen in which cells vary in size and shape and are haphazardly arranged in a hyaline or variable protein matrix. These may represent desquamation from different or separate portions of the renal tubule. The epithelial cell cast does not remain constant once formed but undergoes a series of changes from epithelial cell to cellular, granular, and finally waxy.

Red Blood Cell Casts (Blood and Hemoglobin Casts). The presence of red blood cell casts in the

Figure 6-122

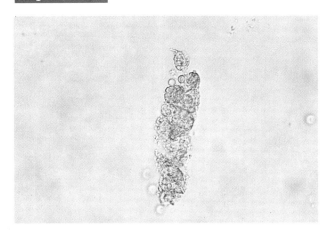

Epithelial cell cast. Pyridium stained, ×400.

Figure 6-123

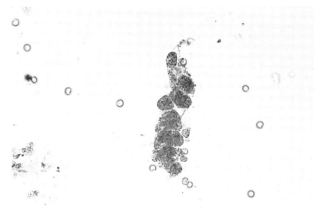

Epithelial cell cast and red cells. Sedi-Stain, ×400.

Figure 6-124

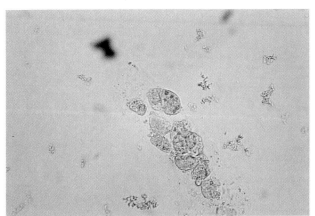

A

B

Epithelial cell cast. Cells stained by bilirubin in the urine, ×400. A, Brightfield.
B, Same cast as A with phase contrast.

urine sediment is an important pathologic finding that should not be missed. Red blood cells may enter the nephron and be incorporated into a cast at any point along the nephron. However, most red cell casts are the result of glomerular disease with entry of red blood cells into the urine leaking at the glomerulus such as in acute glomerular nephritis and lupus nephritis.

Once red cells are present in the lumen of the nephron, they can clump together to form red cell casts. This may be enhanced by the proteinuria associated with glomerular damage. Red cell casts are probably the most fragile of all the casts that might be found in the urine sediment. This may explain their rarity, especially as fully intact casts. They are often observed as fragments or portions of casts, as seen in Figs. 6-126 and 6-127.

Figure 6-125

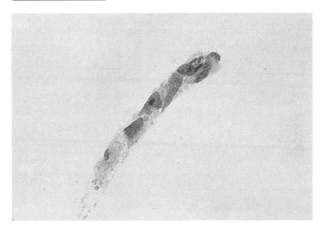

Epithelial cell cast, from cytocentrifuged preparation.
Papanicolaou stain, ×400.

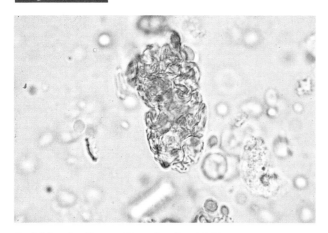

Red blood cell cast. Unstained, ×1000.

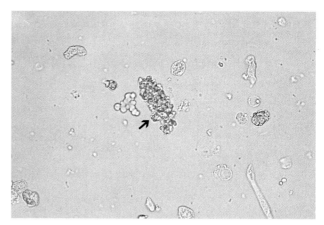

Red blood cell cast (*at arrow*). Unstained, ×400.

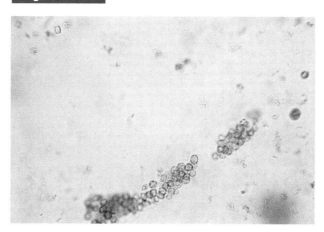

Red blood cell cast. Sedi-Stain, ×450.

Discovery of red cell casts may depend on special handling—the urine should be absolutely fresh and handled gently so that the casts remain intact.

The presence of hemoglobin gives the red cell cast a characteristic orange yellow color unlike anything else seen in the urine sediment (Figs. 6-126, 130, and 135). This color is best appreciated with brightfield microscopy, and any sediment suspected of containing red cell or blood pigment casts should be observed unstained with brightfield illumination as well as other microscopic techniques. Color from hemoglobin should not be confused with staining from bilirubin or Pyridium present in the urine specimen. These substances will stain all cell forms present in the urine sediment.

Supravital stains may be useful in the identification of red blood cell casts. The cast may be seen to contain red cells that stain colorless or lavender in a pink matrix, as shown in Fig. 6-128.

Phase contrast may also be helpful in the identification of red cell casts, as shown in Figs. 6-129, A and B, and 6-130, A, B, and C.

Cytocentrifugation may also be helpful. The number of red cells present in a cast varies from only a few in a generally hyaline matrix (Fig. 6-131) to a cast packed with so many cells that no matrix is visible (Fig. 6-132).

Red cell casts may also be associated with the conversion of fibrinogen (present because of glomerular damage and leakage from the blood) to fibrin in the renal tubules. The red cell casts may result from trapped erythrocytes in a fibrin matrix.

Like other cellular casts, the red cell cast changes once formed. Cells degenerate and become unrecognizable resulting in a **blood cast**, as in Figs. 6-133 and 6-134.

A blood cast probably begins as a red cell cast and results from the degeneration of red cell structure. Although cellular remnants can be seen as granules that become progressively smaller, the red cell outline cannot be seen. The blood cast has similar clinical significance to the waxy cast, implying renal stasis and is seen with chronic renal disease, especially affecting the glomerulus. It may be recognized by its yellow or red brown color, which is best appreciated in the unstained sediment with brightfield microscopy. This should not be confused with pigmentation and coloration in the urine caused by bilirubin or from Pyridium therapy. When stained with Sedi-Stain, the granules usually stain dark purple, and the cast appears to be a granular cast.

A **hemoglobin cast** consisting of a totally waxy matrix stained with hemoglobin is extremely rare. More often a mixed cast consisting of remnants of red cells in the form of granules in at least part of the waxy matrix is seen (Fig. 6-135).

Bacterial Cast. Casts made up of bacteria in a protein matrix have been described. They are an important finding, and according to Haber, are only associated with **pyelonephritis** or intrinsic renal infections.[4]

Figure 6-129

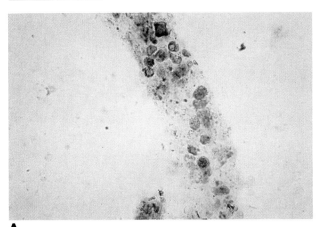
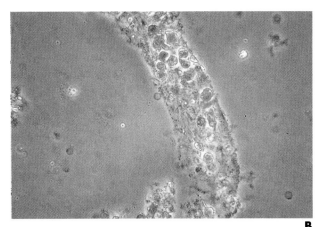

A

B

Red blood cell cast. Sedi-Stain, ×400. **A,** Brightfield. **B,** Same cast as in A with phase contrast.

Figure 6-130

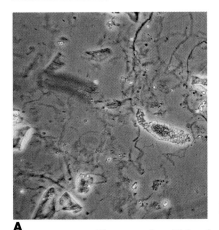
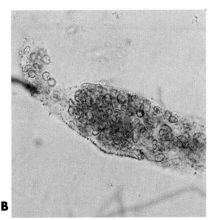
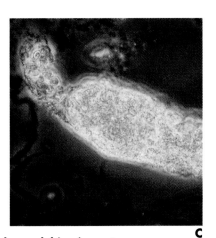

A

B

C

Pigmented red blood cell cast, showing typical coloration from hemoglobin pigment. **A,** Squamous epithelial cells and mucus also present. Phase contrast, ×100. **B,** Same cast as in A at higher magnification. Brightfield, ×400. **C,** Phase contrast, ×400.

Figure 6-131

Figure 6-132

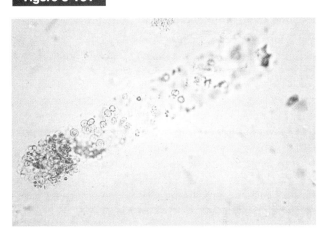
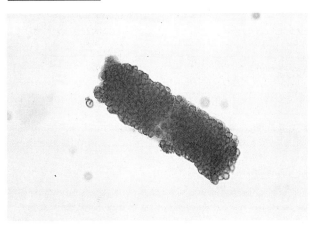

Hyaline red blood cell cast. Unstained, ×450.

Red blood cell cast, completely filled with red cells. Sedi-Stain, ×400.

Figure 6-133

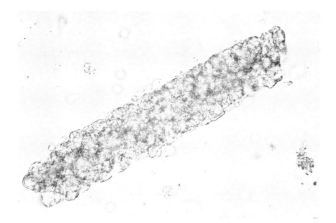

Blood cast. Unstained, ×400.

Figure 6-134

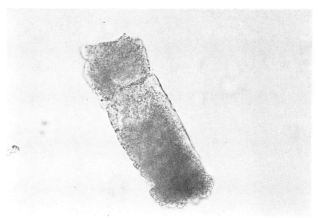

Blood (pigment) cast. Unstained, ×400.

Figure 6-135

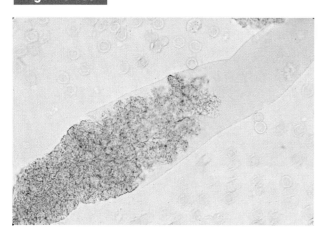

Combination blood and hemoglobin cast. Unstained, ×512. (From Ward PCJ: Urinary sediment. Image Premastering Services, Ltd., 1992, Mosby.)

Figure 6-136

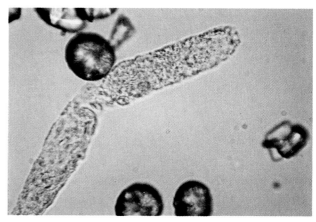

Granular cast. Unstained ×400.

They are probably mistaken for granular casts, which they resemble. Examination with phase or interference contrast microscopy and supravital stain is helpful. Bacterial casts are more easily recognized if a dry or cytocentrifuged preparation is stained with Gram stain. The bacteria in the cast may be packed closely together, sparsely distributed throughout, or concentrated in an area of a cast matrix. They may be seen along with white blood cells in the cast. Bacterial casts should be suspected in urine specimens with significant (moderate to large) proteinuria, white blood cells, bacteria, and casts, possibly resulting from untreated pyelonephritis.

Mixed Cell Cast. A variety of mixed cell casts may be seen in the urine sediment. They may appear as a cast made up of two different cell types, almost like two different casts in one. Or they may consist of a

cast of a predominant cell type with additional cellular inclusions. Examples include a white cell cast with bacteria or a mixed cast of renal tubular epithelial cells and neutrophils.

Granular Casts

A few granular casts may be present in the urine sediment of normal healthy persons, especially after vigorous exercise. However, increased numbers are not normal and may represent serious pathology. The granules seen in these casts may result from breakdown of cells within the cast or the renal tubules, or aggregates of plasma proteins, including fibrinogen, immune complexes, and globulins in a Tamm-Horsfall matrix. Once cells have completely degenerated into granules within the cast, it is impossible to be certain of cell origin. The

Figure 6-137

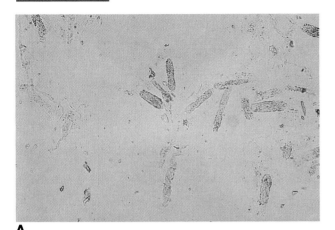

A

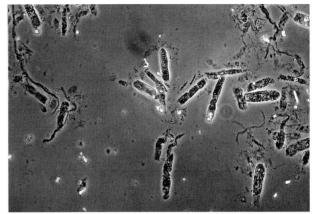

B

Several hyaline finely granular casts. Unstained, ×100. **A,** Brightfield. **B,** Same field as A with phase contrast showing improved visualization of casts and mucus.

presence of only one or two recognizable cells within an otherwise granular matrix may suffice for correct identification. Identification is clinically useful, since red cells within casts usually indicate glomerular injury, epithelial cells show renal tubular damage, and leukocytes are seen with interstitial inflammation or infection. Granular casts may be seen in both renal glomerular and tubular disease and are associated with interstitial tubular disease and renal allograft rejection.

The size of granules within a cast varies; the granules become progressively smaller as they degenerate to a waxy cast. The number of granules within a cast also varies from only a few granules within a basically hyaline matrix to a cast that seems to be completely filled with (usually coarse) granules. Granular casts have been further classified as being coarsely or finely granular. Although such distinction is subjective, it is unnecessary, and the term **granular** is sufficient (Figs. 6-136 and 6-137, *A* and *B*).

Again, if the cast has a definite hyaline matrix with only a few fine granules, primarily visible with phase contrast microscopy, it should be reported as hyaline rather than granular.

The use of supravital stains, such as a Sternheimer-Malbin stain, is especially useful in visualizing granular casts. The granules have an affinity for stain and show as dark purple granules in a matrix that may or may not be clearly visible, depending on the number of granules present. A variety of granular casts, unstained and stained, are seen in Figs. 6-138, 6-139, 6-140, 6-141, and 6-142.

Phase contrast microscopy is also helpful and may be used with or without supravital staining (Figs. 6-143, *A* and *B*, 6-144, *A*, *B*, and *C*, and 6-145, *A* and *B*).

When several somewhat shortened granular casts are seen, especially with phase contrast microscopy,

Figure 6-138

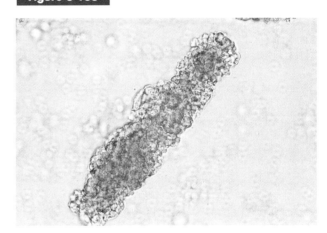

Granular cast with coarse granules (almost cells). Sedi-Stain, ×400.

Figure 6-139

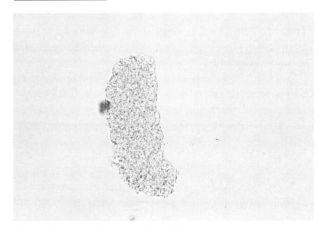

Granular cast. Unstained, ×400.

Figure 6-140

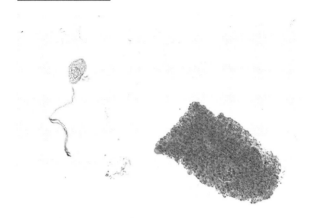

Stained granular cast like the cast in Fig. 6-139. Also, mucus, and renal epithelial cell. Sedi-Stain, ×400.

Figure 6-141

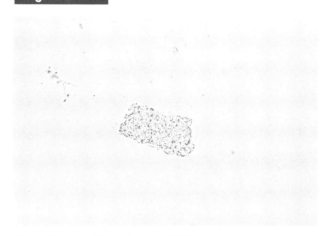

Granular cast. Unstained, ×400.

Figure 6-142

Granular cast, like the cast in Fig. 6-141. Sedi-Stain, ×400.

Figure 6-143

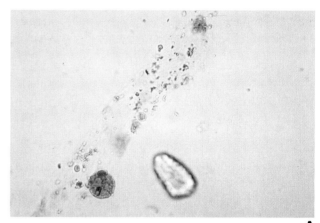

A

B

Granular cast (hyaline with fine granulation). Sedi-Stain ×400. A, Brightfield. B, Same field as A with phase contrast.

the possibility that these are actually proximal renal tubular epithelial cells should be considered (see also Renal Epithelial Cells). They are better visualized with brightfield microscopy when stained with a supravital stain, as was shown in Figs. 6-58, 6-59, and 6-60.

Cytocentrifugation and stain with either Wright's or Papanicolaou stain is most helpful in differentiating a possible granular cast (Fig. 6-146) from proximal renal tubular epithelial cells as shown in Figs. 6-147 and 6-148.

Waxy Casts

Waxy casts have already been mentioned as the final stage of degeneration—from cellular to granular and finally waxy casts. They are not normally seen in urine but are a serious, pathologic finding and imply

Figure 6-144

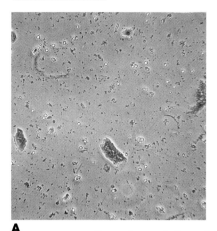

A

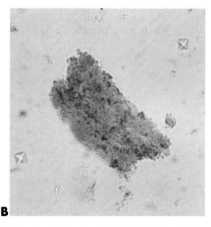

B

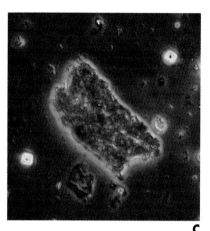

C

Granular cast (broad, broken) stained with Sedi-Stain. **A**, Low power with phase contrast, ×100. **B** and **C**, Same cast as **A**, at higher magnification, showing the presence of red cells and calcium oxalate. **B**, Brightfield, ×400. **C**, Phase contrast, ×400.

Figure 6-145

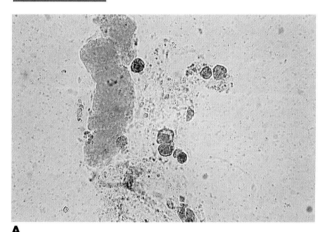

A

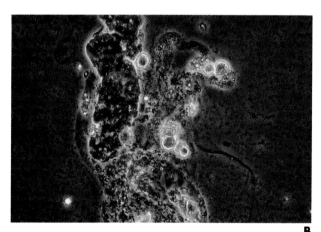

B

Granular (almost waxy) cast. Sedi-Stain, ×400. **A**, Brightfield. **B**, Phase contrast.

Figure 6-146

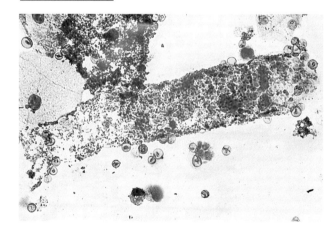

Figure 6-147

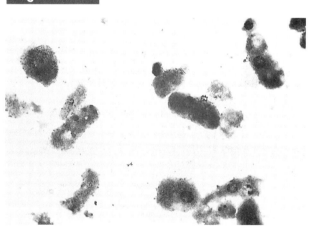

Granular cast in Wright's stained cytocentrifuged preparation. Squamous epithelial cell, white blood cells, and many red blood cells also present, Cytospin, ×400.

Renal tubular epithelial cells (proximal) appearing like granular casts. Cytospin, Wright's stain, ×400.

Figure 6-148

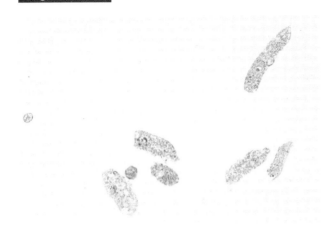

Renal tubular epithelial cells (proximal) appearing like granular casts. Cytospin, Papanicolaou stain, ×400.

Figure 6-149

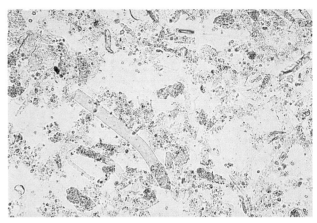

Telescoped urine sediment with mixture of casts ranging from hyaline to waxy. Unstained, ×100.

Figure 6-150

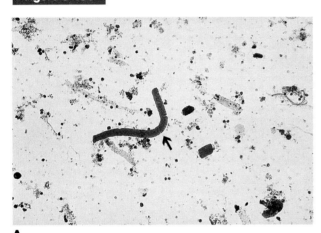

A

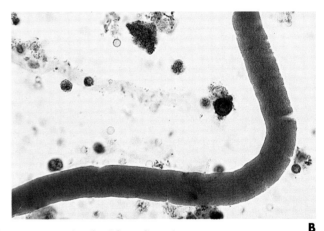

B

Mixture of casts from same specimen as Fig. 6-149, stained with Sedi-Stain. A, Large waxy cast at arrow, ×100. B, Same cast as A at higher magnification, ×400.

renal stasis. Waxy casts are associated with severe chronic renal disease and renal amyloidosis and are only rarely seen in acute renal disease. Since they are associated with renal stasis, waxy casts are often of greater diameter than most casts and referred to as **broad casts**. Such broad, waxy casts have been called **renal failure casts**. The range of casts that might be encountered as they degenerate with renal stasis may be appreciated in the **telescoped sediment**, which is seen when the kidney resumes function after a period of renal shutdown. Such specimens are seen in Figs. 6-149 and 6-150, A and B.

Waxy casts are homogeneous, like hyaline casts; however, they are easier to visualize since they are more refractile with sharper outlines, as shown in Figs. 6-151, 6-152, and 6-153.

As already mentioned, waxy casts tend to be wider than hyaline casts and usually have irregular broken or blunt ends and fissures or cracks (Fig. 6-154).

They may have a completely homogeneous, waxy appearance, but often have a portion or end of another type such as the granular end seen in Fig. 6-155, A and B.

Although phase and interference contrast microscopy are useful tools in visualizing waxy casts, brightfield microscopy with supravital staining is especially helpful (Figs. 6-156 and 6-157, A and B). Waxy casts tend to stain more readily than hyaline casts and are easily visualized when stained.

Cytocentrifugation and staining with Wright's or Papanicolaou stain may also be useful, especially in differentiation of casts from fibers (Fig. 6-158).

Figure 6-151

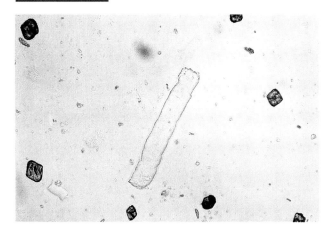

Waxy cast. Unstained, ×100.

Figure 6-152

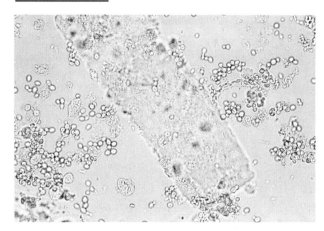

Broad waxy cast (note blunt end), many yeast. Unstained, ×400.

Figure 6-153

Broad waxy cast (broken and degenerating, with fat inclusions). Unstained, ×400.

Figure 6-154

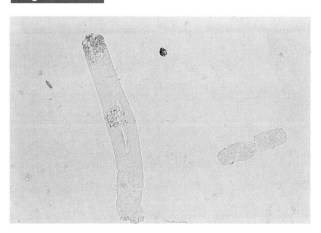

Waxy cast with fissure and granular end (left), granular to waxy cast (right). Unstained ×160.

Figure 6-155

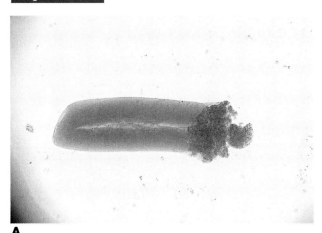

A

B

Broad waxy cast with central fissure and granular end. Sedi-Stain. A, Low-power, ×160. B, Higher magnification of same cast as in A, showing granular end and fat inclusions, ×400.

Care must be taken not to confuse waxy casts with fibers from disposable diapers or other contaminating fibers present in the urine sediment. These may closely resemble the classic waxy cast but are of no diagnostic significance. The presence of contaminating fibers should be suspected when the urine is essentially negative in respect to chemical and other sediment findings, yet contains structures that resemble waxy casts. A helpful tool in such cases is polarizing microscopy. Most fibers are birefringent; that is, they will polarize light, whereas waxy casts (or any protein-based constituents such as cells) are not birefringent, as shown in Fig. 6-159 (see also Figs. 6-182 and 6-238).

Figure 6-156

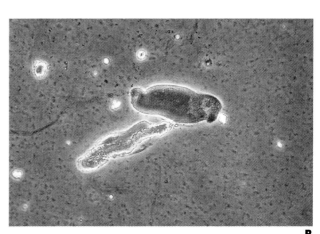

Waxy casts (broad, degenerating). Sedi-Stain, ×400.

Figure 6-157

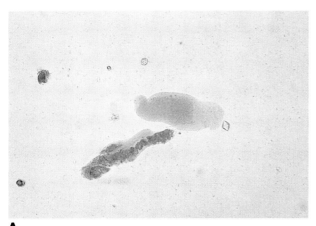

A   B

Waxy casts, one partially granular. Sedi-Stain, ×400. **A,** Brightfield. **B,** Same field as A with phase contrast showing the presence of mucus and bacteria.

Figure 6-158

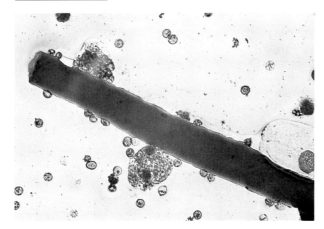

Waxy cast. Red cells and epithelial cells also present. Wright's stain Cytospin, ×400.

Figure 6-159

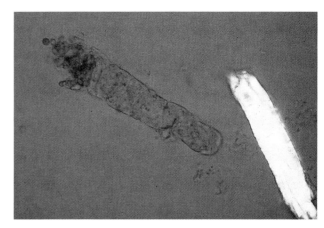

Waxy cast with fatty end (**left**) and strongly birefringent contaminating fiber (**right**). Compensated polarized light, ×400.

Figure 6-160

Fatty cast, unstained, ×400.

Figure 6-161

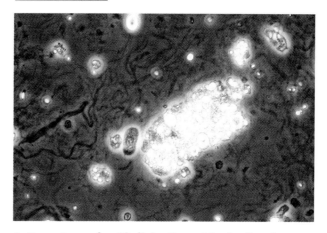

Fatty cast, renal epithelial cell, oval fat bodies, fat and mucus. Phase contrast, ×400.

Figure 6-162

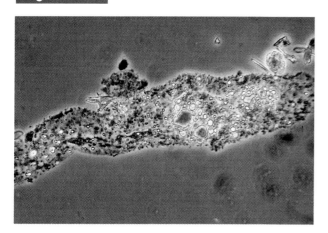

Large fatty cast with oval fat body inclusion, stained with Sudan III for fat. Phase contrast, ×400.

Figure 6-163

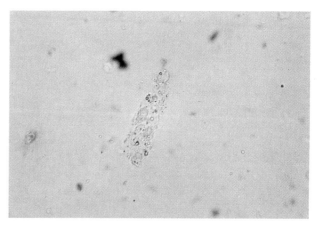

Fatty cast showing weak staining with Sudan III for neutral fat or triglyceride, ×400

Fatty Casts

Fatty casts are another important abnormal pathologic finding in the urine sediment that often indicates severe renal dysfunction. They are related to oval fat bodies, described in the section on renal tubular epithelial cells. Oval fat bodies are renal tubular epithelial cells or macrophages with ingested lipid (fat). They are often seen with, and have similar significance to, fatty casts and free fat droplets in the sediment. The presence of these three structures is associated with the nephrotic syndrome, where the urine contains an extremely large amount of protein (>500 mg/dL). Such a urine specimen is typically pale with a foamy appearance, (especially when mixed or shaken) because of very high albumin content. Fatty casts are also seen in cases of diabetes mellitus with renal degeneration and toxic nephrosis such as from ethylene glycol or mercury poisoning.

Fatty casts contain droplets of fat that are highly refractile when observed microscopically, especially with the normal brightfield microscope (Fig. 6-160).

In the case of fatty casts, phase contrast microscopy may actually detract, since fat and fat-containing cells may be mistaken for other cells or crystals (Fig. 6-161).

If the lipid consists of neutral fat or triglyceride, it will stain orange or red with fat stains such as Sudan III or oil red O (Figs. 6-162 and 6-163).

If the lipid droplets are made up of cholesterol esters, they will show a typical Maltese cross pattern when viewed with polarized light, as seen in Fig. 164, A, B, and C. (These should not be confused with the presence of starch granules.)

When stained with a supravital stain such as Sedi-Stain, the matrix of the fatty casts and other cellular elements or debris will stain, whereas the refractile fat

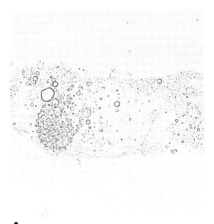

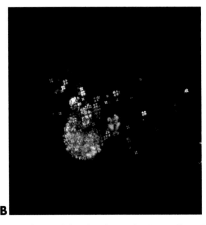

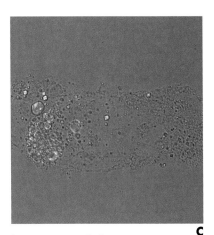

A

B

C

Large fat-filled fatty cast with oval fat body inclusion, showing the presence of cholesterol as a Maltese cross, ×400. **A**, Brightfield. **B**, Polarized light, showing Maltese cross formation. **C**, Compensated polarized light showing Maltese cross formation in the cast matrix.

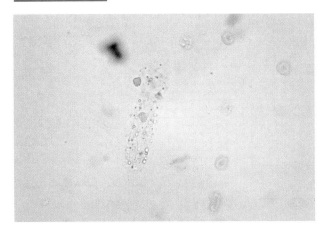

Fatty cast (fat globules in hyaline matrix). Sedi-Stain, ×400.

A

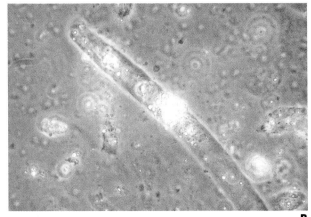

B

globules will remain unstained but stand out in the purple matrix, as seen in Fig. 6-165.

Although cytocentrifugation may be helpful, the fat droplets are dissolved in the staining process and seen merely as vacuoles or holes where lipid was previously present.

The number of lipid droplets seen within a fatty cast varies, and casts containing fat have been described with various names, depending on the number and/or distribution. In some cases the cast is basically hyaline with only a few fatty inclusions. This is seen in Fig. 6-166, *A* and *B*. A few fat globules may also be seen within what is basically a granular or cellular cast (Figs. 6-167 and 6-168).

Fatty cast (hyaline with oval fat body inclusion). Unstained, ×400. **A**, Brightfield. **B**, Phase contrast.

Or, the cast may appear to be completely filled with droplets of fat. Care must be taken not to confuse such fatty casts with red cell casts.

Finally, fatty casts may be seen with oval fat bodies enclosed within the cast. These are sometimes referred to as **oval fat body** or **renal tubular fat casts**. These may be seen in Figs. 6-162, 6-164, and 6-167.

Pigmented Casts

Hemoglobin (and blood) Casts. Blood and blood pigment casts were discussed with red blood cell casts. As stated, a blood cast probably began as a red cell cast that degenerated. Although cellular remnants remain as granules, the red cell outline cannot be seen. The blood cast has similar clinical significance to the waxy cast, implying renal stasis and is seen with chronic renal disease, especially affecting the glomerulus.

A **hemoglobin cast** is made up of hemoglobin pigment contained within a protein matrix. It is extremely rare. Such a cast might be seen following severe intravascular hemolysis and might be followed by the presence of hemosiderin granules in the urine, epithelial cells, and possibly within casts (hemosiderin casts) about 2 days after the severe hemolytic episode.

Myoglobin Casts. These are extremely rare, may occur in cases of myoglobinuria, as a result of acute muscle damage, and may be associated with acute renal failure. Myoglobin casts resemble hemoglobin casts; however, the color is darker (red brown).

Bilirubin and Drug Pigment Casts. These casts occur when bilirubin or highly-colored drugs such as phenazopyridine (Pyridium) are present in the urine. Pathology depends on the type of cast present and therefore stained. These highly-colored pigments stain any structures present in the urine—casts or cells. This staining is helpful since the pigments serve to emphasize structures that might otherwise be missed in an unstained urine sediment. Examples are seen in Figs. 6-169, *A* and *B* and 6-170.

Inclusion Casts

These are casts that contain various inclusions within a protein (hyaline) matrix. Strictly speaking, any cast could be called an inclusion cast. This is certainly the case with granular and fatty casts already described. However, a few very rare examples not described elsewhere will now be discussed.

Hemosiderin Cast. Casts may be seen that contain granules of hemosiderin 2 to 3 days after an acute hemolytic episode. These coarse yellow-brown granules might appear much like other granules in a granular cast (Fig. 6-171). Unlike granules of other origin, hemosiderin will stain blue with a Prussian blue stain

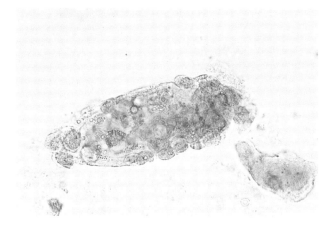

Figure 6-167

Cellular cast with fat inclusions. Sedi-Stain, ×400.

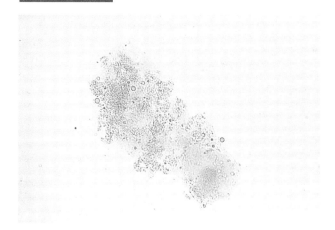

Figure 6-168

Waxy cast with fat inclusions. Sedi-Stain, ×400.

for iron as shown in Figs. 6-172 and 6-173. See also Procedure 6-1, Rous Test for Hemosiderin in Urine.

Hemosiderin should be considered as a possible urine sediment constituent when unusual granules are seen in the urine, in renal epithelial cells and macrophages, and in so-called granular casts, especially after a clinical history of possible intravascular hemolysis.

Crystal Cast. There is some disagreement as to whether or not there is such a thing as a crystal cast or if crystals present in the urine are merely adhering to a cast form. According to the College of American Pathologists Surveys Glossary of Terms, "they have no clinical importance . . . (and) arise from the adherence of crystals to a preexistent hyaline cast matrix, usually after refrigeration of urine."[1] According to Schumann, "Casts containing **urates**, calcium **oxalate**, and **sulfonamides** (sulfamethoxazole) are occasionally seen. A matrix is visible in a true crystal cast."[8]

Figure 6-169

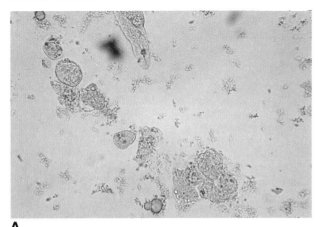

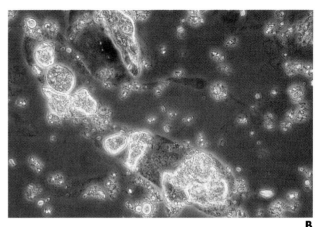

A **Bilirubin-stained epithelial cell cast, ×400. A, Brightfield. B, Phase contrast.** B

Figure 6-170

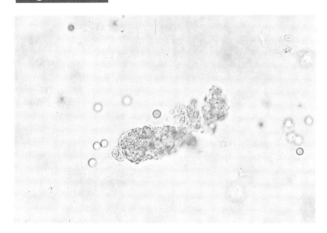

Pyridium-stained cellular cast, many red cells, ×400.

Figure 6-171

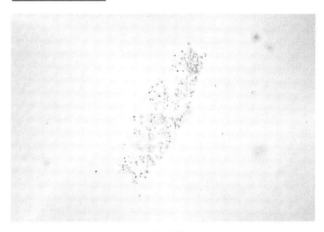

Hemosiderin cast, appearing like a granular cast. Unstained, ×400.

A sulfonamide cast is seen in Fig. 6-174, *A* and *B*. In any case, crystalline casts should not be confused with more pathologic forms. For example, a crystalline cast consisting of a rare ovoid form of calcium oxalate resembling red blood cells should not be reported as a red blood cell cast. Similarly, a pseudocast of crystals aligned along a strand of mucus or other exogenous fibers that might be present in the urine should not be reported as a crystal cast (Figs. 6-175 and 6-176). In such cases, the use of polarizing and compensated polarizing microscopy is helpful in separating crystals from protein-based inclusions. However, crystal-containing casts or pseudocasts must not be mistaken for fatty casts showing the presence of cholesterol esters as a Maltese cross formation (Fig. 6-174, *A* and *B*)

Pseudocasts and Structures Confused With Casts

Many structures occurring in urine sediment may be mistaken for casts. As a general rule, they are easier to visualize than a true cast and are most often misidentified by the student or inexperienced microscopist. Such structures include unusual aggregates of various substances referred to as pseudocasts, mucus threads, rolled squamous epithelial cells, hyphae of molds, disposable diaper fibers, and bits of hair, threads, or scratches. Whenever a cast is suspected, other chemical and microscopic findings should be noted. In general, casts occur together with proteinuria, although hyaline and granular casts may be seen with negative or small amounts of protein. When casts are seen in an otherwise negative urine, **pseudocasts** or other artifacts should be considered.

Figure 6-172

Hemosiderin cast (hyaline with inclusions of blue green hemosiderin granules) (Prussian blue stain for iron), ×400.

Figure 6-173

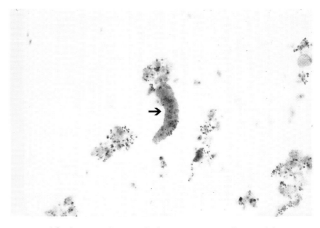

Hemosiderin cast (*arrow*), in very strongly positive Rous Test. Prussian blue stain for iron, ×400.

Figure 6-174

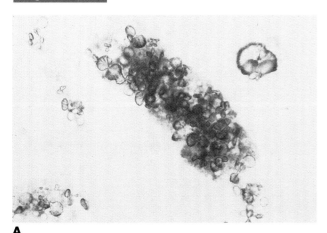

A

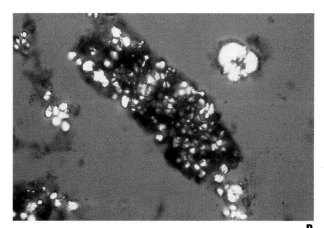

B

Sulfonamide Cast. Sedi-Stain, ×400. **A**, Brightfield. **B**, With polarized light.

Pseudocasts. These are structures or aggregates of material within the urine specimen that assume the general shape of a cast. They are not of diagnostic significance and should not be misinterpreted and reported as a cast. Large amounts of amorphous urates in the sediment may assume cast-like aggregates and appear to be granular casts. The use of polarized and compensated polarized microscopy is helpful in distinguishing such aggregates from a granular cast. Urates are birefringent and polarize light, whereas protein granules do not.

Cells, crystals, or amorphous materials seen adhering to mucus or fibers in the urine may resemble a cast (Figs. 6-175 and 6-176). Careful microscopic observation for the protein matrix of a cast, the use of stains, phase and interference contrast,

and polarizing microscopy are all helpful distinguishing techniques.

Clumping of white cells into a cast-like form or adherence of cells to mucus should not be mistaken for the true white cell cast (Fig. 6-177) (see also Fig. 6-121).

Exogenous fibers may closely resemble casts, as shown in Fig. 6-178, where one fiber is seen along with many granular casts.

Mucus Threads. Mucus threads, sometimes mistaken for hyaline casts, have been discussed. However, mucus strands or threads are long and ribbonlike with undefined edges and pointed, split, or frayed ends. Mucus, a common constituent in the urine sediment, is secreted by glands in the lower urinary tract and vagina. It may be increased with various inflammato-

Figure 6-175

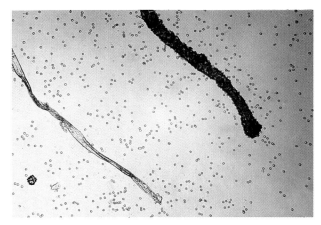

Fiber (*left*) and calcium oxalate crystals arranged on a long fiber, appearing to be a possible cast (*right*). Many red blood cells also present. Unstained, ×100.

Figure 6-176

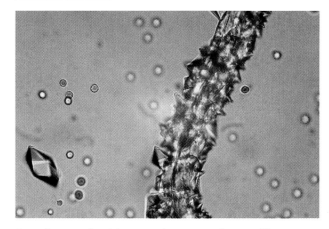

Pseudocast of calcium oxalate crystals on a fiber. Unstained, ×400.

Figure 6-177

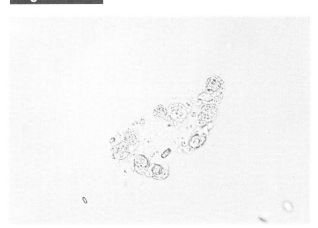

Pseudocast; clump of white cells resembling a cast. Unstained, ×400.

Figure 6-178

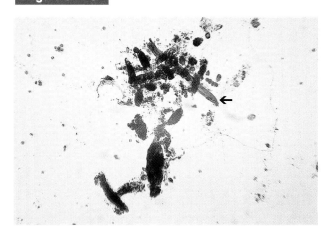

Low-power field showing many granular casts and a fiber (*arrow*). Sedi-Stain, ×100.

Figure 6-179

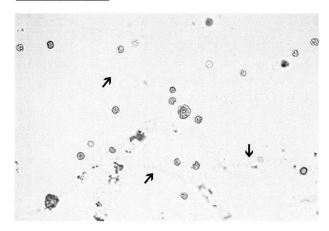

Stained urine containing mucus (*arrows*), also white cell and several red cells, including many dysmorphic forms. Sedi-Stain, ×400.

ry conditions. Mucus is easily overlooked with bright-field microscopy but becomes very apparent with phase and interference contrast microscopy. Mucus stains pale pink or pale blue with Sternheimer-Malbin stain much like hyaline casts which may stain slightly darker than mucus (Figs. 6-179, 6-180, and 6-181).

Rolled Squamous Epithelial Cells. Occasionally **squamous epithelial cells** that have folded or rolled into a cigar shape may be mistaken for hyaline or hyaline finely granular casts. Careful examination will show pointed rather than rounded ends, a single round nucleus, which appears like a white blood cell, and generally short length.

Disposable Diaper Fibers. These were discussed in the section on waxy casts. The fibers are almost identical to waxy casts: highly refractile with blunt ends.

Figure 6-180

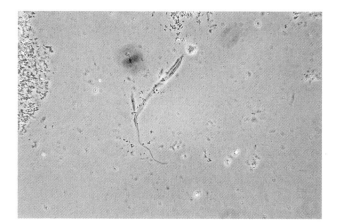

Mucus, like hyaline cast. Phase contrast, ×100.

Figure 6-181

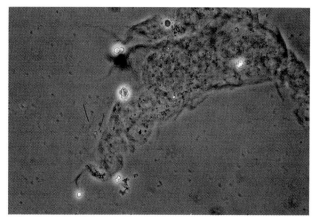

Mucus, also bacteria and yeast. Phase contrast, ×400.

Figure 6-182

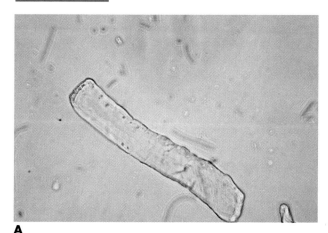

A

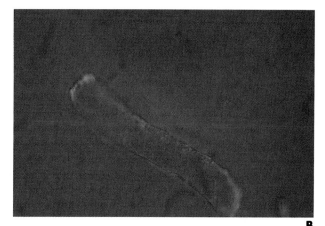

B

Disposable diaper fiber, resembling a waxy cast, ×400. A, Brightfield.
B, Compensated polarized light showing the presence of weak birefringence.

They may be present in specimens from infants or adults wearing disposable diapers. The presence of diaper fibers is suspected when waxy casts are seen in the absence of other pathologic findings, especially without proteinuria. Polarizing microscopy is particularly helpful in the identification of diaper fibers. Most fibers are at least weakly birefringent; that is, they will polarize light, whereas waxy casts do not (Fig. 6-182, *A* and *B*). See also Fig. 6-238 under Contaminants and Artifacts.

Other Structures. Various artifacts such as hair, clothing fibers or thread, and even scratches on the microscope slide may be seen in the urine sediment and mistaken for casts. The appearance of these highly refractive and visible structures are soon learned and ignored by the microscopist.

Occasionally yeast or fungus may be present with mycelia or pseudohyphae that might be mistaken for hyaline casts. See Fig. 6-100 and the section on Yeast and Fungus.

CRYSTALS AND AMORPHOUS MATERIAL

Clinical Significance

Crystals and **amorphous** (shapeless and formless) microcrystalline deposits are often the most apparent constituents seen in the urinary sediment. They may be strikingly beautiful, especially when viewed with polarized or compensated polarized light. However, they are also the least important of the urine sediment constituents normally encountered. They represent a nuisance as they distract from more important pathologic findings, such as cells and casts, which might be obscured or overlooked by their presence. The use of a supravital stain and phase contrast microscopy is helpful in visualizing these more important constituents. Rarely, pathologic crystal forms may be present in the urine sediment, and these must be recognized. Crystals and amorphous material represent what is sometimes referred to as the **unorganized** urine sediment.

The presence of crystals in the urine sediment is called **crystalluria**. As the urine cools to room temperature or is refrigerated, many specimens will become cloudy or show some lack of clarity, because of the precipitation of crystals and amorphous materials. Generally, crystals are important only when present in urine when voided (at body temperature). Clinical importance is limited, although the presence of crystals may imply the chemical composition of urinary **calculi** (stones) in cases of **lithiasis** (kidney stone formation). However, stone formation may exist without the presence of crystals in the urine, as do crystals without stone formation. Abnormal forms may indicate metabolic disorders, such as the presence of cystine crystals in the urine of persons with cystinuria, an inherited metabolic condition. Finally crystals of some drugs used in medication (such as sulfonamides), especially in high dosage, may precipitate and be found in the urine. These should be recognized since their presence may reflect renal damage caused by blockage if they precipitate in the kidney tubules. Other drugs may cause allergic reactions and should be discontinued to prevent renal damage. These allergic reactions are associated with the presence of eosinophils, and crystalluria is unlikely.

Crystals precipitate out of solution when the salt concentration in solution (in this case, the urine) is greater than the solubility threshold for that salt. It should be apparent, therefore, that crystals are more likely to be found in a more concentrated urine specimen as reflected by specific gravity. However, it should be remembered that certain crystals in the urine, such as radiographic media, do not ionize; therefore the specific gravity by reagent strip may be relatively low, whereas the specific gravity by refractometer is extremely high (>1.035).

Crystal forms encountered in the urine are usually classified as being **normal** or **abnormal**. These are further subclassified as normal **acid crystals** (crystals seen in normal urine of an acidic pH), normal **alkaline crystals** (crystals seen in normal urine of an alkaline pH), **abnormal crystals** of metabolic origin, and abnormal crystals of **iatrogenic** origin. Iatrogenic refers to crystals that result from medication or treatment—that is, inadvertently caused by the physician. Crystals are summarized in Box 6-2 and arranged in approximately the order of importance or frequency in which they are encountered.

Crystals are usually identified on the basis of morphology. The identification is aided by knowledge of the urinary pH. This is because certain forms are seen in urine of an acidic pH (generally 6.5 or less), whereas others are associated with urine of an alkaline pH (generally 7.0 or more). Although pH 7 is neutral, crystals present in urine of pH 7 are generally normal alkaline crystal forms.

Normal crystals are generally reported on the basis of morphology alone. They are observed with low-power and high-power objectives (depending on size) and usually reported as few, moderate, or many per high-power field. It should be understood that it is shape, not size, that is considered for a given crystal form, although some crystals are typically large or small. Color of the urine specimen itself and the microscopic view of the crystal are also helpful. In some uncertain situations, solubility in heat, acids, or alkalis is considered, as shown in Table 6-1.

The abnormal crystals may represent serious pathology and generally require confirmation before they are reported to the clinician. They are observed under low and high power (depending on size) and enumerated and reported as average number per low-power field. This confirmation may be a chemical test, such as a

---

Box 6-2

CRYSTALS FOUND IN THE URINE SEDIMENT

Normal Acid Crystals
Amorphous urates
Uric acid
Acid urates
Monosodium urate or sodium urates
Calcium oxalate (also neutral and alkaline urine)

Normal Alkaline Crystals
Amorphous phosphates
Triple phosphates
Ammonium biurate
Calcium phosphate
Calcium carbonate

Abnormal Crystals of Metabolic Origin
Cystine
Tyrosine
Leucine
Cholesterol
Bilirubin
Hemosiderin

Abnormal Crystals of Iatrogenic Origin (Drugs)
Sulfonamides
Ampicillin
Radiographic contrast media
Acyclovir

Table 6-1

NORMAL CRYSTALS IN THE URINE SEDIMENT: DESCRIPTION AND COMMON SOLUBILITIES

Crystal	pH	Color	Shape	Heat	Alkali (10% NaOH)	Acetic Acid (Glacial)
Normal Acid Crystals						
Amorphous urates (Na, K, Mg, Ca) (common)	Acid	Pink or red	Amorphous (are very small crystals)	Soluble at 60° C	Soluble	Changed to uric acid
Uric acid (common)	Acid (low)	Yellow or red-brown (rarely, colorless hexagons)	Large variety— rhombic, rosettes, 4-sided plates, "whetstones" lemon-shaped	Soluble at 60° C	Soluble	Insoluble
Acid urates (Na, K, NH₄) (uncommon)	Acid (or neutral)	Brown	Small spheres, clusters, resemble biurates	Soluble at 60° C		Changed to uric acid
Monosodium urate (uncommon)	Acid	Colorless	Slender needles or amorphous ppt.			
Calcium oxalate (dihydrate) (common)	Acid or alkaline	Colorless	Octahedral, "envelopes"			Insoluble (soluble dilute HC1)
Calcium oxalate (monohydrate) (uncommon)	Acid or alkaline	Colorless	Oval, ovoid rectangle, dumbbell			
Normal Alkaline Crystals						
Amorphous phosphates (Mg, Ca) (common)	Alkaline	Colorless	Amorphous granules	Insoluble		Soluble
Triple phosphate (NH₄, Mg) (common)	Alkaline or neutral	Colorless	3 to 6 sided prisms— "coffin lids" (common) flat, fern-leaf, sheets, flakes (less common)			Soluble
Calcium phosphate (uncommon)	Alkaline	Colorless	Slender prisms with 1 wedgelike end, often in rosettes, flat plate (rare)	Insoluble		Soluble
Ammonium biurate (common in "old urine")	Alkaline	Dark yellow or brown —like uric acid/urates	Spheres or "thorn apples"	Soluble 60° C with acid		Slowly change to uric acid
Calcium carbonate (uncommon)	Alkaline	Colorless	Tiny spheres in pairs or fours (crosses)			Soluble effervesces

Modified from Schumann GB, Schweitzer SC: *Examination of urine*. In Henry JB, ed: *Clinical diagnosis and management by laboratory methods*, ed 18, Philadelphia, 1991, WB Saunders, p. 429-430.

diazo reaction used for the sulfonamides or a cyanide nitroprusside reaction for **cystine**. In addition, knowledge of medications or procedures such as intravenous pyelograms in cases of suspected radiographic media will help to confirm an abnormal crystal form. Common confirmatory tests are included in Table 6-2.

Normal Acid Crystals

These are crystals that might be encountered in normal urine of an acidic pH. In most cases, if the urine is of pH 6.5 or less, crystalline deposits are some form of uric acid or calcium oxalate. Uric acid is an especially pleomorphic crystal; thus, when unusual crystal forms are encountered, they are often found to consist of uric acid or a salt of this acid. Unfortunately most of the abnormal crystals of drugs or medications are also associated with an acidic pH and these must be ruled out before unusual forms are assumed to be a form of uric acid.

Amorphous Urates. Concentrated urine of an acidic pH is often found to contain amorphous urates, especially when cooled to room temperature or refrigerated. These are often seen in the concentrated urine associated with dehydration and fever.

Amorphous means without shape or form, and amorphous urates are a salt of uric acid (sodium, potassium, magnesium, or calcium). The urates are generally yellow-red or red-brown in color and are seen as a shapeless granulation of very small microcrystals that polarize light if present in sufficient numbers (Fig. 6-183).

When sufficient urates are present, the urine specimen is characteristically highly colored (amber) and shows a fluffy precipitate that is sometimes referred to as "brick dust." The gross appearance of the urine may be mistaken for blood, but the nature of the precipitate is quite different—fluffy and pink or orange (like ground-up red construction bricks)—rather than the characteristic red button seen with red blood cells.

When the urine specimen is neutral or alkaline, amorphous deposits are amorphous phosphates. These are microscopically indistinguishable from amorphous urates, although the gross appearance is of a white precipitate. Although pH is usually sufficient in making this distinction, reactions with heat and acid differ. Amorphous urates will dissolve when the sediment or urine-containing tube is heated to 60° C in a hot water bath. Urates will change to uric acid when acidified with glacial acetic acid (Fig. 6-184). They are soluble in 10% sodium hydroxide but change to ammonium biurate when treated with ammonium hydroxide.

Uric Acid. Together with amorphous urates, uric acid crystals are the most common form of crystalline material seen in normal urine of an acidic pH. To be

Figure 6-183

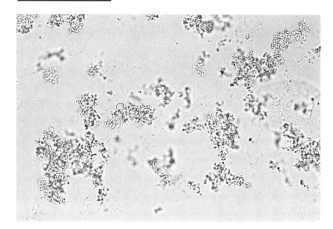

Amorphous urates, ×400.

Figure 6-184

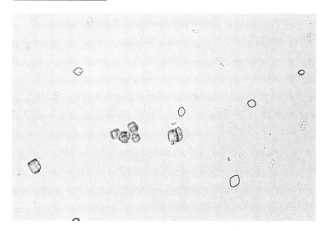

Amorphous urates converted to uric acid with acetic acid, ×400.

present as a crystal of uric acid, the pH usually needs to be less than pH 6. Although of little clinical significance, the presence of urates or uric acid and elevated serum uric acid may be associated with gout. When large numbers are seen together with evidence of epithelial injury of the kidney, such as the presence of renal epithelial cells and epithelial cell casts, they may indicate stone formation and gouty nephropathy. Most urine specimens will eventually precipitate out crystals of uric acid if allowed to remain at room temperature for sufficient time.

They are pathologic only when seen in fresh urine immediately after it is voided. The uric acid concentration in urine depends on dietary intake of purines and breakdown of nucleic acids. For this reason, large amounts of urates or uric acid are often seen in patients with leukemia or lymphoma receiving chemotherapy.

Beside being the most common crystal seen in acidic urine, uric acid is the most varied morphologically. It is troublesome in that it may assume a form that mimics most of the abnormal crystals also seen in acidic urine. Uric acid crystals are typically colored either yellow or reddish brown, but colorless forms may also be seen. They are often seen as a four-sided plate or "whetstone," which may be relatively thin or thick and laminate (Fig. 6-185 and Fig. 6-186). These may be turned into rosettes. Rhombic plates or prisms (Fig. 6-187 and 6-188), barrel-shaped forms (Fig. 6-189), thick cubes, oval forms with pointed lemon-shaped ends (Fig. 6-190), and wedges are also seen. Occasionally colorless hexagonal (six-sided) forms resembling cystine are seen (Fig. 6-191, *A* and *B*). Other rare forms encountered are shown in Figs. 6-192 and 6-193, *A* and *B*.

Uric acid is strongly birefringent and gives a beautiful play of colors when viewed with polarized and compensated polarized light, as shown in Figs. 6-191, B and 6-193, B). Like urates, uric acid is soluble at 60° C and in 10% sodium hydroxide. However, it is insoluble in glacial acetic acid.

Acid Urates. These are an uncommon form of uric acid seen in acidic or neutral urine. They may be sodium, potassium, or ammonium urates and are small brown spheres or clusters that resemble ammonium **biurate** (ammonium urate). They are often seen in urine together with amorphous urates appearing as larger forms of the amorphous granules and have no special or additional significance. They might be mistaken for sulfamethoxazole and are important to recognize for this reason (Fig. 6-194, *A* and *B*).

Like amorphous urates and uric acid, acid urates are soluble at 60° C and in 10% sodium hydroxide and changed to uric acid with glacial acetic acid (Fig. 6-195, *A* and *B*).

Figure 6-185

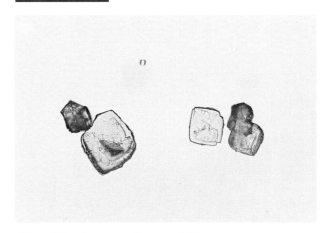

Uric acid, whetstone shape, ×160.

Figure 6-186

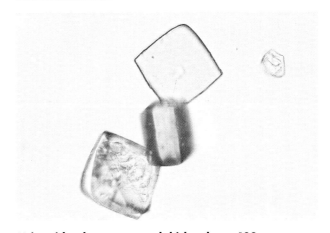

Uric acid, whetstones, and thick cube, ×400.

Figure 6-187

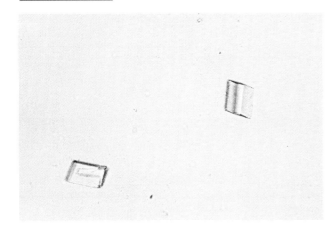

Uric acid, as rhombic prisms, ×400.

Figure 6-188

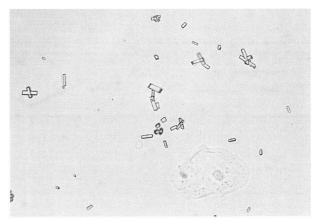

Uric acid, tiny rectangles or rhomboids, ×400.

Figure 6-189

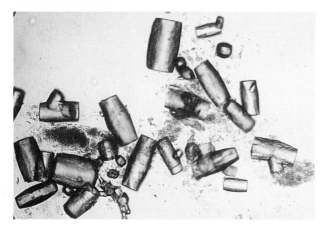

Uric acid, large, barrel-shaped, ×100

Figure 6-190

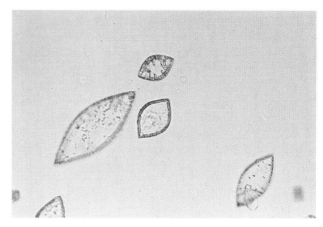

Uric acid, large, lemon-shaped, ×400.

Figure 6-191

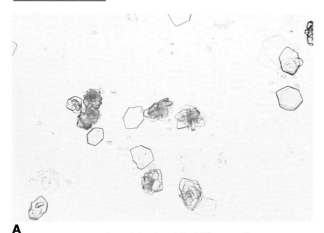

A

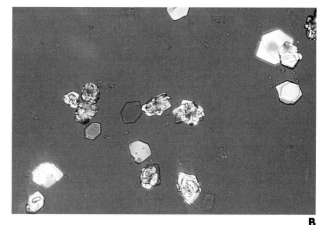

B

Uric acid, six-sided like cystine, ×160. **A,** Brightfield. **B,** Compensated polarized light showing strongly birefringent (polarizing) crystals.

Monosodium Urate or Sodium Urates. These are another uncommon form of uric acid seen in acid urine. Monosodium urates are the form of uric acid seen in the synovial fluid in cases of gout. If present in the urine, they appear as slender, colorless needles (Fig. 6-196). They may also be seen as an amorphous precipitate, part of the amorphous urates.

Calcium Oxalate. The other normal crystal seen in normal urine of an acidic pH is calcium oxalate. Although usually classified as a normal acid crystal, calcium oxalate may also be seen in neutral and alkaline urine. It may be present as a dihydrate or monohydrate of calcium oxalate. The dihydrate form is common and easily recognized. The monohydrate form is uncommon and may be confused with red blood cells or other forms.

Figure 6-192

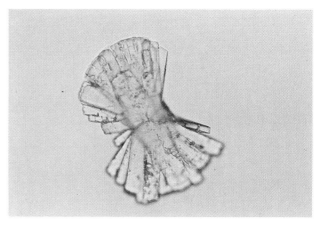

Uric acid, rare form, ×400.

Figure 6-193

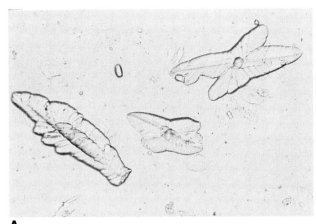
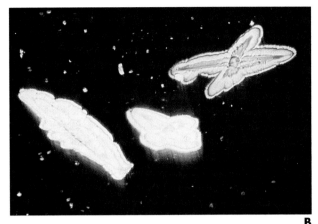

A

B

Uric acid, very unusual star-shaped form, ×160. **A**, Brightfield. **B**, Polarized light, showing strong birefringence.

Figure 6-194

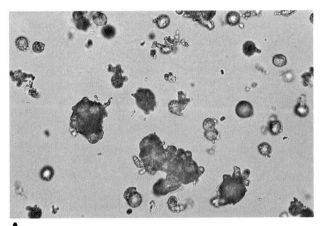
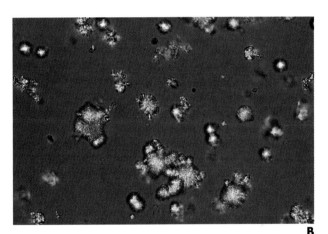

A

B

Acid urates, like ammonium biurate and sulfonamides (sulfamethoxazole), ×400. **A**, Brightfield. **B**, Compensated polarized light showing strong birefringence.

Figure 6-195

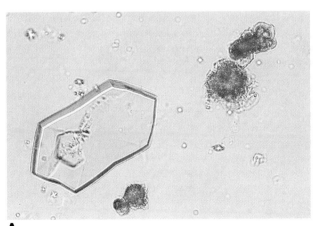
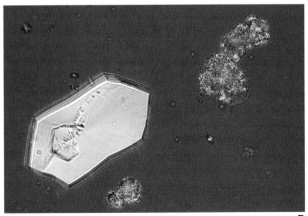

A

B

Acid urates from Fig. 6-194 converted to uric acid with acetic acid, ×400. **A**, Brightfield. **B**, Compensated polarized light.

Figure 6-196

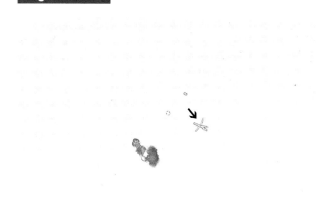

Monosodium urate, tiny needles or rod-shaped crystals (*arrow*), ×400.

Figure 6-197

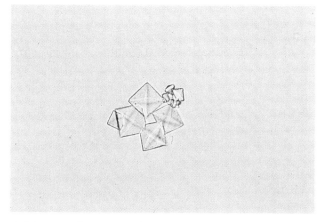

Calcium oxalate, typical envelope shape (octahedral), ×400.

Figure 6-198

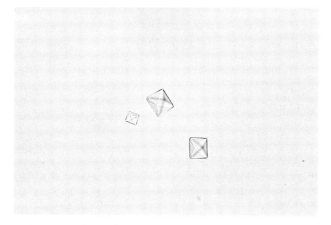

Calcium oxalate, three typical octahedrals, ×160.

The presence of calcium oxalate crystals without other symptoms is of little clinical significance. However, when associated with symptoms of lithiasis, the crystals may give indirect evidence of the composition of urinary stones. Most urinary stones contain calcium, and about 75% are composed of calcium oxalate.[2] The presence of large typical calcium oxalate crystals in clusters may be associated with stone formation. There also is a correlation between calcium stones and excess oxalate and uric acid in the urine. Uric acid may provide the nidus for stone formation. Excess oxalate may result from ingestion of foodstuffs containing oxalic acid such as spinach and rhubarb. Excessive ingestion of Vitamin C may result in increased formation of calcium oxalate crystals, since oxalic acid is a breakdown product of ascorbic acid. Calcium oxalate crystals may also be seen in cases of ethylene glycol or methoxyflurane poisoning.

Calcium oxalate (dihydrate) is typically seen as a colorless octahedron—an eight-sided form that may be thought of as two four-sided pyramids joined at the base, as shown in Figs. 6-197 and 6-198. These have been described as envelopes, or squares with a cross. They vary somewhat in size but are typically small, colorless, glistening octahedrons. Large forms may also be seen. Occasionally, they may be seen as rectangular forms with pyramidal ends (Fig. 6-199, *A* and *B*).

Occasionally, calcium oxalate is present as a monohydrate. This is seen as an ovoid, oval, or dumbbell form that is usually a very small crystal. The ovoid shape is troublesome, since the size and shape are essentially like a red blood cell. It may be distinguished by its ability to polarize light, as shown in Fig. 6-200, *A*, *B*, and *C*. All forms of calcium oxalate are strongly birefringent when viewed with polarized and compensated polarized light. This fact is helpful in distin-

guishing unusual forms of calcium oxalate from possible red cells or other cells that do not polarize light.

Large ovoid forms of calcium oxalate monohydrate have been associated with ethylene glycol (antifreeze) poisoning. These are shown in Fig. 6-201, *A* and *B*.

Normal Alkaline Crystals

These are the crystals that might be encountered in normal urine of an alkaline pH (generally pH 7.0 and above). They are generally a phosphate or calcium-containing crystal, although the alkaline counterpoint of uric acid, ammonium biurate, is also seen. Phosphates in general have little significance clinically. They are associated with an alkaline pH and infection.

Amorphous Phosphates. The amorphous material seen in urine of an alkaline pH are amorphous phosphates. These cannot be distinguished from amor-

Figure 6-199

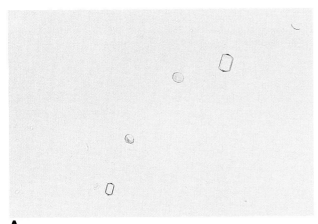

A

B

Calcium oxalate, elongated with pyramidal end, plus two red blood cells, ×400.
A, Brightfield. B, Compensated polarized light. Note that the red cells do not
polarize light.

Figure 6-200

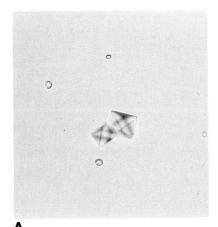
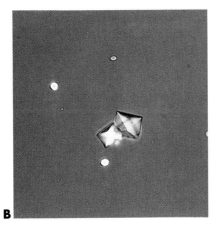
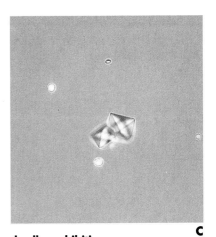

A

B

C

Calcium oxalate, typical and oval forms appearing like red blood cells, exhibiting
strong birefringence with polarized and compensated polarized light, ×400.
A, Brightfield. B, Polarized light. C, Compensated polarized light.

Figure 6-201

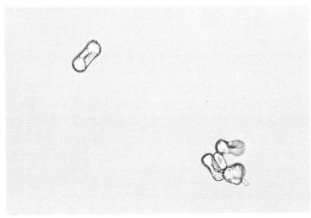
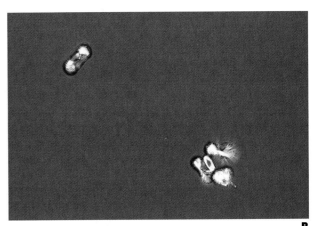

A

B

Calcium oxalate, rare large ovoid form of a type associated with ethylene glycol
poisoning, ×400. A, Brightfield. B, Compensated polarized light.

Figure 6-202

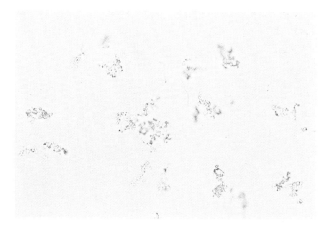

Amorphous phosphates, seen as a fine, lacy precipitate difficult to distinguish from bacteria, ×400.

Figure 6-203

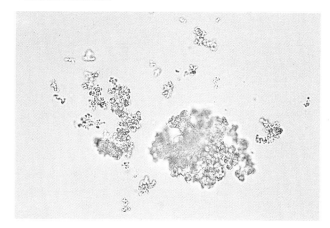

Amorphous phosphates, ×400.

Figure 6-204

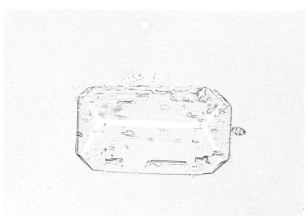

A
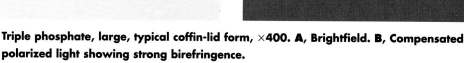
B

Triple phosphate, large, typical coffin-lid form, ×400. **A,** Brightfield. **B,** Compensated polarized light showing strong birefringence.

phous urates microscopically, although phosphates lack color and tend to be seen as a finer, more lacy precipitate (Fig. 6-202 and 6-203). Unlike urates, phosphates are insoluble when heated to 60° C and dissolve when treated with acetic acid and dilute hydrochloric acid.

Amorphous phosphates, seen as a fluffy white precipitate, are a common cause of cloudiness in alkaline urine. They appear like, and are often seen with, bacteria. Care must be taken not to overlook bacteria when they are present. Supravital stain and phase or interference contrast microscopy will usually make this distinction apparent. Unfortunately, polarized microscopy is not helpful in distinguishing phosphates from bacteria, since phosphates usually fail to polarize light.

Triple Phosphates. Crystals of triple (ammonium magnesium) phosphate (also referred to as struvite)

are a striking finding when seen in the urine sediment. Although relatively common, the occurrence of triple phosphate crystals is of limited clinical significance. However, 10 to 20% of urinary stones contain struvite resulting from infection with urease-positive bacteria.[2] Thus stones consisting of struvite have been referred to as infection stones.

Morphologically, triple phosphate appears as a colorless crystal of a characteristic three- to six-sided prism referred to as a coffin lid, as seen in Fig. 6-204, *A* and *B*. They vary greatly in size from tiny to relatively huge crystals; large forms are common. Various shapes are seen in Fig. 6-205, *A* and *B*. Triple phosphates are birefringent when viewed with polarized or compensated polarized light. Long prism forms may be difficult to distinguish from calcium phosphate (Fig. 6-206). They have similar clinical significance and either may be reported as phosphates.

Figure 6-205

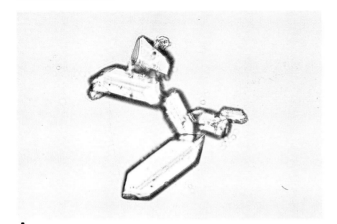 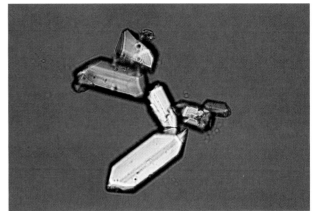

A   B

Triple phosphate, various forms, ×400. A, Brightfield. B, Compensated polarized light, showing birefringence.

Occasionally, an unusual fern-leaf form of triple phosphate is seen. These occur when the typical forms dissolve into solution (Fig. 6-207).

Triple phosphates are soluble in acetic acid.

Ammonium Biurate. These crystals are very rarely seen in a freshly voided urine specimen; however, they are often present in old specimens, especially those that have been retained for the purpose of teaching students or staff members. Ammonium biurate, also called ammonium urate, is the alkaline counterpoint of uric acid, and like uric acid and amorphous urates, tends to precipitate as the urine stands or is stored.

Ammonium biurates are dark yellow or brown in color, like uric acid. They are seen as spheres with radial or concentric striations, often with long prismatic spicules referred to as "thorn apples," as shown in Figs. 6-208, 6-209, and 6-210, *A* and *B*.

Biurates are important in that they may be mistaken for certain forms of sulfonamides, especially sulfamethoxazole (see Figs. 6-226 and 6-227). However, biurates are seen in alkaline urine, and the sulfonamides are usually limited to urine of an acidic pH. Very rare exceptions may occur.

Like other urates and uric acid, ammonium biurates are soluble at 60° C and will eventually convert to uric acid when treated with concentrated hydrochloric acid or glacial acetic acid.

Calcium Phosphate. These colorless crystals are uncommon in normal alkaline urine. Calcium monohydrogen phosphate is also known as *brushite* and *hydroxyapatite.* Calcium phosphates are typically a slender prism with a wedge-like end occurring either singly or arranged in rosettes (Figs. 6-211 and 6-212, *A* and *B*). They may appear like and with triple phosphate crystals as elongated lath-shaped brushite crystals and have similar clinical significance. Calcium phosphates are weakly birefringent when viewed with

Figure 6-206

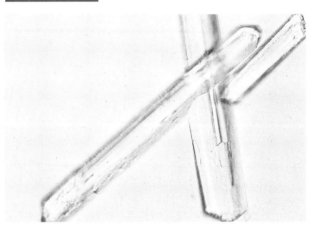

Triple phosphate, large long prisms appeaing like calcium phosphate, ×400.

Figure 6-207

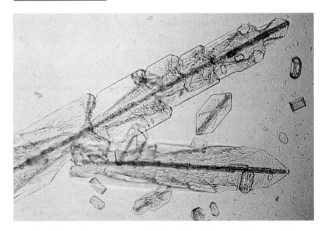

Triple phosphate, unusual fern-leaf form of crystals going into solution, ×400.

Figure 6-208

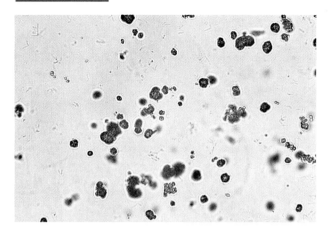

Ammonium biurates and bacteria, ×400.

Figure 6-209

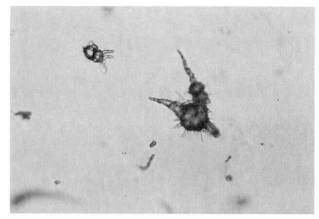

Ammonium biurate, large "thorn apples," ×400.

Figure 6-210

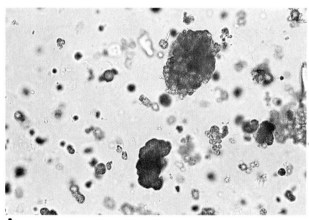

A

B

Ammonium biurates, like sulfonamides, and acid urates, ×400. **A,** Brightfield.
B, Compensated polarized light showing strong birefringence.

polarized and compensated polarized light. They may be mistaken for certain forms of sulfonamides, also seen as long slender prisms or needles. However, these particular sulfonamides are rarely clinically used and are associated with an acidic urine pH.

Flat plate-like forms of calcium phosphate have also been described. These are rare and may be mistaken for large degenerating squamous epithelial cells (Fig. 6-213).

Calcium phosphate, as other phosphates, is insoluble when heated to 60° C, slightly soluble in dilute acetic acid, and soluble in dilute hydrochloric acid.

Calcium Carbonate. Crystals of calcium carbonate are another crystalline form uncommon in normal urine of an alkaline pH. They are typically tiny colorless spheres or granules that occur in pairs or fours and are seen as small crosses (Fig. 6-214).

These tiny forms are of little clinical significance. They appear like—and are probably mistaken for—

Figure 6-211

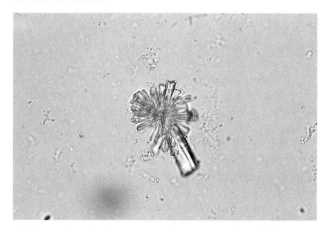

Calcium phosphate, arranged as a rosette, ×400.

Figure 6-212

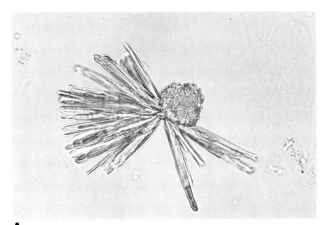

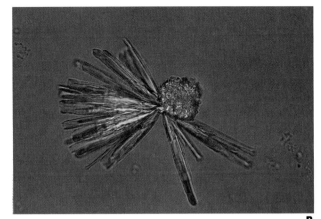

A

B

Calcium phosphate, slender prisms arranged in a rosette, ×400. A, Brightfield. B, Compensated polarized light showing weak birefringence.

amorphous phosphates, of which they might be part. They are morphologically very similar to the dumbbell form of calcium oxalate. Unlike phosphates, both calcium carbonate and calcium oxalate are strongly birefringent when viewed with polarized and compensated polarized light.

Calcium carbonate crystals are soluble in acetic acid and show effervescence as carbon dioxide is released. This may be demonstrated by adding glacial acetic acid to a small amount of sediment in a small test tube to produce bubbling. Or, acetic acid may be flowed under the coverslip of the wet preparation to form bubbles.

Abnormal Urinary Crystals–Introduction

With only a few, very rare exceptions, the abnormal crystals encountered in the urinary sediment are seen in urine specimens of an acid pH—6.5 or less. As already mentioned, the normal crystals may be reported on the basis of morphology or microscopic evidence, together with the urine pH. However, abnormal crystalline forms require further confirmation. Whenever possible, this should be chemical confirmation; however, a history of medications or treatment procedures may be the only possible confirmation. Appropriate confirmation is included in Box 6-2 and the descriptions that follow. Like casts, they are reported as the number seen per average low-power field.

Abnormal crystals may be further classified as being of metabolic (physiologic) or iatrogenic origin (Table 6-2). The abnormal crystals of metabolic origin are the result of certain disease states or inherited metabolic conditions. Abnormal crystals of metabolic (physiologic) origin include cystine, tyrosine, leucine, cholesterol, bilirubin, and hemosiderin. Abnormal crystals of iatrogenic origin are the result of medication or treatment,

Figure 6-213

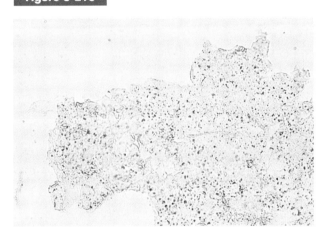

Calcium phosphate plate. Sedi-Stain, ×400.

Figure 6-214

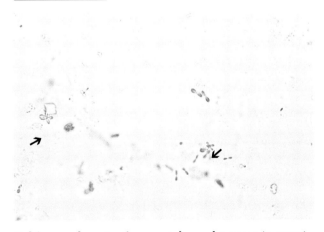

Calcium carbonate, tiny crystals, and crosses (*arrows*), ×400.

Table 6-2

ABNORMAL CRYSTALS IN THE URINE SEDIMENT: DESCRIPTION AND CONFIRMATORY TESTS

Crystal	pH	Color	Shape	Confirmatory Test
Crystals of Physiologic (Metabolic) Origin				
Cystine (most common physiologic/ abnormal crystals)	Acid	Colorless	Transparent, usually refractile six-sided plates. May polarize (depending on thickness)	Cyanide nitroprusside reaction—red purple color
Tyrosine (rare)	Acid	Colorless (usually appear black w/focusing)	Fine silky needles arranged in sheaves or rosettes usually occur with leucine	Nitrosonaphthol test— orange color
Leucine (extremely rare)	Acid	Yellow	Oily-appearing spheres with radical and concentric striations usually occur with tyrosine	Amino acid separation
Cholesterol (rare)	Acid or neutral	Colorless	Flat plate with corner notch (seen with large proteinuria and after refrigeration)	
Bilirubin (uncommon)	Acid	Reddish brown	Amorphous needles, rhombic plates or cubes; may color uric acid crystals	
Hemosiderin	Acid or neutral	Golden brown	Granules, in clumps, in cells, casts	Blue with Prussian blue reaction (Rous Test)
Crystals of Iatrogenic Origin (Drugs)				
Sulfonamides (most common drugs seen)	Acid	Yellow to brown	Various—depends on the drug. Mimics various forms of uric acid/urates/biurates.	For all forms: Hydrolyze with heat and acid. Apply diazo reaction— magenta color.
Acetylsulfa- diazine	Acid	Yellow-brown	Sheaves of wheat with eccentric bindings	
Sulfadiazine	Acid	Brown	Dense globules	
Acetylsulfa- methoxazole	Acid	Brown	Dense spheres or irregularly divided spheres	
Ampicillin (Penicillins)	Acid	Colorless	Long slender needles, form clusters. Sheaves after refrigeration.	
Radiographic media (meglumine diatrizoate)	Acid	Colorless	Flat plates, some with corner notch like cholesterol; elongated crystals	Specific gravity >1.035 False-positive SSA protein test
Acyclovir (rare)	Alkaline (7.5)	Colorless	Fine slender needles	Infrared analysis and/or clinical history

Note: Abnormal crystals must be confirmed by chemical test or clinical history before reporting.

Modified from Schumann GB, Schweitzer SC: *Examination of urine.* In Henry JB, ed: *Clinical diagnosis and management by laboratory methods*, ed 18, Philadelphia, 1991, WB Saunders, p 429-430.

Figure 6-215

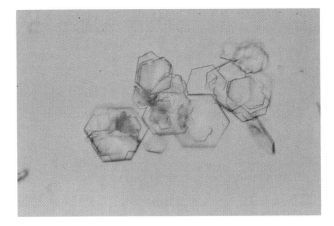

Cystine, thin colorless hexagons with laminations, ×640.

Figure 6-216

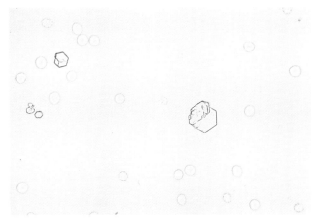

Cystine crystals and red blood cells, ×400.

Figure 6-217

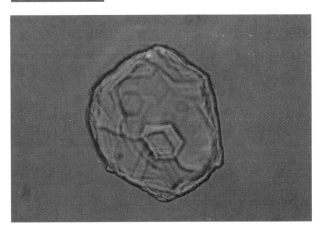

Cystine, relatively thin crystal that does not polarize light. Cytospin, Wright's stain, compensated polarized light, ×1000.

Figure 6-218

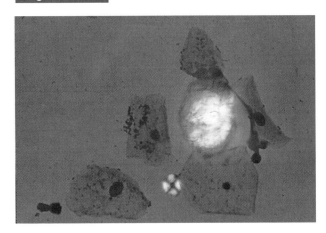

Cystine, relatively thick crystal that polarizes light. Also present, squamous epithelial cells, starch granule, and yeast. Cytospin, Wright's stain, compensated polarized light, ×400.

inadvertently caused by the physician. Examples include various sulfonamides, ampicillin, radiographic contrast media, and acyclovir (Table 6-2).

Abnormal Crystals of Metabolic Origin

Cystine. Crystals of cystine are probably the most important of the abnormal crystals of physiologic origin found in the urine. They may be seen in the urine of patients with cystinuria, inherited amino acid transport disorder affecting cystine, ornithine, lysine, and arginine. Of these, only cystine crystals are seen in the urine. Patients with cystinuria are apt to form cystine stones, which may cause kidney damage. Although cystine stones represent less than 1% of all kidney stones, they are important pathologically. Unlike stones consisting primarily of calcium oxalate, cystine stones (also struvite and uric acid stones) may fill the renal collecting system, resulting in **staghorn calculi.** These are particularly damaging, causing renal stasis and shutdown and require removal by shock-wave lithotripsy or surgery, since the calculi are too large to be passed by the patient.

Cystine crystals are colorless and show a characteristic refractile, hexagonal (six-sided) plate, which is often laminated (Fig. 6-215 and 6-216). The ability to polarize light depends on the thickness of the crystal. The thin form will not polarize light, but thicker crystals will, as shown in Figs. 6-217 and 6-218.

Cystine crystals may be confused with a colorless, hexagonal form of uric acid seen in Fig. 6-191. Like uric acid, cystine crystals are most insoluble at an acid pH. However, they remain insoluble until pH 7.4. They are soluble in dilute hydrochloric acid and alkali (especially ammonia) and are destroyed by the presence of bacteria with formation of ammonia. They are insoluble in acetic acid, alcohol, ether, and boiling water.

CYSTINE CONFIRMATORY TEST: NITROPRUSSIDE REACTION

Reagents:

Ammonium hydroxide, 10%
Dilute 17 mL concentrated ammonium hydroxide to 100 mL with distilled or deionized water.

Sodium cyanide, 5% (w/v)
Dissolve 5 g sodium cyanide in distilled or deionized water and dilute to 100 mL. Add 200 μL 28% ammonium hydroxide (1:2 dilution of concentrated ammonium hydroxide, as a preservative).

Sodium nitroprusside (sodium nitroferricyanide), 5% (w/v)
Dissolve 0.5 g finely crushed sodium nitroprusside crystals in distilled or deionized water and dilute to 10 mL. Stable 1 week at 2° C-8° C.

Procedure:

1. Place 3-4 drops of urine sediment in a small test tube.

2. Add 1 drop 10% ammonium hydroxide.

3. Add 1 drop 5% sodium cyanide: wait 5 minutes.

4. Add 2-3 drops 5% sodium nitroprusside.

5. Read immediately.

Positive Result: A stable beet-red (red-purple) color. Color may fade to orange-red upon standing.

Confirmation of cystine may be done with the cyanide-nitroprusside reaction. In this reaction, cystine is reduced to cysteine by sodium cyanide. The resulting free sulfhydryl group will react with nitroprusside to give a red purple color. (Procedure 6-2).

Tyrosine. Tyrosine crystals in urine are rare but may occasionally be seen (together with leucine) in urine from patients with severe liver disease. Tyrosine is also associated with hereditary tyrosinosis and oasthouse disease.

Tyrosine crystals are colorless needles that usually appear black as the microscope is focused. They are fine, silky needles, which are usually arranged in sheaves or rosettes (Fig. 6-219).

Tyrosine is seen in urine of an acidic pH. It is soluble in alkali, dilute mineral acids, and, relatively, in heat. It is insoluble in alcohol and ether. Chemical confirmation may be done with the nitrosonaphthol test; positive reactions are seen as an orange color.

Leucine. These are extremely rare. They are associated with severe liver disease and certain rare hereditary disorders of amino acid metabolism and seen together with tyrosine.

Leucines are described as yellow, oily-looking spheres with radial and concentric striations that may be found in urine of an acidic pH. It is said to be birefringent and seen as a pseudo Maltese cross when viewed with polarized light. Confirmation may be made by amino acid separation by high performance ion exchange liquid chromatography.

Cholesterol. Droplets of cholesterol are seen in the urine as free fat, in renal epithelial cells (oval fat bod-

Figure 6-219

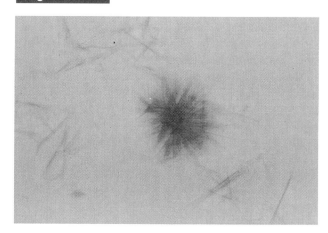

Tyrosine, fine silky needles, ×400.

ies), and fatty casts in cases of nephrotic syndrome and lipoid nephrosis. However, cholesterol crystals or plates are extremely rare in freshly voided urine sediment. They may be seen, rarely, after the specimen has been refrigerated. When they are seen, they have the same significance as the more common globules or droplets of cholesterol ester. When cholesterol crystals are seen alone, especially in large numbers, another drug or crystal should be suspected.

Like most abnormal crystals, cholesterol crystals are associated with urine of an acidic or neutral pH. They are seen as colorless, large, flat, rectangular plates with one or more corners notched out (Figs. 6-220, *A* and *B*, 6-221).

Figure 6-220

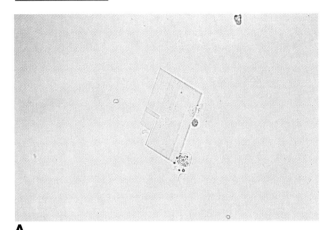

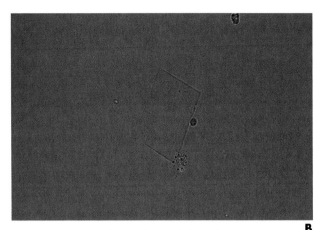

A

B

Cholesterol, large, flat, rectangular with notched corner. Oval fat body, and shrunken, crenated red cell also present, ×400. A, Brightfield. B, Compensated polarized light showing very weak birefringence.

Figure 6-221

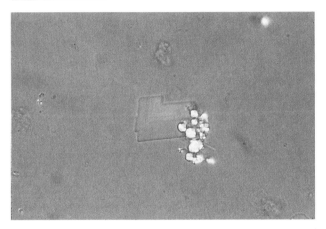

Cholesterol crystal and fat globules showing Maltese cross formation of cholesterol. Compensated polarized light, ×400.

Crystals of cholesterol may be mistaken for radiographic media, such as meglumine diatrizoate used in intravenous pyelograms or other imaging techniques (see Fig. 6-232). These are morphologically similar to cholesterol but are associated with very high specific gravity (>1.035 by refractometer) and a false-positive delayed sulfosalicylic acid test for protein. Whenever large numbers of possible cholesterol crystals are encountered, radiographic media or another drug form clinically unrelated to cholesterol should be suspected. One such crystal without any other evidence of lipiduria is seen in Fig. 6-222, A and B. These crystals were not present in the original urine at room temperature, but precipitated after refrigeration.

Absolute confirmation of cholesterol crystals may be difficult. However, they are very soluble in chloro-

form, ether, and hot alcohol. Their presence is associated with heavy proteinuria, free fat, oval fat bodies, and fatty casts, and they should not be reported in the absence of any of these findings.

Bilirubin. Rarely, crystals of precipitated bilirubin are seen in the urine of patients with bilirubinuria. Their significance is the same as for the chemical detection of bilirubin in the urine. Bilirubin crystals are seen as reddish-brown needles that cluster in clumps, or as spheres (Fig. 6-223).

When present, cells or casts in the sediment will be stained with the bilirubin pigment.

Hemosiderin. Hemosiderin was discussed in the section on renal epithelial cells. However, it is included in this section on abnormal crystals because of the morphologic resemblance to amorphous urates.

Hemosiderin may be seen in acid or neutral urine a few days after a severe intravascular hemolytic episode. Hemosiderin granules are coarse yellow-brown granules that occur as free granules in the urine, in renal epithelial cells or macrophages, or in casts (Fig. 6-224).

Hemosiderin may be confirmed with the Rous Test, a wet Prussian blue stain for iron described in Procedure 6-1 (Fig. 6-225). (See also Figs. 6-75, 6-76, 6-171, 6-172, and 6-173).

Abnormal Crystals of Iatrogenic Origin (Drugs)

Sulfonamides. The presence of sulfonamides in the urine is an important, though iatrogenic, pathologic finding. Many morphologic forms may be encountered, depending on the type of sulfonamide administered. Their importance is due to the likelihood of renal damage as the crystals precipitate in the nephron, causing bleeding (hematuria) and oliguria because of blockage. The physician must be alerted to this crystallization, so

Figure 6-222

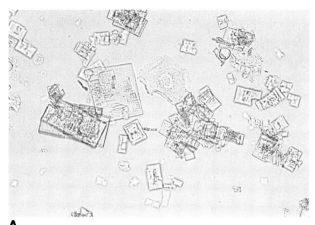

A

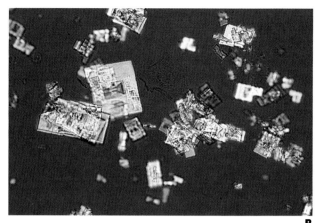

B

Unidentified crystals (probably a drug) appearing like cholesterol after refrigeration of the specimen, ×400. **A,** Brightfield. **B,** Compensated polarized light showing strong birefringence.

Figure 6-223

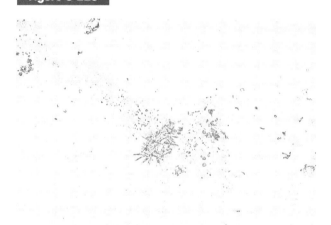

Bilirubin crystals. Cytospin, ×400.

Figure 6-224

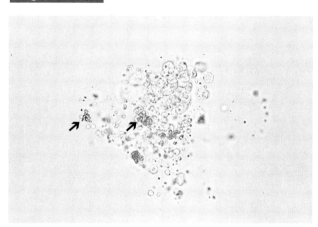

Hemosiderin, yellow brown granules (*arrows*). Unstained, ×400.

that the patient is given sufficient fluid for adequate hydration, and the urine made alkaline to dissolve and keep them in solution. In the past much attention was given to the various forms of sulfonamides that might be encountered in the urine. However, current pharmacology has more soluble forms of sulfonamides. Nevertheless, adequate hydration is essential, and maintenance of an alkaline pH will help prevent precipitation of crystals most insoluble at a very acid pH (5 or less).

The sulfonamides are seen to precipitate at low acid pH. They are generally yellow to brown, but sometimes colorless. Shape varies, and sulfonamides mimic various forms of uric acid, urates, and biurates. They have been seen as colorless needles in sheaves or rosettes, arrowheads or whetstones; as brownish shocks of wheat with central binding or rosettes with radial striations; colorless needles as shocks of wheat with eccentric binding;

colorless to greenish-brown fan-shaped needles; and dense brown or irregularly divided spheres. A few of the more commonly encountered forms that precipitate in the urine will now be described.

SULFAMETHOXAZOLE. The most commonly encountered sulfonamide in urine specimens is acetylsulfamethoazole, which is formulated with trimethoprim and supplied as Bactrim or Septra. These have been seen in the urine after an unusually high dosage. Sulfamethoxazole is seen as a dense brown sphere or irregularly divided sphere (Figs. 6-226, 6-227, *A* and *B*, and 6-228).

ACETYLSULFADIAZINE. This is now a rarely used yet dangerous form of sulfonamide seen as yellow-brown sheaves of wheat with eccentric binding (Fig. 6-229).

SULFADIAZINE. Another rarely used form of sulfonamide, sulfadiazine appears as dense brown globules

Figure 6-225

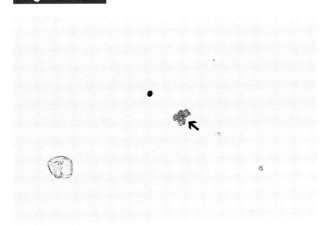

Hemosiderin, blue green granules (*arrow*) stained with Prussian blue stain for iron (positive Rous Test), ×400.

Figure 6-226

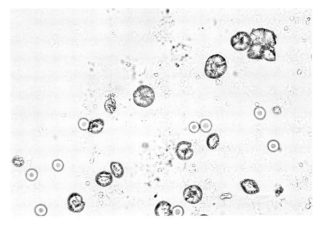

Sulfamethoxazole (Bactrim), and red blood cells, ×400.

Figure 6-227

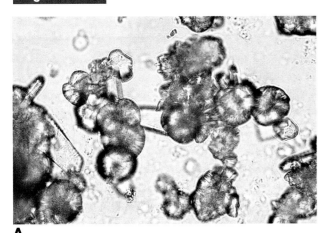

A

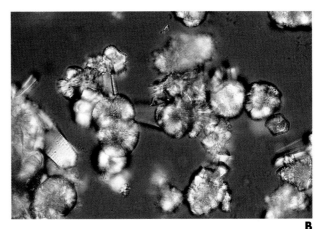

B

Sulfonamide, ×400. A, Brightfield. B, Compensated polarized light showing strong birefringence.

like the crystals in Figs. 6-227, A and B. These are morphologically similar to, and might be confused with, ammonium biurates or acid urates. Although biurates are found in alkaline urine, acid urates are seen in urine of an acid pH.

All forms of sulfonamides may be confirmed by hydrolysis with heat and acid, and application of a diazo reaction (Procedure 6-3).

The Lignin test is not a reliable method of confirmation. Further confirmation may be made by requesting a list of medications administered to the patient.

Ampicillin. Although the penicillins are commonly used antibiotics, they are seldom seen as precipitated crystals in the urine. Rarely, ampicillin crystals may be encountered after administration of high doses, such as in the treatment of bacterial meningitis.

Ampicillin crystals are thin colorless needles that appear in urine of an acidic pH (Fig. 6-230). After the

Figure 6-228

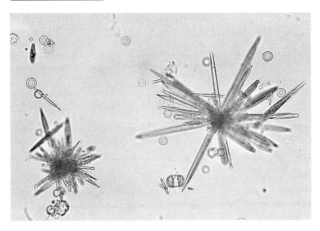

Sulfamethoxazole (Septra) rosette, and red blood cells, ×400.

Procedure 6-3

SULFONAMIDE CONFIRMATORY TEST: DIAZO REACTION

Reagents:

Hydrochloric acid, 10%
Dilute 5 mL concentrated HC1 to 500 mL with distilled or deionized water.

Sodium nitrite, 0.1% (w/v)
Dissolve 0.1 g sodium nitrite in distilled or deionized water; dilute to 100 mL. Stable 2 weeks at 2° C-8° C.

Ammonium sulfamate, 0.5% (w/v)
Dissolve 0.50 g ammonium sulfamate in distilled or deionized water; dilute to 100 mL.

Sulfa dye reagent, 0.1% (w/v)
Dissolve 0.10 g N-(1-naphthyl ethylenediamine dihydrochloride) in distilled or deionized water; dilute to 100 mL.

Procedure

1. Place 3-4 drops of urine sediment in a small test tube.

2. Add 2 drops 10% hydrochloric acid; wait 3 seconds.

3. Add 2 drops 0.1% sodium nitrite; wait 30-60 seconds.

4. Add 2 drops 0.5% ammonium sulfamate.

5. Add 2-3 drops sulfa dye reagent.

6. Read immediately.

Positive result: Magenta color.

Figure 6-229

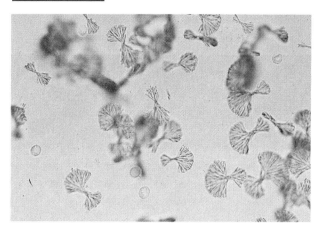

Acetylsulfadiazine, as sheaves of wheat with eccentric binding and red blood cells, ×400.

urine has been refrigerated, the crystals tend to form clusters and sheaves (Fig. 6-231).

Radiographic Contrast Media. Crystals of **radiographic contrast media** such as meglumine diatrizoate (Renografin, Hypaque) may occasionally be seen in the urine of patients for a brief period after injection of these compounds for diagnostic radiographic procedures (see also the sulfosalicylic acid test for urine protein and cholesterol crystals.) Their importance is primarily one of false identification: they may be mistaken for crystals of cholesterol. Occasionally, their presence may be of clinical importance, especially in dehydrated elderly patients who may experience renal blockage from crystalline precipitation.

Crystals of meglumine diatrizoate may be seen in urine as flat rectangular plates, often with a notched corner. They closely resemble cholesterol plates (Fig. 6-232).

They may also occur as long, thin prisms or rectangles. They are strongly birefringent when viewed with polarized and compensated polarized light. The presence of radiographic media should be suspected when many crystals resembling cholesterol plates are seen; the gross urine specimen appears cloudy, and the specific gravity by refractometer is extremely high (greater than 1.035). Since it does not ionize, the specific gravity by reagent strip is unaffected by the presence of radiographic media, however. When present, the urine may show a delayed false-positive sulfosalicylic acid precipitation test for protein. This should not be mistaken for true protein precipitation, as shown in Fig. 6-233 and Fig. 4-1, A-D.

The presence of radiographic media may be confirmed by a clinical history of recent radiographic imaging procedures. This is further confirmed by the observation of an abnormally high specific gravity by refractometer and false-positive sulfosalicylic acid test for protein.

Acyclovir. Other drug forms are occasionally seen in the urine sediment. One of these seen at the University of Minnesota Hospital and Clinic was the antiviral drug acyclovir. Unlike most abnormal crystals seen in acidic urine, these crystals were present in urine at pH 7.5. They were seen as colorless slender needles that polarized light and exhibited negative

Figure 6-230

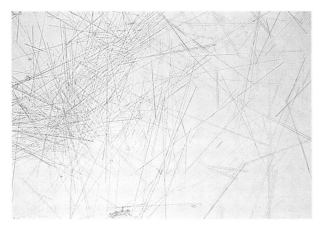

Ampicillin, thin colorless needles, ×100.

Figure 6-231

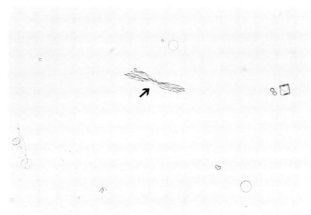

Ampicillin (*arrow*), appearing after refrigeration. Red cells and calcium oxalate also present, ×400.

Figure 6-232

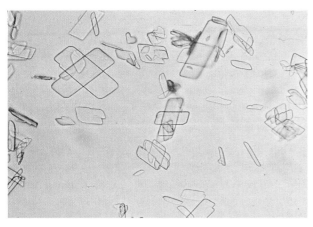

Radiographic contrast media, meglumine diatrizoate (Renografin), appearing somewhat like cholesterol, ×400.

Figure 6-233

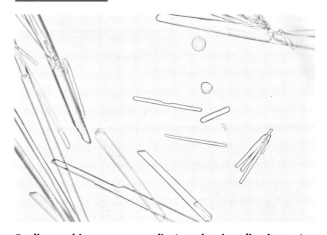

Radiographic contrast media (meglumine diatrizoate) from false-positive sulfosalicylic acid protein precipitation test, ×400.

Figure 6-234

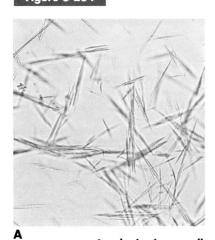

A

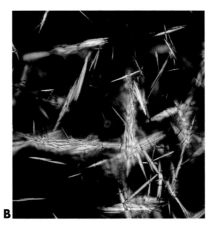

B

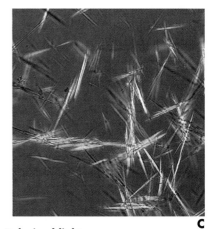

C

Acyclovir, tiny needle-shaped crystals, ×400. **A,** Brightfield. **B,** Polarized light.
C, Compensated polarized light showing strong negative birefringence. (Slow wave orientation north-south).

birefringence, appearing like crystals of monosodium urate in synovial fluid. These are seen in Fig. 6-234, *A, B,* and *C*.

In the case described, the patient had acute lymphocytic leukemia in remission and was treated with high doses of acyclovir for recurrent herpes infections. The acyclovir crystals were confirmed by infrared analysis.

■ CONTAMINANTS AND ARTIFACTS

The presence of various contaminants and artifacts encountered in the urine sediment are most important in that their presence may distract from more important findings. They are most noticed by the inexperienced microscopist, who with experience will ignore them. As a general rule, those structures most apparent at first glance are unimportant.

Starch

Because of the use of barrier protective gloves in all areas of the laboratory and medical care, the presence of granules of **starch** in the urine sediment is common. Starch refers to cornstarch, a carbohydrate commonly used to line surgical or barrier protective gloves. It is sometimes referred to as talc, which was formerly used in surgical gloves. Talc is actually talcum, or hydrated magnesium silicate, a chunky, irregular crystal that is not starch.

Starch is an ubiquitous structure that is easily recognized but must not be confused with globules or droplets of cholesterol, as shown in Fig. 6-71, 6-72, and 6-74. Both cholesterol globules and starch are birefringent and polarize as a Maltese cross (white cross on a black background) when viewed with polarized light and as a beach ball of opposed yellow and blue quadrants when viewed with compensated polarized light. The term beach ball is meant to describe spherulites of urate crystals in synovial fluid. However, similar appearing forms are seen with starch and with cholesterol droplets.[3] Starch is most easily recognized with brightfield microscopy, as shown in Fig. 6-235, *A*. It is seen as an irregular, generally round granule with a central dimple or slit. Even when polarized, the Maltese cross formation produced by starch is more irregular and fuzzy than the very round, regular formation produced by droplets of cholesterol (Fig. 6-235, *B* and *C*).

Fibers (Including Disposable Diaper Fibers)

Contaminants may be introduced into the urine specimen at the time of collection or by laboratory personnel at the time of specimen processing or examination. Cotton threads, wool fibers, synthetic fibers, or hair may enter the urine at the time of collection. They are all highly refractile structures, which should not be mistaken for casts (Figs. 6-236 and 6-237). They are typically large, long, and may be twisted.

The presence of disposable diaper fibers are especially troublesome since they closely resemble waxy casts (Fig. 6-238, *A*). Diaper fibers may be seen in the urine of both infants and incontinent adults and should be suspected when other findings associated with waxy casts, such as protein, are absent. The appearance with polarized light differs. Diaper fibers are birefringent and will polarize light, but waxy casts will not (Figs. 6-238, *B* and *C*).

Figure 6-235

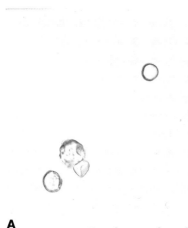 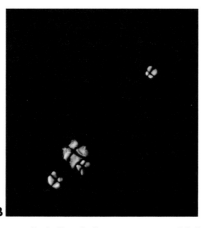 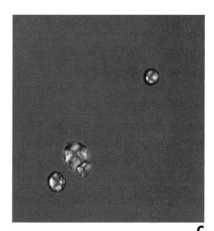

A   B   C

Starch granules, showing typical dimpled appearance with brightfield illumination, unlike cholesterol esters of fat, and Maltese cross formation with polarized and compensated polarized light, ×400. **A,** Brightfield. **B,** Polarized light showing Maltese cross formation and similarity to fat as cholesterol. **C,** Compensated polarized light showing so-called beach-ball appearance (like spherulites of urate crystals in synovial fluid).

Figure 6-236

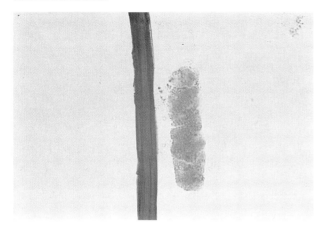

Fiber, probably hair (*left*), waxy cast (*right*), Sedi-Stain, ×400.

Figure 6-237

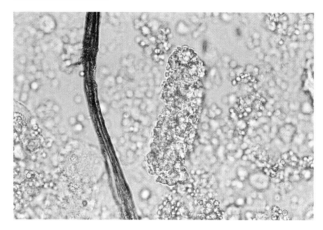

Fiber (*left*), granular cast (*right*), and many yeast, ×400.

Figure 6-238

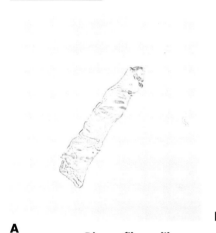 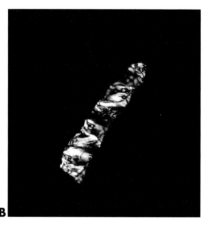 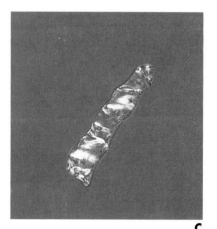

A   C

Diaper fibers, like waxy casts, showing birefrigence with polarized and compensated polarized light, ×400. **A**, Brightfield. **B**, Polarized light. **C**, Compensated polarized light.

Air Bubbles

Air bubbles are introduced in the laboratory as the coverslip is applied to the sediment or sediment introduced into the standardized slide. They are highly refractile and structureless and easily recognized (Figs. 6-239 and 6-240).

Oil Droplets

Oil droplets may be the result of contamination from lubricants such as vaginal creams, catheter lubricant, or mineral oil. They may be confused with red blood cells or fat globules of physiologic origin. Oil droplets are highly refractile and structureless as seen in Fig. 6-241.

Contaminating oil should be distinguished from fat of physiologic origin. Unusual and spectacular fat of probable exogenous origin arranged along fibers is seen in Fig. 6-242, *A* and *B*.

True lipiduria is usually associated with other findings such as proteinuria, fatty casts, and oval fat bodies as described previously. The presence of cholesterol esters that polarize as a Maltese cross will rule out fat from contamination. It is noteworthy that oil may float, both on top of the urine specimen or sediment and onto the underside of the coverglass. This is especially troublesome when standardized slides are employed, as the depth of the preparation is generally greater than with the applied coverslip on a regular microscope method. Therefore, when searching for fat or oil, care should be taken to focus on the underside of the coverglass.

Glass Fragments

Fragments of glass may be seen in the urine sediment, probably from very small pieces of coverglass. These are colorless and highly refractile but are

Figure 6-239

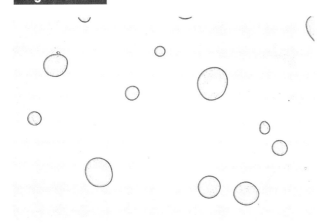

Air bubbles, ×400.

Figure 6-240

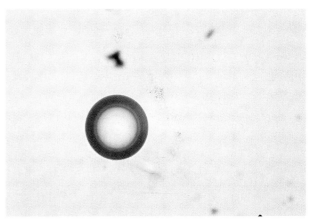

Air bubble, (large), ×400.

Figure 6-241

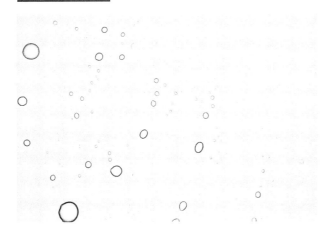

Immersion oil, ×400.

extremely pleomorphic. They may appear like crystals, as shown in Fig. 6-243.

Stains

The various supravital stains used with urinary sediment may precipitate, especially when added to urine of an alkaline pH. This precipitate may be seen as amorphous purple granulation or brown to purple needle-shaped crystals in clusters.

Similarly, Sudan III fat stain may precipitate as clusters of needle-shaped crystals that are bright red or red-orange.

Pollen Grains

These may be seen as a urinary contaminant, especially on a seasonal basis. They are fairly large and regularly shaped with a thick cell wall. They may resemble the eggs of some parasitic worms (Fig. 6-244).

Figure 6-242

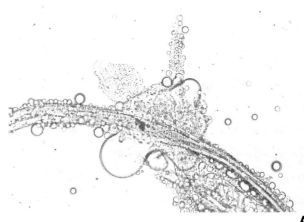

A

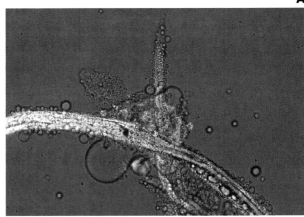

B

Fat of exogenous origin, arranged on fibers, ×400.
A, Brightfield. B, Compensated polarized light.

Fecal Contamination

This is usually the result of contamination of the urine specimen with feces during collection. However, if there is a **fistula** (an abnormal connection) between the

Figure 6-243

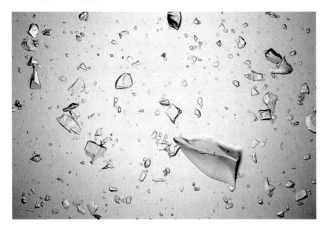

Glass fragments from coverslip, appearing like crystals, ×100.

Figure 6-244

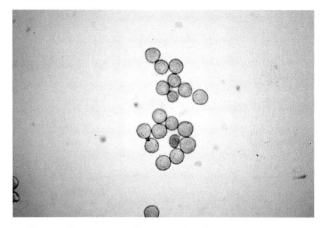

Pollen grains, seasonal contamination, ×100.

Figure 6-245

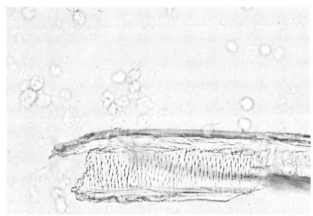

A

B

Plant fiber, from fecal contamination. Cells and bacteria also present, ×400.
A, Brightfield. B, Compensated polarized light showing birefringence.

Figure 6-246

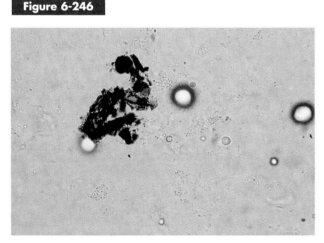

Charcoal in urine, indicating fecal contamination due to a fistula, ×400.

Figure 6-247

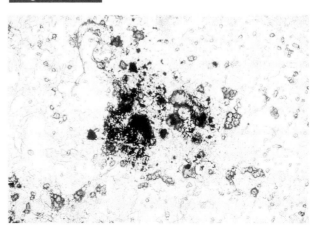

Charcoal, from same specimen as Fig. 6-246. Cytospin, unstained, ×63 (very low-power).

colon and urinary tract, fecal constituents may be seen in the urine. This is a serious pathologic condition. The presence of feces in urine is usually observed as an overall yellow-brown color of the gross urine specimen. Microscopic findings include plant fibers, skeletal muscle fibers, and microorganisms (Fig. 6-245, *A* and *B*).

Rarely, columnar epithelial cells from the gut mucosa or squamous epithelial cells from the anal mucosa are seen.

When detection of a fistula is clinically necessary, patients may be fed activated charcoal, which is carefully searched for in the urine. The presence of charcoal in the urine demonstrates an abnormal connection between the gut and urinary tract (Figs. 6-246 and 6-247).

REVIEW QUESTIONS

CELLS

1 Which of the following constituents present in urine sediment is a sensitive early indicator of renal disease?
 a. crystalluria
 b. hematuria
 c. lipiduria
 d. pyuria

2 What are dysmorphic red cells and what is their significance?

3 What are ghost or shadow red cells and what do they indicate?

4 A useful technique to differentiate ovoid calcium oxalate from red blood cells is:
 a. brightfield microscopy
 b. interference contrast microscopy
 c. phase contrast microscopy
 d. polarizing microscopy

5 Which of the following statements concerning pyuria is false?
 a. Pyuria indicates inflammation somewhere in the urogenital tract.
 b. Pyuria is always accompanied by the presence of bacteria.
 c. Pyuria is associated with acute pyelonephritis.
 d. Pyuria may indicate urinary tract infection.

6 What are glitter cells and what do they indicate?

7 The presence of eosinophils in the urine is associated with:
 a. acute glomerular nephritis
 b. drug-induced interstitial nephritis
 c. nephrotic syndrome
 d. renal transplant rejection

8 The presence of lymphocytes in the urine is associated with:
 a. acute glomerular nephritis
 b. drug-induced interstitial nephritis
 c. nephrotic syndrome
 d. renal transplant rejection

9 What are clue cells and what do they indicate?

10 Of the following epithelial cell types, which provides strong evidence of active kidney disease or tubular injury when 15 or more cells are found using 10 high-power fields?
 a. parabasal
 b. renal
 c. squamous
 d. transitional

11 Renal epithelial fragments originate from the
 a. collecting ducts
 b. distal convoluted tubules
 c. loop of Henle
 d. proximal convoluted tubules

12 What are oval fat bodies and what syndrome are they associated with?

13 The nephrotic syndrome is associated with all of the following except:
 a. albuminuria
 b. edema
 c. hyperalbuminemia
 d. hyperlipidemia
 e. lipiduria

14 Useful microscopic techniques in the detection of fat globules, oval fat bodies, and fatty casts include:
 a. brightfield examination
 b. polarized and compensated polarized microscopy
 c. Sudan staining
 d. more than one of the above
 e. all of the above

15 Match the following urinary constituents and special techniques:
A. Gram stain
B. Hansel's stain
C. phase contrast microscopy
D. polarizing microscopy
E. Rous test (Prussian blue stain)
F. Sudan stain
____ bacteria
____ cholesterol
____ eosinophils
____ hemosiderin
____ neutral fat/triglycerides
____ oval fat bodies
____ Trichomonas
____ yeast

CASTS

1 Which of the following conditions is most likely to result in cast formation?
a. proteinuria, high specific gravity, acid pH
b. proteinuria, low specific gravity, alkaline pH

2 What is a cylindroid and what does it indicate?

3 Which of the following microscopic techniques is most helpful in the detection of hyaline casts?
a. brightfield
b. polarized light
c. phase contrast
d. supravital staining

4 Match the following disease states or conditions and type of cast found in the urine sediment:
A. bacterial cast
B. epithelial cell cast
C. fatty cast
D. hemosiderin cast
E. hyaline/granular cast
F. myoglobin cast
G. red blood cell cast
H. waxy cast
I. white blood cell cast
____ acute glomerulonephritis
____ acute pyelonephritis
____ chronic renal disease/renal failure
____ heavy metal/nephrotoxic poisoning
____ nephrotic syndrome
____ severe crushing injury
____ severe hemolytic episode
____ strenuous exercise

5 Which of the following microscopic techniques is **most** helpful in the visualization of hemoglobin pigment in red cell and blood pigment casts?
a. brightfield
b. phase contrast
c. polarizing
d. supravital staining

6 A blood pigment cast is analogous to which of the following casts:
a. fatty
b. granular
c. hemosiderin
d. hyaline
e. waxy

CRYSTALS

1 The presence of uric acid crystals in the urine sediment is most significant in:
a. Absolutely freshly voided urine
b. Any sediment; they are pathologic whenever present
c. Concentrated urine
d. Dilute urine
e. Urine preserved by refrigeration

2 Indicate which of the following constituents of the urine sediment are birefringent (i.e., they polarize light) by placing an **X** in the space provided.
____ calcium oxalate
____ red blood cells
____ casts
____ diaper fibers
____ cholesterol
____ neutral fat
____ uric acid
____ triple phosphate
____ radiographic contrast media
____ calcium carbonate
____ sulfonamides
____ renal tubular epithelial cells
____ glitter cells
____ clue cells
____ yeast
____ starch

3 Most normal crystals seen in urine of an acid pH are made up of what two chemical compounds?
a.
b.

4 Which of the following is the most common chemical constituent found in renal or bladder stones?
   a. calcium oxalate
   b. cystine
   c. triple phosphate
   d. uric acid/urates

5 Urinary stones referred to as infection stones contain which of the following?
   a. calcium oxalate
   b. cystine
   c. triple phosphate
   d. uric acid/urates

6 Abnormal urinary crystals are most likely to be seen in which of the following urine specimens:
   a. pH 5
   b. pH 7
   c. pH 8
   d. specific gravity 1.010

7 Which of the following abnormal crystals is associated with stone formation:
   a. cystine
   b. hemosiderin
   c. leucine
   d. meglumine diatrizoate
   e. sulfonamide

CONTAMINANTS

1 Which of the following does **not** show a so-called Maltese cross formation when viewed with polarized light?
   a. calcium oxalate
   b. fat as cholesterol
   c. starch
   d. urate spherulites

2 The presence of which of the following chemical constituents will help differentiate waxy casts and disposable diaper fibers:
   a. acid pH
   b. glucose
   c. ketones
   d. leukocyte esterase
   e. protein

3 The presence of a fistula between the urinary and gastrointestinal tract is associated with which of the following in the urine?
   a. activated charcoal
   b. red blood cells
   c. waxy casts
   d. white blood cells

◆ CASE #1

A urine specimen is obtained from a 14-year-old boy with a history of a sore throat. Three weeks ago he was cultured and treated for a streptococcal throat infection with a single intramuscular dose of penicillin. Two weeks after his initial visit, he showed no abnormal physical findings; however, his urinalysis revealed microscopic hematuria and he was told to rest. Currently he has weakness and anorexia. He woke up with a headache and puffy eyelids and says his urine is dark and there is very little of it.

Urinalysis Results:

Physical Appearance:
   color: red (red-brown)
   transparency: cloudy

Chemical Screening:
   pH   6
   specific gravity   1.025
   protein (strip)   300 mg/dL   protein (SSA) 3+
   blood   large
   nitrite   negative
   leukocyte esterase negative
   glucose   negative
   ketones   negative
   bilirubin   negative
   urobilinogen   normal

Because of the results of the protein test by reagent strip, the urine was tested with the sulfosalicylic acid test for protein. A microscopic examination of the urine sediment was also performed.

Microscopic examination of the urine sediment:
   Red blood cells   10-25/hpf (dysmorphic forms present)
   White blood cells   0-2/hpf
   Casts   2-5 red blood cell casts/lpf
   Crystals   few amorphous urates

1. What urinalysis findings are abnormal or discrepant?
2. What is the significance of dysmorphic red cells in the urine sediment of this patient?
3. Proteinuria is an important indication of renal disease. Match the following protein tests (a and b) with the proteins they measure:
   a. Reagent strip test for protein?
   b. Sulfosalicylic acid test for protein?
   ___ albumin
   ___ plasma globulins
   ___ Tamm-Horsfall glycoprotein
4. What is the significance of red blood cell casts in this patient?
5. Why don't you see bacteria in the microscopic examination of the sediment in this patient?
6. What is the likely diagnosis for this patient?

CASE #2

A urine specimen is collected from a 7-year-old girl with a history of several recent infections. She is seen because of lethargy, pallor, and facial edema and is found to have generalized edema. The urine specimen is pale but noticeably foamy.

Urinalysis Results:

Physical Appearance:
color:	pale
transparency:	hazy
foam:	large quantity, white

Chemical Screening:
pH	6
specific gravity	1.010
protein (strip)	>2000 mg/dL protein (SSA) 4+
blood	negative
nitrite	negative
leukocyte esterase	negative
glucose	negative
ketones	negative
bilirubin	negative
urobilinogen	normal

Microscopic examination of the urine sediment:
red blood cells	0-2/hpf
white blood cells	0-2/hpf
casts	2-5 fatty casts/lpf
	5-10 hyaline casts/lpf
epithelial cells	moderate oval fat bodies
	few renal
	few squamous
other	moderate fat globules

1. What urinalysis findings are abnormal or discrepant?
2. What is causing the large amount of white foam in this urine specimen?
3. Explain the edema exhibited by this patient in terms of the urinalysis findings.
4. What are oval fat bodies and what do they signify in this patient?
5. What is the name of the syndrome exhibited by this patient?

 CASE #3

A midstream clean-catch urine specimen is collected for culture and urinalysis from a 23-year-old mother of two children. She is presently in the sixth month of pregnancy. She is being seen because of back pain, fever, chills, and vomiting.

Urinalysis Results:

Physical Appearance:
color:	yellow
transparency:	cloudy

Chemical Screening:
pH	6
specific gravity	1.010
protein (strip)	100 mg/dL protein (SSA) 2+
blood	negative
nitrite	positive
leukocyte esterase	positive
glucose	negative
ketones	negative
bilirubin	negative
urobilinogen	normal

Microscopic examination of the urine sediment:
red blood cells	0-2/hpf
white blood cells	25-50/hpf (glitter cells present)
casts	5-10 granular/lpf
	2-5 cellular/lpf
epithelial cells	few transitional
	few squamous
bacteria	many (rods)

1. What urinalysis findings are abnormal or discrepant?
2. Are these findings consistent with an upper or a lower urinary tract infection? Explain.
3. In this case the white cells are most likely to consist of what cell type? Explain.
4. The cellular casts are most likely to consist of what type of cells? Explain.
5. The disease exhibited by this patient is acute pyelonephritis. What portion of the kidney is affected by this disease? (choose one.)
   a. glomerulus
   b. interstitium

CASE #4

A 76-year-old man complains of difficulty when urinating. He has trouble initiating urinary flow and has terminal dribbling. His physical examination reveals an enlarged, firm prostate. After the patient is instructed to empty his bladder, he is catheterized and 50 mL of residual urine is collected for culture and urinalysis.

Urinalysis Results:

Physical Appearance:

color:	yellow
transparency:	cloudy

Chemical Screening:

pH	7.5	
specific gravity	1.010	
protein (strip)	trace	protein (SSA) trace
blood	negative	
nitrite	positive	
leukocyte esterase	positive	
glucose	negative	
ketones	negative	
bilirubin	negative	
urobilinogen	normal	

Microscopic examination of the urine sediment:

red blood cells	0-2/hpf
white blood cells	10-25/hpf
casts	none seen
epithelial cells	moderate transitional
bacteria	many (rods)

1. What urinalysis findings are abnormal or discrepant?
2. Are these findings consistent with an upper or a lower urinary tract infection? Explain.
3. In this case the white cells are most likely to consist of what cell type? Explain.
4. Explain the presence of epithelial cells in this patient?
5. The disease exhibited by this patient is acute cystitis. What is the likely source of infection in this patient?

 CASE #5

A urine specimen is obtained from a 35-year-old man complaining of acute pain in the right flank radiating into the groin. He has experienced similar pain in the past, together with the passage of small calculi in the urine. His sister was also known to suffer from urolithiasis (stone formation).

Urinalysis Results:

Physical Appearance:

color:	pink
transparency:	cloudy

Chemical Screening:

pH	5	
specific gravity	1.025	
protein (strip)	trace	protein (SSA)trace
blood	large	
nitrite	negative	
leukocyte esterase	negative	
glucose	negative	
ketones	negative	
bilirubin	negative	
urobilinogen	normal	

Microscopic examination of the urine sediment:

red blood cells	10-25/hpf
white blood cells	0-2/hpf
casts	none seen
crystals	5-10 cystine/lpf

Additional (confirmatory) tests:

Nitroprusside Reaction for Cystine	positive

1. What urinalysis findings are abnormal or discrepant?
2. Radiography showed bilateral, radiopaque renal pelvic opacities in this patient. This finding and a family history of renal stones suggests a genetically influenced condition. Recognizing this, what are the stones composed of in this patient? Explain.
3. Explain the presence of red cells in the urine of this patient.
4. What is the significance of the urinary pH and specific gravity in this patient.
5. What normal crystal do cystine crystals resemble, and how do they differ?

CASE #6

A first-morning, midstream urine specimen is collected as part of an annual physical examination. The patient has no clinical evidence of urinary tract or kidney disease and is taking no medications.

Urinalysis Results:

Physical Appearance:

color:	yellow
transparency:	cloudy

Chemical Screening:

pH	6.5
specific gravity	1.025
protein (strip)	negative
blood	negative
nitrite	negative
leukocyte esterase	negative
glucose	negative
ketones	negative
bilirubin	negative
urobilinogen	normal

Microscopic examination of the urine sediment:

red blood cells	10-25/hpf
white blood cells	0-2/hpf
casts	none seen
epithelial cells	few squamous
crystals	few calcium oxalate

1. What urinalysis findings are abnormal or discrepant?
2. This laboratory performs microscopic analysis of the urine sediment only when abnormal physical or chemical results are obtained. Why was the microscopic done on this specimen?
3. How would you investigate the apparent discrepancy between the chemical screening test for blood and the finding of red cells in the urinary sediment?

REFERENCES

1. *CAP surveys manual, section II: appendix II glossary of terms for urine sediment, vaginal fluids, stool and miscellaneous specimens*, Northfield, Ill., 1993, College of American Pathologists, p 44.
2. Coe FL, Parks JH, Asplin JR: *The pathogenesis and treatment of kidney stones*, NEJM 327(16):1141, 1992.
3. Fiechtner JJ, Simkin PA: *Urate spherulites in gouty synovia*, JAMA 245(15):1533, 1981.
4. Haber MH: *Urinary sediment: a textbook atlas*, Chicago, 1981, American Society of Clinical Pathologists, p 90-91.
5. Rous P: Hemosiderin, *J Exp Med* 18:645, 1918.
6. Schumann GB, Schweitzer SC: *Examination of urine*. In Henry, JB, ed: *Clinical diagnosis and management by laboratory methods*, ed 18, Philadelphia, 1991, WB Saunders, p 421.
7. Schumann GB, Schweitzer SC: *Examination of urine*. In Henry JB, ed: *Clinical diagnosis and management by laboratory methods*, ed 18, Philadelphia, 1991, WB Saunders, p 424.
8. Schumann GB, Schweitzer SC: *Examination of urine*. In Henry, JB, ed: *Clinical diagnosis and management by laboratory methods*, ed 18, Philadelphia, 1991, WB Saunders, p 426.
9. Schumann GB: *Urine sediment examination*, Baltimore, 1980, Williams & Wilkins, p 83.

BIBLIOGRAPHY

Bradley GM, Linne JJ: *The University of Minnesota hospital and clinic laboratory handbook*, ed 2, Hudson, Ohio, 1992, Lexi-Comp.

Bradley M: *Urine crystals—identification and significance. Laboratory Medicine*, June 1982; 13:348-353.

CAP surveys manual, section II: appendix II glossary of terms for urine sediment, vaginal fluids, stool and miscellaneous specimens, Northfield, Ill., 1993, College of American Pathologists.

Graff L: *A handbook of routine urinalysis*, Philadelphia, 1983, JB Lippincott.

Haber MH: *A primer of microscopic urinalysis*, ed 2, Garden Grove, Calif., 1991, Hycor Biomedical.

Haber MH: *Urinary sediment: a textbook atlas*, Chicago, 1981, American Society of Clinical Pathologists.

Haber MH: *Urine casts: their microscopy and clinical significance*, ed 2, Chicago, 1976, American Society of Clinical Pathologists.

Linne JJ, Ringsrud KM: *Basic techniques in clinical laboratory science*, ed 3, St. Louis, 1992, Mosby.

Physician's office laboratory guidelines, tentative guidelines, ed 2, Villanova, Pa., June 1992, National Committee for Clinical Laboratory Standards, 12(5) POL1-T2.

Routine urinalysis and collection, transportation, and preservation of urine specimens, tentative guidelines, Villanova, Pa., December 1992, National Committee for Clinical Laboratory Standards, 12(26) GP16-T.

Schumann GB, Schumann JL: *A manual of cytodiagnostic urinalysis*, Salt Lake City, 1984, Cytodiagnostics Co.

Schumann GB, Schumann JL: *Cytodiagnostic urinalysis urine sediment entities transparencies and explanatory test*, Salt Lake City, 1984, Cytodiagnostics Co.

Schumann GB, Schweitzer SC: *Examination of urine*. In Henry JB, ed: *Clinical diagnosis and management by laboratory methods*, ed 18, Philadelphia, 1991, WB Saunders.

Schumann GB, Weiss MA: *Atlas of renal and urinary tract cytology and its histopathologic bases*, Philadelphia, 1981, JB Lippincott.

Schumann GB: *Urine sediment examination*, Baltimore, 1980, Williams & Wilkins.

Ward PCJ: *The urinary sediment*, Image Premastering Services, 1992, Mosby.

Synovial fluid from joint after injection with Aristocort®. Compensated polarized light, slow-wave orientation (N-S).

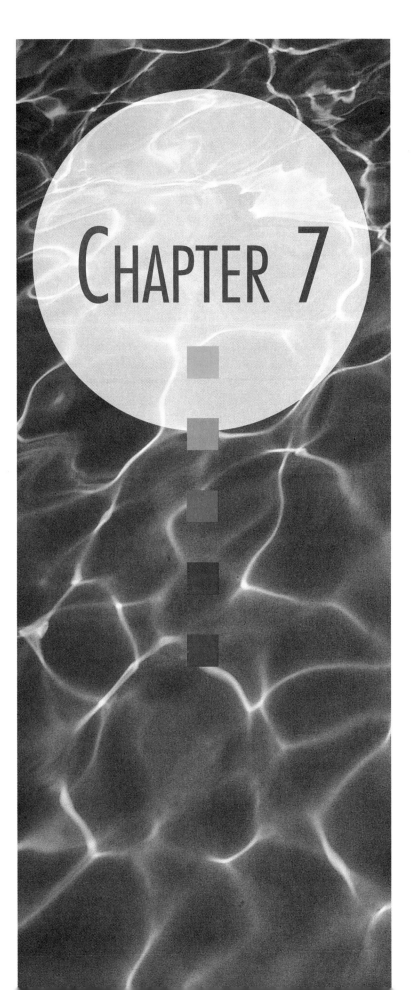

CHAPTER 7

BODY FLUIDS

CHAPTER OUTLINE

● **Introduction**

● **Cerebrospinal Fluid Analysis**
 Lumbar Puncture
 Collection of Cerebrospinal Fluid Specimen—Cell
   Counts and Differential
 Laboratory Assays
 Microscopic Examination
 Microbiologic tests
 Chemistry Assays

● **Synovial Fluid Analysis**
 Differential Diagnosis of Joint Diseases Using
   Synovial Fluid Assays
 Collection of Synovial Fluid Specimen
 Laboratory Assays

● **Serous Fluid Analysis (Pleural, Pericardial And
 Peritoneal Fluids)**
 Transudates Versus Exudates
 Pleural Fluid
 Pericardial Fluid

 Peritoneal Fluid (Ascitic Fluid)
 Collection of Serous Fluid Specimen
 Laboratory Assays

● **Semen Analysis**
 Collection of Semen Specimen
 Laboratory Assays

● **Amniotic Fluid Analysis**
 Collection of the Amniotic Fluid Specimen
 Laboratory Assays

● **Morphologic Characteristics Of Cells Seen In
 Body Fluids**
 Cells from Peripheral Blood
 Phagocytic (Mononuclear) Cells
 Lining Cells
 Miscellaneous Cells
 Miscellaneous Other Findings

● **References**

LEARNING OBJECTIVES

▶ Understand the importance of unique **specimen
 collection requirements** and/or challenges upon
 which valid laboratory assays depend, including
 the use of proper anticoagulants or additives for
 preservation.

▶ Understand the importance of **following laboratory protocol for specimen handling** before performing the assay or study.

▶ Understand the importance of the initial **observation of the gross appearance** of the specimen.

▶ Understand the necessity for **use of universal precautions** when handling specimens.

▶ Recognize **patterns of infection** as illustrated by
 protein and glucose levels, leukocyte counts and
 cell types, along with gram-staining reactions
 seen in body fluid specimens.

▶ Recognize **patterns of characteristic changes in
 gross appearance** of synovial fluid, along with
 microscopic changes occurring in the various
 crystal-induced arthritides.

▶ Understand the **use of compensated polarized
 light microscopy** techniques to differentiate birefringent crystals in synovial fluid.

▶ Recognize the **usefulness of cytocentrifugation
 techniques** to provide a good yield of cellular
 material for body fluid cytologic studies.

▶ Understand the basic **concepts of the "routine
 tests"** often ordered for many of the body fluids.

▶ **Classify serous fluids as transudates or exudates**
 based on laboratory findings—specimen appearance, total protein levels, and absence or presence of cells.

▶ Understand the **usefulness of classic cell counting techniques using hemocytometry** for many
 body fluids in which cell numbers are of varying
 numbers.

▶ Understand how to recognize **patterns of varying
 cell types (morphology) as seen microscopically**
 in various pathologic states where assay of body
 fluid specimens is helpful.

▶ Understand **clinical correlations of laboratory
 test results with diseases or conditions** in which
 body fluid specimens are collected and examined.

INTRODUCTION

Fluids such as cerebrospinal, serous (pleural, pericardial, peritoneal/ascitic), gastric, nasal, synovial, seminal, sweat, saliva, tears, vitreous humor, and amniotic are examples of body fluid specimens, other than blood or urine, that can be analyzed by the medical laboratory. Laboratory testing of these miscellaneous body fluids is usually done to aid in the diagnosis of specific conditions or diseases.

Depending on the nature of the tests to be done, various divisions of the laboratory are involved in handling the specimens. Since cell counts are usually done in the hematology laboratory, the entire specimen can often first be sent to this laboratory section. From there it is sent to microbiology, chemistry, or to other specialized testing areas, as needed.

Some facilities have specimen receiving laboratories, which receive, process, and disperse specimens to the proper area for testing. Some of these specimens require specialized testing procedures in addition to the more routine laboratory testing procedures done on blood and urine. Routine tests are ordered on most body fluid specimens. Cell counts, morphologic studies on stained cytocentrifuged smears, Gram stain and culture, and total protein levels are some of the most commonly ordered laboratory assays. When certain chemistry tests are performed on body fluids (analytes such as glucose or protein, for example), it is customary to simultaneously include a collection of venous blood to measure blood levels for the same constituent. Many of the body fluids are difficult to collect, and the amounts collected are small in volume. Because some of the specialized laboratory tests using these body fluid specimens are infrequently done, as compared with the great numbers of routine tests done using blood and urine, there is need for availability of and adherence to clearly written procedures explaining the details of specimen requirements for each test ordered using each of the specific body fluids being tested.

Obtaining body fluids other than blood or urine usually involves unique collection requirements necessitating a careful review of what is needed for the specific laboratory test ordered. Requirements can include proper patient preparation before collection, temperature of collection, use of preservatives, transport time limitations, specimen container specifications, and specimen processing and handling criteria. If specimens are not collected, preserved, transported, and processed correctly, the reported analytic result for the test may be inaccurate, thus possibly adversely affecting the patient's diagnosis or treatment plan.

The adherence to infection control policies is important in collecting, handling, and testing body cavity fluids. Universal precautionary procedures should be applied to all body fluid specimens. These precautions recognize the infectious potential of any patient specimen. Body fluids included in the specimens posing the greatest risk for persons handling them are blood, semen, vaginal secretions, cerebrospinal fluid, synovial fluid, serous fluids, and amniotic fluid (see Chapter 1). The essence of any policy employing universal precautions is the avoidance of direct contact with any patient specimen in general, but when contact is necessary, health care workers should use the appropriate barrier precautions to prevent cross-transmission and exposure of their own skin and mucous membranes to the infectious agent. The best precaution is frequent handwashing, the most important way of interrupting the transmission of infectious pathogens. Personal protective equipment such as gloves, gowns, and masks are additional means of providing barrier protection.

In this chapter, there will be a brief overview of specimen collection and handling requirements as well as a limited discussion of routine tests done for the following specimens: cerebrospinal fluid, synovial fluid, serous fluids (pericardial, pleural, and peritoneal), seminal fluid (semen), and amniotic fluid. Other miscellaneous fluids will not be specifically addressed.

CEREBROSPINAL FLUID ANALYSIS

Cerebrospinal fluid (CSF) is found in the space known as the subarachnoid space between the arachnoid mater and the pia mater—two of the three membranes comprising the meninges covering the brain and spinal cord. From the outside in, the three membranes making up the meninges are the dura mater, the arachnoid mater, and the pia mater. The cerebrospinal fluid circulates upward over the central hemispheres of the brain and downward around the spinal cord. Most of the fluid is formed by the choroid plexuses in the ventricles of the brain through processes of ultrafiltration of plasma and active secretion or transport. Approximately 20 mL of fluid per hour is produced in the choroid plexuses and reabsorbed by the villi in the arachnoid. There is normally a total volume of 90-150 mL of cerebrospinal fluid in adults and 10-60 mL in neonates.

Cerebrospinal fluid serves to protect the underlying tissue of the central nervous system. It acts as a mechanical buffer to prevent trauma, to regulate the volume of intracranial pressure, to circulate nutrients, to remove metabolic waste products from the central nervous system, and to generally act as a lubricant for the system. The normal intact blood-brain barrier prevents the passage of certain plasma constituents from the blood to the brain. The blood-brain barrier consists of two morphologically distinct components: the endothelium of the capillaries acts as a tight junction between adjacent cells and the epithelium of the choroid plexus. The endothelium of the capillaries regulates passage of constituents such as glucose, urea, or creatinine. These diffuse freely but require several hours for equilibration. Proteins diffuse slowly at rates decreasing with increasing size of the protein molecule. Many drugs do not enter the spinal fluid from the blood. Because of the blood-brain barrier, cerebrospinal fluid is not an ultrafiltrate of plasma. There is active transport between the blood, cerebrospinal fluid, and brain in both directions, giving varying concentrations of substances in each. Normally there is less glucose, bicarbonate, and urea in the spinal fluid than in the blood. Electrolytes such as sodium, magnesium, and chloride are more concentrated in the spinal fluid than in the blood. There is very little protein in spinal fluid.

Analysis of the cerebrospinal fluid can provide essential diagnostic information in some conditions. Cerebrospinal fluid is usually collected by **lumbar puncture (spinal tap)**. There are four major categories of disease that indicate performing a lumbar puncture: infections of the meninges, subarachnoid hemorrhage, malignancies of the central nervous system, and demyelinating disorders. Newer diagnostic procedures such as imaging techniques—CT scan or magnetic resonance imaging (MRI)—have changed some of the former indications for a lumbar puncture. Only for a few conditions (e.g., meningitis) is the lumbar puncture essential and often diagnostic. In other situations the use of the lumbar puncture for analysis of CSF aids in making the diagnosis by ruling out certain other specific disorders. The specimen must always be collected and handled carefully and appropriately, observing an extremely critical collection procedure. The physician must obtain a complete clinical history and perform a physical examination of the patient before any collection is attempted. One absolute contraindication for the lumbar puncture is the presence of infection at the puncture site, since the puncture could spread the infection to the meninges.

Lumbar Puncture

Cerebrospinal fluid is normally collected by lumbar puncture in one of the spaces between the third, fourth, or fifth lumbar vertebrae, depending on the age of the patient. The puncture is done in this location to avoid damage to the spinal cord. When a cerebrospinal fluid analysis is being considered, the benefits to the patient versus the potential harm from the collection process must be weighed.

The greatest risk of complications for the patient after a lumbar puncture is headache. Other potential complications include bleeding, or brain herniation caused by elevated intracranial pressure resulting in

paralysis or death. Some bleeding may result from a **traumatic tap (bloody tap)** where there has been trauma to the blood vessels during the collection process. This is recognized as blood in the spinal fluid specimen, with more blood being seen in the first tube collected than in the last. This condition is usually minor and self-limiting for the patient.

Collection of Cerebrospinal Fluid Specimen

The most important indication for doing the lumbar puncture is to diagnose **meningitis** of bacterial, fungal, mycobacterial, and amebic origin. Laboratory examination of the cerebrospinal fluid in these cases can often provide the needed diagnostic information. These conditions are very serious ones and require immediate diagnosis and treatment.

Specimens are collected under strictly sterile conditions by using specific precautions during the collection process, and only by experienced individuals, usually the attending physician. The skin must be disinfected carefully before the puncture to avoid contaminating the specimen or the patient with the normal flora residing on the skin surrounding the site. If iodine has been used as a disinfectant, it is important to remove it after the cleansing process before performing the tap, since contamination with iodine has been associated with false-positive results for bacterial antigen tests done on cerebrospinal fluid. The cerebrospinal fluid specimen is collected and divided into three or four sterile tubes for culture and Gram stain, cell counts and cell differential, and chemistry and immunologic tests. Normal cerebrospinal fluid is sterile, crystal-clear, and has the appearance of water.

Use of Infection Control—Precautions Employed. Cerebrospinal fluid is considered an infectious substance, and universal precautionary measures must be employed during the collection and handling process. Since one of the primary indications for collection of the cerebrospinal fluid is to diagnose various infectious menigitides, there is always the danger of spreading these infectious pathogens if the cerebrospinal fluid is not handled carefully. Proper use of sterile technique during the collection process itself, along with the wearing of personal protective equipment, is essential. The use of barrier precautions during collection, processing, and testing of the specimen cannot be overemphasized.

Skin Preparation. The skin site should be prepared as for a blood culture using a solution of iodine such as povidone-iodine. The skin around the site should be draped with a sterile material and the site scrubbed for 30 seconds with the disinfectant solution, applying the solution in a concentric, outward moving circle. This process should be repeated a second time for another 30 seconds and the iodine solution left on the skin 2 to 4 minutes for maximum effectiveness. The iodine can be removed with 70% isopropyl alcohol. The site must not be touched before or during the collection of the specimen, and any contamination with normal flora from surrounding body surfaces must be avoided. If the patient is allergic to iodine, a solution of chlorhexidine may be used, removing it with sterile water and then with 70% isopropyl alcohol.

Measurement of Intracranial Pressure. After performing the lumbar puncture and before any fluid is withdrawn the **intracranial pressure** must be measured by allowing some of the fluid to rise in a sterile, graduated, manometer tube. The normal opening pressure varies between 90 and 180 mm of CSF, measured with the patient in a recumbent, lateral position. Pressure normally varies from 5 to 10 mm with variations in the patient's respirations, coughing, or straining. Only 1 to 2 mL of fluid is removed if the pressure is greater than 200 mm. There are several disorders that can give increased or decreased cerebrospinal fluid pressures. If the pressure falls markedly after 1 to 2 mL of fluid is removed, the physician should suspect cerebellar herniation or spinal cord compression above the puncture site. In this case, no more fluid should be removed, and the patient should be watched carefully for several hours. If the pressure is normal and no marked drop in pressure is noted after removal of 1 to 2 mL of fluid, the collection process may continue.

Collecting the Specimen and General Specimen Handling. Once the pressure has been determined to be normal, the spinal tap can continue by removing 10 to 20 mL of fluid slowly into three or four sterile, screw-capped, leakproof tubes. Usually about 3 to 5 mL is placed in each tube. The tubes are collected sequentially, with the order of collection noted on the containers themselves. The first 3 to 5 mL of fluid removed is placed in a tube labeled #1, the next 3 to 5 mL is placed in tube #2 and so forth. Normal closing pressure after removal of 10 to 20 mL of cerebrospinal fluid is about 45 to 90 mm. After the fluid is collected and before the needle is withdrawn, the opening pressure, closing pressure, and total volume of the fluid collected should be recorded.

The first tube is used for chemistry and immunology tests, the next tube for microbiologic tests, and the last tube for cell counts and cell differential studies. The tubes of cerebrospinal fluid are all examined for their appearance as they are collected. Abnormalities in appearance of the specimen are noted and recorded.

After collection, the specimen tubes must be properly labeled and transported to the laboratory immediately for processing and handling to ensure the optimum information from the analyses. Cell counts and glucose determinations are especially affected by a time lapse since these constituents begin to deteriorate quickly. Specimens used for these tests must be assayed as soon as possible after collection. Any excess specimen tubes not needed for testing purposes should be saved for future retesting use, if needed.

TRAUMATIC PUNCTURE. A traumatic lumbar puncture (traumatic tap) gives a pink or red color to the fluid caused by the presence of red blood cells from trauma to the blood vessels in the spinal canal during the puncturing process. The color clears as the fluid continues to drip into the collection tubes. The first tube appears the most red and subsequent samples appear less red. There is a clearing of blood between the first tube and the third tube, and usually, complete clearing is noted in the last tube collected. A clot may be seen in fluids that are extremely bloody from a traumatic tap.

Laboratory Assays

Laboratory tests are most useful when the results are used in conjunction with clinical findings and results of other diagnostic procedures. The most important laboratory tests are done to diagnose bacterial meningitis, followed by fungal and mycobacterial infections. If these disorders are suspected, the use of Gram stains, stains for acid-fast organisms, cultures, and tests for bacterial or fungal antigens are the most important. Cytologic examinations, immunophenotypic studies, and biochemical tumor marker tests are done on cerebrospinal fluid to diagnose some malignancies and for demyelinating disorders. The finding of immunoglobulin G (IgG) abnormalities is important because of the association between them and the presence of multiple sclerosis.

Some tests are done routinely on all cerebrospinal fluids, whereas others are done only when indicated. The routine tests should include cell count, differential count, glucose level, and protein level, in addition to the opening CSF pressure reported during the collection process itself. When glucose and protein tests are done on cerebrospinal fluid, it is important to compare those results with the accompanying blood chemistry levels for glucose and protein. Some investigators feel that if the results for opening pressure, CSF protein, cell count, and cytospin differential are normal, no further tests are necessary for that fluid (Table 7-1).

When the volume of the specimen collected is insufficient for the usual specimen handling/processing protocol to be followed, a decision as to prioritizing of tests to be done must be made in conjunction with the patient's primary attending physician. Cerebrospinal fluid is categorized as a difficult-to-recollect specimen, so every attempt must be made to provide the best information with the specimen collected.

Gross Examination for Color, Clarity, and Clotting. All tubes collected are examined for their color and clarity. Normal cerebrospinal fluid is clear and colorless. In the presence of disease, the fluid becomes hazy or cloudy because of the presence of cells, microorganisms, increased protein, or lipids. It can also appear bloody, viscous, or clotted. Cerebrospinal fluid appears hazy or cloudy with leukocyte counts greater than 0.20×10^9/L or erythrocyte counts greater than 0.40×10^9/L. Fluid that appears pink-red usually indicates the presence of red blood cells. This pink-red color can be caused by a **subarachnoid hemorrhage**, an intracerebral hemorrhage, an infarct, or from a traumatic puncture.

DIFFERENTIATION OF SUBARACHNOID HEMORRHAGE FROM A TRAUMATIC PUNCTURE. It is important to differentiate color caused by pathologic bleeding from that caused by trauma during the collection process. Specimens collected sequentially from patients with a subarachnoid hemorrhage will appear evenly red in all tubes collected as compared with the subsequent clearing of the red color in tubes as they are collected from a traumatic puncture (tap).

After centrifugation, the supernatant fluid is clear with a traumatic tap, whereas the supernatant fluid appears **xanthochromic** (a faint pink, orange, or yellow color caused by the release of hemoglobin from hemolyzed red blood cells) from a subarachnoid hemorrhage. The centrifuged supernatant can be compared to a tube of distilled water, using a white sheet of paper as a background. Lysis of the red cells present in the cerebrospinal fluid begins about 2 hours after a subarachnoid hemorrhage. The supernatant from a subarachnoid hemorrhage can be clear if the bleeding is less than 2 hours old or if there has been only minimal red cell lysis. Examination for xanthochromasia should be done within 1 hour or less after collection of the specimen to avoid false-positive reports. At about 1 to 4 hours after a subarachnoid hemorrhage, a pale pink to pale orange xanthochromasia appears in the spinal fluid because of the presence of oxyhemoglobin. The color reaches a peak at about 24 to 36 hours and gradually disappears in 4 to 8 days. In specimens from a bloody tap, red cells also begin to lyse within 1 to 2 hours, so it is always important to process the spinal fluid specimens within 1 hour or less for any xanthochromasia interpretations. Twelve hours after a subarachnoid hemorrhage,

Table 7-1

REFERENCE VALUES FOR CEREBROSPINAL FLUID[4]

Component	Conventional Units	SI Units
Erythrocyte count	0	0
Leukocyte count*		
Adults	0-5 mononuclear cells/μL	$0\text{-}0.005 \times 10^9$/L
Neonates	0-30 mononuclear cells/μL	$0\text{-}0.003 \times 10^9$/L
Leukocyte differential		
Adults:		
lymphocytes	60% ± 20%	0.60 ± 0.20
monocytes	30% ± 15%	0.30 ± 0.15
neutrophils	2% ± 4%	0.02 ± 0.04
Neonates:		
lymphocytes	20% ± 15%	0.20 ± 0.15
monocytes	70% ± 20%	0.70 ± 0.20
neutrophils	4% ± 4%	0.04 ± 0.04
Total Protein		
Adults	15-45 mg/dL	150-450 mg/L
Adults, >60 y	15-60 mg/dL	150-600 mg/L
Neonates	15-100 mg/dL	150-1000 mg/L
Glucose	50-80 mg/dL	2.75-4.40 mmol/L
Lactate	9-26 mg/dL	1.13-3.23 mmol/L

Children have intermediate leukocyte values, <20/μL the first year of life and <10/μL until adolescence.

there will be a **yellow xanthochromia** caused by the presence of bilirubin in the spinal fluid. This color will peak at about 2 to 4 days and will gradually disappear within 2 to 4 weeks.

In spinal fluid specimens from a subarachnoid hemorrhage, **erythrophagia** may be seen when the specimen is observed microscopically. Erythrophagia is the ingestion of erythrocytes by macrophages present in the fluid. Macrophages containing large brown black **hemosiderin** granules may be seen approximately 48 hours after a hemorrhage. The hemosiderin arises from the iron of the ingested red cells. It may remain for up to 4 months. The presence of hemosiderin is another diagnostic aid in distinguishing a true hemorrhage in the central nervous system from blood in the spinal fluid caused by a bloody tap. A **Prussian blue stain** will confirm the identity of the iron within the cytoplasm of cells.

A more sensitive and specific test to aid in differentiating the origin of blood in the specimen is an immunoassay for D-Dimer Fibrin, which gives a positive reaction in cerebrospinal fluid from patients with a subarachnoid hemorrhage. It is not present in specimens associated with a traumatic tap. It is possible, however, to have a subarachnoid hemorrhage concurrently with a traumatic tap.

CLOTTING. Normal cerebrospinal fluid does not clot. Specimens collected from a traumatic tap can clot because of the presence of fibrinogen from the blood. In cases of suppurative meningitis, tuberculous meningitis, or when the protein content of the fluid is sharply elevated, clotting may be seen. There usually are no clots present in specimens from patients with a subarachnoid hemorrhage.

Microscopic Examination—Cell Counts and Differential. Red and white cell counts are routinely done using a manual **counting chamber (hemocytometer)** method (Procedures 7-1 and 7-2 and Fig. 7-1). Electronic cell counts are generally not done for spinal fluid specimens because of poor precision in the normal ranges. There are normally only very few white cells and no red cells present in spinal fluid, and the electronic counting devices are not standardized for these low numbers (see Table 7-1). Occasionally, an electronic cell counter can be used for bloody specimens.

Cell morphology, including a differential count, is examined on a concentrated, stained smear made from the cerebrospinal fluid and not from the cells seen in the counting chamber. The use of a concentrating method that yields the maximum number of cells with their morphologic appearance intact is recommended for preparation of the smear. **Cytocentrifugation,** sedi-

Procedure 7-1

CEREBROSPINAL FLUID RED CELL COUNT

1. Insert a disposable Pasteur pipette directly into the well-mixed specimen. Carefully mount both sides of a clean counting chamber (hemocytometer). Discard pipette in biohazard container.

2. With the low-power (10×) objective, quickly scan both ruled areas of the hemocytometer to determine whether red cells are present and to get a rough idea of their concentration.

3. With the high-power (40×) objective, count the red cells in 10 mm². Count five squares on each side, using the four corner squares and the center square (see Fig. 7-1).

4. Red cells will appear small, round, and yellowish. Their outline is usually smooth, although they may occasionally appear crenated.

5. If the number of red cells is fairly high (more than 200 cells per ten squares) count fewer squares and adjust the calculations accordingly.

6. If the fluid is extremely bloody, it may be necessary to dilute it volumetrically with saline or some other isotonic diluent. It is preferable to count the undiluted fluid in fewer than 10 squares, if possible. Adjust the calculations if dilution is necessary.

7. Calculate the number of cells per liter as follows:

Total cells counted × dilution factor × volume factor = cells/μL = cells × 10^6/L

Example: If 10 squares are counted, the volume counted is 1 μL (10 mm² × 0.1 mm) and if the fluid was not diluted, there is no dilution factor. Therefore the number of cells counted in 10 squares is equal to the number of cells per microliter, or × 10^6/L.

8. Decontaminate the hemocytometer by placing it in a Petri dish and flooding it with disinfectant solution. Allow the disinfectant to remain on the hemocytometer for at least 5 minutes, then rinse it well with 70% alcohol and clean it.

From Linne JJ, Ringsrud KM: *Basic techniques in clinical laboratory science,* ed 3, St. Louis, 1992, Mosby., p. 413

CEREBROSPINAL FLUID WHITE CELL COUNT

1. Rinse a disposable Pasteur pipette with glacial acetic acid, drain it carefully, wipe the outside completely dry with gauze, and touch the tip of the pipette to the gauze to remove any excess acid. It is very important that no glacial acetic acid be left on the outside of the pipette because it would contaminate the spinal fluid specimen when the pipette is placed in it.

2. Place the pipette in the well-mixed CSF sample and allow the pipette to fill to about 1 in. of its length. Tilt the CSF tube slightly, if necessary, to allow filling by capillary action. Place a finger over the clean end of the pipette and remove it from the sample.

3. Mix the spinal fluid with the acid coating the pipette by placing the pipette in a horizontal position and removing your finger from the end of the pipette. Rotate or twist the pipette to mix the CSF and acid together. Be careful not to allow any of the fluid to drip from the pipette.

4. Mount the acidified CSF on both sides of a clean hemocytometer. Wait for 3 to 5 minutes to allow time for red cell hemolysis.

5. With the low-power (10×) objective, quickly scan both ruled areas of the hemocytometer to determine whether white cells are present, and to get a rough idea of their concentration. The white cell nuclei will appear as dark, refractile structures surrounded by a halo of cytoplasm.

6. Using the low-power (10×) objective, count the white cells in 10 mm², 5 mm² on each side of the hemocytometer using the four corner squares and the center square (see Fig. 7-1).

7. To estimate the types of white cells present, classify each white cell seen as polynuclear or mononuclear. This chamber differential is inaccurate and a differential cell count on a stained preparation is preferred.
   a. To classify cells, change from the low-power (10×) to the high-power (40×) objective.
   b. Polynuclear white cells have a segmented or twisted, irregular nucleus, and a moderate amount of cytoplasm. They are usually neutrophils.
   c. Mononuclear white cells have a round grainy nucleus, and usually a smaller amount of cytoplasm. They may be lymphocytes, monocytes, or other nucleated cells.

8. If it appears that the number of white cells is more than 200 cells per ten squares, count fewer squares and adjust your calculations accordingly. Dilution may be necessary (see Procedure 7-1).

9. Calculate the white cell count in cells per microliter as described in Procedure 7-1.

10. Decontaminate and clean the hemocytometer as described in Procedure 7-1.

From Linne JJ, Ringsrud KM: *Basic techniques in clinical laboratory science*, ed 3, St. Louis, 1992, Mosby, p. 413.

---

mentation, or filtration methods produce good yields. Ordinary centrifugation methods do not give as good results. Wright's stain is used to show the morphologic characteristics of the blood cells present in the smear. A predominance of **polymorphonuclear white cells** (neutrophils) usually indicates a bacterial infection, whereas the presence of many mononuclear cells (lymphocytes and monocytes) can indicate a viral infection.

RED AND WHITE CELL COUNTS. Cell counts should be performed as soon as possible after collection because cells lyse on prolonged standing, and the cell counts will be invalid. Ideally, cell counts should be performed within 30 minutes of collection. Since these spinal fluid specimens often contain pathogenic organisms, they should be handled carefully, employing good infection control techniques to prevent contamination. The use of special disposable equipment such as disposable counting chambers can be considered. Traditional hemocytometers must be thoroughly disinfected after use. Semiautomatic micropipettes can be used to prepare dilutions, if needed. The dilution needed will depend on the turbidity of the fluid—the more turbid the fluid, the more cells are likely to be present, and the higher the dilution needed.

Red Cell Count. There are normally no red cells present in spinal fluid (see Table 7-1). The red cell count done on spinal fluid is of limited diagnostic use in most instances. If the spinal fluid appears clear (normal), the cell count can be done using an undiluted specimen. For bloody specimens, dilution is necessary with normal saline (see Procedure 7-1).

White Cell Count. There are normally from 0 to 5 white cells (mononuclear cells—lymphocytes and monocytes) per µL in adults. The normal range for neonates is higher (see Table 7-1). In doing a white cell count on a bloody fluid, the red cells must first be lysed with glacial acetic acid, which stains the nuclei of the white cells. The white cell count on cerebrospinal fluid is usually done manually using the hemocytometer method (see Procedure 7-2).

EVALUATION OF CELL MORPHOLOGY (CELL DIFFERENTIAL). Concentration of the fluid is done to provide a larger number of cells for evaluation. The use of Wright's stain allows the accurate identification of the cell types present in the smear. It is advisable to prepare and examine a smear of the spinal fluid for all specimens, even when the total cell counts are within the normal levels.

The white cells seen in the spinal fluid smear are counted and differentiated as mononuclear cells (lymphocytes and monocytes) or polymorphonuclear cells (PMNs or neutrophils) and reported as a percentage (see Table 7-1). The presence of other cells from the central nervous system is also noted. If any tumor cells or unusual cells are seen, the smear should be referred for cytologic examination.

Spinal fluid normally contains only a few leukocytes—lymphocytes and monocytes. The appearance of these cells is similar to those as seen in blood smears. A small number of PMNs may also be present in normal spinal fluid. Cells from the central nervous system may also be seen in the fluid. Cells lining the ventricles (ependymal cells) or choroid plexus cells may be found in both normal and abnormal cerebrospinal fluid (see also Morphologic Characteristics of Cells Seen in Body Fluids).

Cytocentrifugation. The use of cytocentrifugation provides a good yield of cellular material while preserving the cellular morphology. A special cytocentrifuge such as the Cytospin (Shandon, Inc., Pittsburgh, Pa.), is used for this procedure. The cytocentrifuge slowly spins the sample from 200 to 1000 rpm for 5 to 10 minutes. During this process, the fluid portion of the specimen is absorbed into a filter paper, and the cellular portion is concentrated in a circle 6 mm in diameter on a microscope slide. The slide can then be stained with Wright's stain or with a variety of other appropriate stains for hematologic or cytologic studies. Other concentrating methods can also be used if a cytocentrifuge is not available.

Microbiologic Tests. If clinical findings suggest meningitis, a microbiologic examination of the cerebrospinal fluid is essential to diagnose or rule out bacterial meningitis. Bacterial meningitis is a lethal condition if untreated, and early diagnosis and appropriate treatment is curative. Delay in diagnosis or treatment can result in permanent deficiencies in the central nervous system, especially sensorineural deafness. The specific causative microorganism must be found to select the adequate antimicrobial agent for treatment. Susceptibility testing is often required.

Figure 7-1

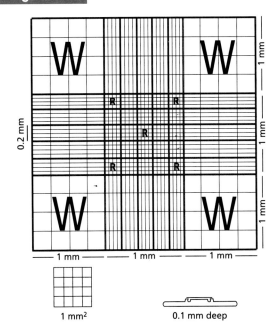

Improved Neubauer ruling for one counting area. Red and white cells in spinal fluid/body fluids are counted in a total of 10 square millimeters using parts of two counting chamber areas—each counting area consisting of 9 square millimeters. *W*, area where white cells in blood are counted (and in body fluids, the red cells are also counted in this area); *R*, area where red cells in blood are counted. (From Bauer JD: *Clinical laboratory methods*, ed 9, St. Louis, 1982, Mosby, p 19.)

Gram stains and culture are done on spinal fluid to aid in the diagnosis of infections of the meninges. For microbiologic examination, the specimen should be tested promptly after collection. Gram stains are done on sediments of the spinal fluid and should be examined only by persons who are experienced in looking at them. It is recommended that the cerebrospinal fluid be centrifuged for 15 minutes at 1500 g to recover the bacteria present. Using the cytocentrifuge will significantly increase this recovery. There are several errors that can affect the interpretation of a Gram-stained spinal fluid. Precipitated dye or stained debris can be mistaken for gram-positive organisms, and stained nuclear fragments or precipitated protein material can be mistaken for gram-negative organisms. One main problem with examination of Gram stains is the high percentage of false-negative results, or the Gram stain's lack of sensitivity. The use of acridine orange, a fluorochrome stain, can improve the sensitivity, especially for direct microscopic examination of clinical specimens, including cerebrospinal fluid. In acute bacterial meningitis, the infecting organisms can actually be seen in Gram stains of the cerebrospinal fluid specimen in 60% to 80% of culture-proven cases. Tuberculosis and cryptococcal infections can also be detected by microscopic examination of the fluid. Where meningitis is suspected, a blood culture should also be done: it will be positive in 40% to 60% of these cases. In some cases, blood cultures may provide the only definitive information about the causative agent, since cultures of cerebrospinal fluid are positive in about 90% of suspicious cases of bacterial meningitis.

Culture of cerebrospinal fluid is done on a sheep blood agar plate, a chocolate agar plate, and in a tube of thioglycolate broth with enhanced CO_2 atmosphere. Recovery of the same organism from all inoculated media can help to distinguish the contaminated specimens from those that are truly positive.

To detect the specific antigens for some of the more common organisms causing meningitis, the use of a rapid screening test using latex agglutination is employed. Single or multiple antigens can be detected. Iodine contamination from the puncture site has been found to give false-positive results, so it is important that all the iodine solution be removed before collecting the specimen when bacterial antigen testing is needed.

Chemistry Assays. Because of the blood-brain barrier, the normal levels of chemical constituents in the cerebrospinal fluid are not the same as for blood. When cerebrospinal fluid chemistry assays are to be performed, accompanying assays on blood from the patient should also be done for comparison purposes. Certain chemistry assays are done more routinely on cerebrospinal fluid—protein levels, glucose, enzymes, lactate, and tumor markers, for example.

PROTEIN. The use of various types of protein tests and protein electrophoresis is common and important in the diagnosis of several conditions and diseases.

An elevated level of protein in fluid collected by lumbar puncture (over 65 mg/dL) is an important abnormal finding in adults. A traumatic puncture can result in an increased level of protein because of contamination with plasma protein. Other causes of increased protein levels are an increase in the permeability of the blood-brain barrier, a decrease in the removal of protein molecules at the arachnoid villi caused by infectious or toxic processes, an obstruction from mechanical blockage (from tumor, abscess, or adhesions), or an increase in the synthesis of immunoglobulins within lymphocytes and plasma cells of the central nervous system.

A decreased level of protein can be seen when there is leakage of cerebrospinal fluid from a tear or trauma in the dura, from removal of large amounts of cerebrospinal fluid during diagnostic procedures such as pneumoencephalography, from increased intracranial pressure, or from hyperthyroidism conditions.

The measurement of **myelin basic protein** (MBP) has been found useful in the diagnosis of multiple sclerosis. An elevated level has been found in about 90%

of multiple sclerosis patients during an acute exacerbation of the disease. This test is not specific for multiple sclerosis, however, and elevated levels of myelin basic protein can be found in other conditions.

C-reactive protein measurements have been done to differentiate a bacterial meningitis from a viral meningitis. Finding C-reactive protein in cerebrospinal fluid is used by many to identify a bacterial meningitis. Its value is not universally established, however.

GLUCOSE. Tests for glucose must be done without delay to prevent falsely low glucose levels because of glycolysis. The normal ratio of glucose in cerebrospinal fluid to that in blood (plasma) is about 0.6; that is, the cerebrospinal fluid glucose level should be about 60% of the plasma level. Glucose levels in cerebrospinal fluid can vary considerably, however. A glucose level in spinal fluid is considered normal when it is over 40 mg/dL in a fasting patient with a normal plasma glucose level. The difference between the level of glucose in blood (plasma) and in cerebrospinal fluid is the important clinical finding.

A decrease in the glucose level in the cerebrospinal fluid is found in acute or chronic meningitis of several etiologies: bacterial, tuberculous, fungal, amebic, or parasitic. Other causes of decreased spinal fluid glucose levels include systemic hypoglycemia, subarachnoid hemorrhage, and neoplasms involving the meninges. Three mechanisms causing the decreased glucose level are impaired glucose transport, increased glycolytic activity in the central nervous system, and increased glucose utilization by the leukocytes and organisms present in the fluid. The decrease in glucose levels in cerebrospinal fluid from patients with bacterial meningitis can be explained by this last mechanism; that is, the bacteria and leukocytes in the spinal fluid specimen utilize the glucose. This explanation is not universally accepted, however, in terms of the amount of glucose that can be metabolized by the numbers of bacteria present. The glucose level in spinal fluid in viral meningitis is usually not reduced. In cases of diabetic coma, the glucose level in the spinal fluid is elevated, whereas in conditions of insulin shock, the glucose level is low, much the same as the levels expected in the blood glucose measurements for these same conditions. A traumatic (bloody) tap can result in an elevated glucose level in the spinal fluid being assayed.

LACTATE. Any condition causing hypoxic injury to the central nervous system tissue can elevate the lactate levels in the spinal fluid. After a severe head injury, there is a high ventricular CSF lactate level occurring within 18 hours of the injury. A return to normal levels is evidence of clinical improvement; continuation of high levels indicates a poor prognosis. Lactate levels are also used in the differential diagnosis of bacterial, tuberculous, and fungal meningitis (more commonly have higher lactate levels) versus viral meningitis (more commonly have lower lactate levels).

ENZYMES. Increased levels of lactate dehydrogenase (LD), creatine kinase (CK), or aspartate aminotransferase (AST) have been reported for many conditions.

Clinical Correlations: Laboratory Assays and Meningitides. The most important disease of the central nervous system needing an immediate diagnosis is infection of the meninges—meningitis. The use of laboratory results from leukocyte counts, cell differentials, protein, and glucose assays are often used in making the diagnosis. If the diagnosis is overlooked, the disease can be rapidly fatal. The infectious agents for these conditions include bacteria, fungi, mycobacteria, and viruses.

BACTERIAL MENINGITIS. In this infection, the cerebrospinal fluid protein level is elevated, the glucose level decreased, with an increase in the number of leukocytes in the fluid, mostly polymorphonuclear leukocytes as differentiated using the stained smear. Pathogenic organisms can be identified using a Gram stain. The most common are *Haemophilus influenzae, Streptococcus pneumoniae, Neisseria meningitides,* and Group B streptococci. The use of Bacterial Antigen Detection tests can screen for specific bacterial pathogens associated with the various common meningitides.

MYCOBACTERIAL MENINGITIS. In meningitis caused by *Mycobacterium tuberculosis,* the cerebrospinal fluid protein levels are elevated and glucose levels are low. The fluid also shows an increase in lymphocytic leukocytes. An increase in polymorphonuclear leukocytes can also be seen, especially in the early stages of the disease.

FUNGAL MENINGITIS. In this meningitis the specific etiologic agent is detected through microscopic examination, culture, or by use of specific fungal antigen tests. There is usually a low or normal level of glucose and an elevated protein level. Usually there is an increased white cell count with a predominance of lymphocytes.

VIRAL MENINGITIS. This type of meningitis is usually associated with a mild or severe leukocytosis predominantly made up of lymphocytes. Neutrophils may predominate in the initial phases of the infection.

■ SYNOVIAL FLUID ANALYSIS

Synovial fluid is the viscous liquid found in the joint cavities. The synovial membranes line the joints, bursae, and tendon sheaths. Synovial fluid supplies nutrients to the articular cartilage and lubricates the joint spaces. Normal synovial fluid generally has the same chemical composition as plasma since it is an ultrafiltrate of plasma with the addition of a high-molecular-weight mucopolysaccharide—a polymer called **hyaluronate** or **hyaluronic acid**. The presence of hyaluronate differentiates synovial fluid from the other body fluids and provides the normal viscosity of the synovial fluid. This viscosity serves as the lubricant for the joints, which must move freely and frequently. Hyaluronate is secreted by the synoviocyte cells lining the joint cavity. The presence of normal synovial fluid viscosity (that of normal egg white) can, however, be a contributing factor to possible difficulties in performing certain laboratory tests, especially in doing cell counts (see more under Laboratory Assays). Normal synovial fluid has a low leukocyte count ($<0.2 \times 10^9$/L), with the majority of the cells being mononuclear (lymphocytes). Red cells and crystals are normally not present, and the fluid is sterile.

Permeability of the synovial membranes and capillaries may be altered by immunological, mechanical, chemical or bacteriologic conditions producing varying degrees of inflammatory responses. Other disorders elicit changes in the chemical constituents of the joint fluid and in the kinds of cells and crystals present in the joint space. Morphologic examination of the fluid for cells and crystals, together with a Gram stain and culture for microorganisms, often are important in establishing a **differential diagnosis** for the type of joint disease (**arthritis**) present. Perhaps the most important assay is the microscopic examination for crystals. Using specific tests, the differential diagnosis may classify the arthritis type and thus provide direction for treatment and management of the condition. It is important that the correct diagnosis be made so the proper therapy can be started and maintained. Urate gouty arthritis, for example, can be treated successfully if diagnosed but may require life-long therapy.

Differential Diagnosis of Joint Diseases Using Synovial Fluid Assays

Conditions affecting the joints (arthritides) may originate from several causes: crystal-induced, degenerative (or noninflammatory), inflammatory, infectious, or hemorrhagic. There is overlap, however, and occasionally more than one diagnostic condition may be present. Some of the conditions in which synovial fluid assay is most useful are included in Table 7-2.

Synovial fluid is examined to help determine the cause of joint disease, as often evidenced by pain or loss of motion noted by the patient. These symptoms are usually accompanied by an effusion, the abnormal accumulation of the joint fluid. The examination of synovial fluid may be especially important in the differential diagnosis if infective arthritis or crystal-induced synovitis is suspected. These two conditions are the ones with the most urgent indications for arthrocentesis and synovial fluid analysis. Variations in white blood cell counts, percentage of neutrophils present, and levels of protein and glucose are helpful in making this differential diagnosis.[3]

Table 7-2

FINDINGS IN SYNOVIAL FLUID BY DISEASE CATEGORY[5]

	Normal	Noninflammatory	Inflammatory	Infectious
Volume (mL) (from knee)	<4	Often >4	Often >4	Often >4
Color/clarity	Clear, colorless to pale yellow	Transparent pale yellow	Translucent to opaque, yellow to white	Opaque, white
Viscosity	Very high	High	Low	Very low
Fibrin clot present	None	Often	Often	Often
WBC × 10⁹/L	<0.15	<3.0	3-50	>50
Neutrophils	<25%	<25%	>70%	>90%

Noninflammatory (Degenerative Diseases) Fluid. Fluid from persons with degenerative joint disorders such as osteoarthritis, traumatic arthritis, and neurogenic joint disease is usually clear and viscous. The white blood cell (WBC) count is less than 3.0×10^9/L with less than 25% neutrophils. Glucose and protein amounts are generally the same as for normal synovial fluid. Fibrils of collagen or fragments of cartilage may be seen, especially if using phase microscopy.

Inflammatory Fluid. This fluid is usually an effusion associated with immunological diseases such as rheumatoid and lupus arthritis. The fluid aspirated is cloudy, yellow, and has a low viscosity. The white cell count is moderately increased: $3.0–50.0 \times 10^9$/L with greater than 70% neutrophils. The glucose content is normal and the protein level is high. Spontaneous fibrin clots may form in the fluid.

Infectious Fluid. Infectious effusions suggest a bacterial infection. This fluid is generally cloudy and has a low viscosity; it may be yellow, green, or milky. The white cell count is very high—greater than 50.0×10^9/L with greater than 90% neutrophils. The glucose content is very low, and the protein content high with fibrin clot formation being common. Most joint infections are bacterial in origin—*Staphylococcus aureus* and *Neisseria gonorrhoeae* are the most common infecting agents. Possible other organisms are streptococci, *Haemophilus*, mycobacterium, fungi, or anaerobic bacteria. The type of organism can vary with the age of the patient.

Crystal-Induced Fluid. These effusions are seen in conditions of gouty arthritis such as urate gout and pyrophosphate gout (pseudogout). The fluid is yellow or turbid and has a fairly high, but variable white cell count of 0.5 to 200.0×10^9/L with an increased number of neutrophils, up to approximately 90%.[3] Crystals of monosodium urate (MSU) are seen with urate gout and calcium pyrophosphate dihydrate (CPPD)

crystals with pyrophosphate gout (pseudogout). These crystals are differentiated by their morphology and appearance when examined using polarized microscopy with the addition of a full wave compensator (compensated polarized microscopy).

Hemorrhagic Fluid. The presence of red blood cells in effusions from bleeding or hemorrhage in the joint characterizes these fluids. This may be as a result of traumatic injury such as a fracture or tumor or from coagulation deficiencies such as hemophilia. Anticoagulant therapy may also result in hemorrhagic effusions.

Collection of Synovial Fluid

The usual sites from which synovial fluid is collected are the large joints: the knee, hip, shoulder, ankle, and wrist. Normal amounts of synovial fluid even in the large joints (such as the knee) can vary between 0.1 to 2.0 mL. The various arthritides produce varying volumes of synovial fluid. Because of the small amount of fluid normally present, it is common to have a "dry tap" unless effusion is present. When effusion is present, it is often possible to aspirate 10 to 20 mL of the fluid for laboratory examination. If no synovial fluid appears in the syringe during the aspiration process, there may be drops present in the needle itself that may be used for laboratory analysis. In these cases the needle should be left on the syringe and transported to the laboratory.

Synovial fluid is collected by needle aspiration called **arthrocentesis**. A sterile disposable needle and plastic syringe should be used for this collection. Only persons experienced in the technique should perform the aspiration procedure. It is done under strictly sterile conditions using the facility's established universal precautions procedure to prevent transfer of possible infectious agents during the collection process. Only rarely do complications occur in joint aspirations.

Synovial fluid is ideally collected into three containers if there is an adequate volume of specimen aspirated: for microbiologic tests, 5 to 10 mL is collected into a sterile tube; for microscopic evaluation of crystals and cells, 5 mL is collected into a sodium heparin—green-topped tube (alternately, liquid ethylenediaminetetraacetic acid or EDTA—purple-topped tube—can be used for examination of cells); and for clot formation, gross appearance, crystal analysis, and chemical or immunologic procedures, 5 mL is collected into a plain, red-topped tube (no anticoagulant added) and allowed to clot. Normal synovial fluid does not clot. Oxalate, powdered (dry) EDTA, and lithium heparin should not be used since some of the constituents in these additives may appear as crystals, confusing the analysis. This can be true, especially when there is only a small volume of synovial fluid collected, giving an excess of anticoagulant in the tube. This excess may crystallize. The red-topped tube should be centrifuged as soon as possible to remove any cells present, since cells may alter the chemical composition of the fluid. Complement tests are particularly affected by cells still present in the synovial fluid specimen. After centrifugation, the supernatant is removed to be used for various biochemical tests, complement tests, and other tests as needed for the differential diagnosis. Biochemical testing is usually done to define inflammatory processes or infectious or systemic diseases.

The viscosity of synovial fluid can be observed at the time the specimen is collected. Normally as the synovial fluid is allowed to drop from the end of the needle, it will form a string 4 to 6 cm in length. If the string breaks before it reaches 3 cm in length, the viscosity is less than normal. Since inflammatory fluids contain enzymes that will break down hyaluronic acid—the viscosity of synovial fluid is caused by the presence of hyaluronic acid—and since anything present in the fluid to decrease its content will affect (lower) viscosity, the viscosity of the fluid will be lowered. Normal synovial fluid is viscous and does not clot, making the use of anticoagulant additives unnecessary for most normal specimens. When infectious and crystal-induced inflammatory processes are present, however, fibrin clots tend to form in the synovial fluid, making the use of an anticoagulant necessary to adequately perform cell counts and analyze crystals morphologically. Because there continues to be some disagreement on the use of anticoagulated versus nonanticoagulated fluid for crystal analysis, it is expedient to have both tubes available; if artifactual anticoagulant crystals are suspected, the plain tube could also be examined.

If only drops of specimen are available, essential tests can still be performed, such as Gram stain and bacteriologic culture, and microscopic examination for cells and crystals. Examination for crystals is perhaps the most vital of all the analyses done on synovial fluid. It ideally employs the use of **compensated polarized light.**

It is important that a complete, well-documented history from the patient is obtained, including the previous administration of any intraarticular drugs. This information will assist the laboratory in assessing and interpreting the microscopic findings.

Laboratory Assays

Routine laboratory examination of synovial fluid should include the following observations (1) gross appearance: description of color, clarity, and viscosity; (2) microbiologic studies: Gram stain and culture; (3) WBC and differential cell counts; (4) crystal analysis using polarizing light microscopy; and (5) other procedures as necessary. For normal findings, see Table 7-3.

Table 7-3

REFERENCE RANGES FOR NORMAL SYNOVIAL FLUID[4]

Laboratory Assay	Reference Range
Leukocytes	0.15×10^9/L (or <150/µL)
Differential WBC:	
Neutrophils	<25%
Lymphocytes	<75%
Monocytes	<70%
Glucose (blood-synovial fluid difference)	<0.55 mmol/L (or <10 mg/dL)
Protein	10-30 g/L (1-3 g/dL)

If only a limited amount of specimen is available, the microbiologic studies (especially the Gram stain) and crystal analysis should be given priority.

If the synovial fluid is highly viscous, it may be difficult to perform microscopic examination of the fluid. An extremely viscous fluid can be pretreated with buffered hyaluronidase, which reduces the viscosity and makes the fluid easier to pipette. The hyaluronidase is added in appropriate volumes and incubated at room temperature for several minutes to obtain a specimen that can be more completely mixed and pipetted to allow a more even cell distribution for performing cell counts.

Results of laboratory assays must always be correlated with the patient's clinical history, physical examination, and radiologic findings.

Gross Appearance—Color, Clarity, and Viscosity. Normal synovial fluid is crystal clear, viscous, and colorless, resembling uncooked egg white. Non-inflammatory fluid is usually clear, viscous, and pale yellow. Fluid from patients with inflammatory arthritides frequently appears cloudy, turbid, and yellow. It clots on standing because of the presence of fibrinogen and other coagulation factors caused by the inflammatory condition. Fluid from patients with infectious disease often appears grossly purulent. The color of the infectious fluid varies depending on the chromogen of the invading bacteria. Fluid containing crystals or debris from cartilage can appear cloudy or turbid. Fluid from patients with a crystal-induced synovitis can appear purulent or opaque white or occasionally green.

If the arthrocentesis results in the presence of blood in the specimen with an unevenly appearing distribution, it probably has resulted from a bloody or traumatic tap. In this instance, as the aspiration continues, the appearance of blood in the fluid diminishes. This situation also can result in streaks of blood appearing in the syringe. This specimen is not truly a hemorrhagic (bloody) specimen which is uniformly bloody and often does not clot. To distinguish a traumatic tap from a true **hemarthrosis** (bleeding into the joint), the specimen can be centrifuged. A dark-red or dark-brown supernatant fluid is evidence of joint bleeding rather than a traumatic tap. A xanthochromic appearance (yellow) in the supernatant fluid indicates prior bleeding into the joint and that the blood has been in the joint for some time. This appearance is difficult to evaluate because of the normal light yellow appearance of synovial fluid.

To test for clarity, read newsprint through a test tube containing the fluid. Turbidity of the specimen will increase as protein and cell content increase and crystals precipitate, making the newsprint more difficult to read through the tube. Turbidity usually indicates an increase in white cells present in the fluid (leukocytosis); turbidity increases with the degree of inflammation present.

Viscosity can be observed at the time of the arthrocentesis itself. Viscosity can also be assessed in the laboratory by tipping the nonanticoagulated (plain red topped) tube and noting whether the fluid appears thick (viscous) or watery (thin). The viscosity of the specimen parallels the test for mucin clot formation—the **Mucin Clot Test.** The use of this test is of questionable value because its result does not usually lead to any significant change in diagnosis or treatment plan. In the Mucin Clot Test, the polymerization ability of the hyaluronate present in normal synovial fluid is observed. This polymerization ability is affected by various arthritides, resulting in changes in the synovial fluid viscosity. In the test for mucin clotting, a dilute acetic acid solution is added to a supernatant of the centrifuged specimen, and the appearance of the clot that forms is described in terms of "good," "fair," or "poor." Normal synovial fluid will result in a "good" clot that remains intact even when the tube is shaken.

Microbiologic Tests. Gram stain of synovial fluid is one of the priority tests done, even on small volumes (drops) of fluid, to aid in the differential diagnosis of infectious agents affecting the joint. The absence of organisms on the Gram-stained smear does not rule out an infectious joint, however. The Gram-stained smear is positive in less than 25% of patients with gonococcal arthritis and in about 75% of patients with staphylococcal infections.[3] Classical microbiologic studies (Gram stain and culture) can be supplemented with immunologic and biochemical techniques currently available in many laboratories.

Fluid for aerobic culture is collected into a sterile container; fastidious anaerobic culture requires special anaerobic collection containers. *Neisseria gonorrhoae, M. tuberculosis,* staphylococcal organisms, and gram-negative organisms can contribute to bacterial infections of the joints.

WBC and Differential Cell Count. The use of the white cell count is important in the classification of synovial fluid effusions as inflammatory, noninflammatory, or infectious, based on the numbers of white cells counted. Considerable overlap may be seen in the white cell counts for the various arthritides.

For examination of cellular morphology (cytology) and white cell differentiation, smears of the synovial fluid are prepared. To prevent cellular distortion and degeneration of any cells present, the smears should be prepared within 1 hour of the arthrocentesis. Cytocentrifugation yields the best preparation for microscopic morphologic examination.

For both cell counts and cellular morphology examination, pretreatment with hyaluronidase may be necessary if the specimen is highly viscous.

WHITE CELL COUNT. To perform the count, a drop of undiluted, well-mixed synovial fluid is usually mounted in a standard hemocytometer and the cells counted as for other body fluids. If the specimen contains a large number of white cells, greater than 50.0 × 10^9/L, it must first be diluted with physiologic saline (0.9 g/dL) or saponified saline, mixed, and then remounted. The addition of methylene blue dye can be used to help identify leukocytes when a brightfield microscope is used. If any dilution is used, the dilution factor must be applied to the cells counted. The usual diluents used for counting white cells in blood, such as those containing acetic acid, cannot be used for synovial fluid since they will precipitate the hyaluronic acid, producing cell clumping and falsely low cell counts. If hypotonic saline (0.3 g/dL) is used, red blood cells will be preferentially lysed, which helps in enumerating white blood cells in a bloody fluid. The cell counts can be done using either a phase contrast microscope or a standard brightfield (light) microscope.

Extremely viscous synovial fluids may be difficult to pipette and must be pretreated with buffered hyaluronidase before being pipetted into the hemocytometer. Incubation with this reagent reduces the viscosity, making the fluid easier to pipette.

Normal synovial fluid contains only a few white cells (0–0.15 × 10^9/L or less than 150 WBC/µL), and these are primarily lymphocytes—neutrophils (polymorphonuclear leukocytes [PMNs]) are only rarely seen (less than 25%). Usually no red cells are seen in normal synovial fluid. Increased white cell counts are seen in noninflammatory, inflammatory, infectious, and crystal-induced arthritis. Increased white counts of 0–3 × 10^9/L (with less than 25% neutrophils) suggest a noninflammatory joint fluid; 3–50 × 10^9/L (with more than 70% neutrophils) suggest an inflammatory fluid, and an extremely high white count of 50–300 × 10^9/L (with more than 90% neutrophils) suggests an infectious fluid.[5] A few red cells may be present in infectious fluids. In fluids from patients with crystal-induced arthritis, increased white cell counts (with fewer than 90% neutrophils) can be seen along with the presence of crystals. Use of leukocyte counts give nonspecific information but can assist in making the differential diagnosis of arthritides.

DIFFERENTIAL CELL COUNT. Cytocentrifuged preparations of the synovial fluid are preferred for the best evaluation of cellular morphology and differentiation of the white cells present. This technique requires the use of a special cytocentrifuge that uses a slow centrifugation process for a better yield of cellular material while preserving the morphology of the cells. During the centrifugation process, the fluid portion of the specimen is absorbed into a filter paper and the cellular portion is concentrated onto a microscope slide. This preparation, sometimes called a **Cytospin**, is then stained with Wright's stain or with a variety of special stains for hematologic or cytologic examination.

If a cytocentrifuge is not available, smears can be made from specimens centrifuged with a traditional type of laboratory centrifuge. After centrifugation, the supernatant is removed and the sediment used to prepare smears on a glass slide. Thinly made smears give the best results. These smears are also stained with Wright's stain for microscopic examination of cellular morphology.

The types of cells seen on smears of abnormal synovial fluid include neutrophils (PMNs), lymphocytes, plasma cells, monocytes, eosinophils, mononuclear phagocytes (monocytes, macrophages, and histiocytes), synovial lining cells, and lupus erythematosus (LE) cells (see also Morphologic Characteristics of Cells Seen in Body Fluids). The morphology of the neutrophils and lymphocytes seen in synovial fluid resembles the corresponding blood cells. The presence of synovial lining cells does not appear to have any diagnostic significance. If a high percentage of neutrophils is seen (greater than 80%), a Gram stain should always be done.

Crystal Analysis. The identification of specific crystals is particularly important in differentiation of crystal-induced arthritides. The crystals that can be seen in synovial fluid include **monosodium urate (MSU)**, **calcium pyrophosphate dihydrate (CPPD)**, **cholesterol**, **steroids**, **apatite (hydroxyl)**, and other phosphates, oxalate, and **artifacts**. The crystals may precipitate in or around the joints and cause symptoms of clinical gouty arthritis. The type of gout, or specific clinical arthritis, is determined by the type of crystal being deposited. Deposits of monosodium urate crystals result in urate gout, calcium pyrophosphate dihydrate crystals result in pyrophosphate gout (or pseudogout), cholesterol crystals result in cholesterol gout, and so forth. The identification of specific crystals can confirm diagnosis of a particular crystal-induced joint disorder, underlining the particular importance of careful and accurate microscopic analysis and interpretation in this assay. **Exogenous crystals** can also cause symptoms of clinical arthritis. Crystals from powder in gloves introduced into the joint during surgery or from contamination during intraarticular injection of corticosteroid preparations can cause clinical arthritis but also can make crystal analysis confusing.

There is still incomplete understanding of the mechanism for crystal deposition in the joints, but certain factors appear to predispose to this condition. Aging, familial predisposition, and damage to joints are some of these factors. There are metabolic diseases closely associated with the deposition of specific types of crystals: hypothyroidism, hemochromatosis, and hyperparathyroidism are associated with calcium pyrophosphate dihydrate crystals. Local changes in tissue chemistry or loss of specific inhibitors may also contribute

Figure 7-2

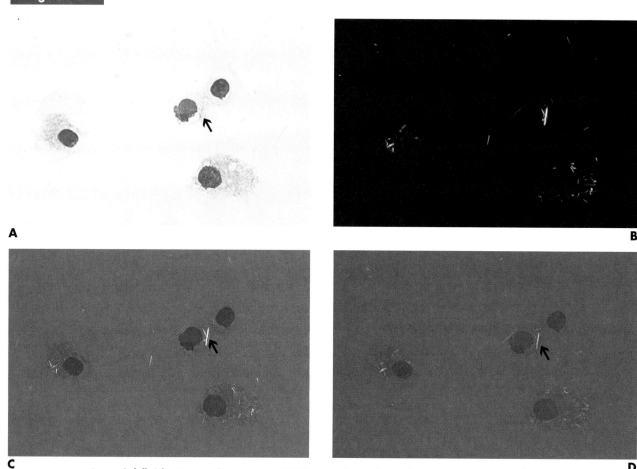

A

B

C

D

Synovial fluid. Monosodium urate (MSU) crystals in Cytospin preparation, Wright's stain, ×640. **A,** Brightfield illumination. Shows cells with intracellular needle-shaped crystals (*arrow*) morphologically resembling MSU. **B,** Same field with polarized light. Shows strongly birefringent crystals, morphologically resembling MSU. **C,** Same field with compensated polarized light, slow wave orientation N-S. Shows cells with intracellular crystals (*arrow*) that are yellow when the long axis of the crystal lies parallel to the direction of the slow wave vibration of the compensator (N-S). Consistent with MSU crystals. **D,** Same field with compensated polarized light, slow wave orientation E-W. Shows cells with intracellular crystals (*arrow*) that are blue when the long axis of the crystal lies perpendicular to the direction of the slow wave vibration of the compensator (E-W). Consistent with MSU crystals.

to crystal deposits. Some of these crystals may be present in the joint for several years before any symptoms of arthritis are noticed by the patient.

MICROSCOPIC ANALYSIS FOR CRYSTALS. A drop of unclotted synovial fluid is placed on a glass slide, a coverglass applied, and initially examined with a **phase contrast microscope**, preferably. The coverglass can be sealed with colorless nail polish to retard evaporation. If nail polish is used, the preparation should be allowed to dry for 15 minutes before any microscopic examination is begun. The microscope objectives may be damaged if they come in contact with the nail pol-

ish before it is dry. A **brightfield microscope** can also be used for the initial evaluation, but should be used with reduced light (by closing the iris diaphragm and lowering the condenser *slightly* to increase the contrast) to more easily find any crystals present. The initial examination is followed by further evaluation using **polarized light microscopy**.

Slides and coverglasses should be cleaned carefully with alcohol and dried with gauze or lens paper before application of the specimen to avoid possible confusion with extraneous fibrous particles that might also polarize. If examination is done too close to the edge

Figure 7-3

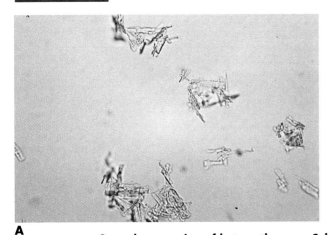
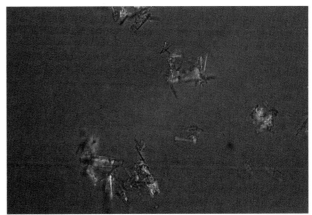

A ... B

Control suspension of betamethasone, Celestone® Soluspan® (Schering Corp.)—a corticosteroid suspension used for intraarticular injections—Cytospin preparation, ×400. **A,** Brightfield illumination. Many needle-shaped crystals, morphologically similar to MSU. **B,** Compensated polarized light with slow wave orientation N-S. Crystals with long axis parallel to slow wave (N-S) are yellow and those with long axes lying perpendicular to the direction of the slow wave vibration of the compensator (E-W) may appear blue; crystals are exhibiting characteristics similar to that of MSU.

of the coverglass where nail polish has been placed to seal the specimen, artifactual confusion may also arise. Artifacts usually have indistinct, amorphous edges or jagged, nonparallel edges, in contrast to the well-defined edges characteristic of monosodium urate or calcium pyrophosphate dihydrate crystals.

BRIGHTFIELD OR PHASE CONTRAST MICROSCOPY. Monosodium urate crystals (MSU) are needle-shaped, may be intracellular, extracellular, or both, and are seen in the initial wet synovial fluid preparation in **urate gout.** Rarely, other crystalline forms may be seen; spherulites or "beachball-like" crystals of MSU have been reported.[2] The presence or absence of intracellular crystals should be noted on the report. Intracellular MSU deposits are characteristic of acute urate gout. Using polarized light MSU crystals appear as birefringent needles or rods (Fig. 7-2). The presence of MSU is a characteristic finding in approximately 90% of patients during acute attacks of gout and are seen in 75% of patients between acute attacks. A control slide with known MSU crystals present should be used for comparison purposes. Some crystalline corticosteroid preparations—betamethasone acetate, for example—appear morphologically identical to MSU and may be used as a control (Fig. 7-3).

Calcium pyrophosphate dihydrate (CPPD) are rhomboid, chunky crystals characteristically seen in the synovial fluid of patients with disorders collectively called **CPPD deposition disease** (Fig. 7-4). Other terms used for this condition are **pseudogout** or **pyrophosphate gout.** This is a distinctively different disease from urate gouty arthritis. These crystals are more commonly seen in patients with degenerative arthritis. CPPD crystals are more difficult to distinguish than MSU since they are only weakly birefringent with polarized light.

Cholesterol crystals are flat, clear, and rhombic with one corner punched out. They are found only rarely in synovial fluid in persons who have had a rheumatoid arthritis condition for a long time but are not normally seen in synovial fluid. **Lipid crystals** exhibiting a Maltese cross formation when observed with polarized light have also been reported in patients with acute arthritis conditions. Crystal deposits of **hydroxyapatite (HA)** can occasionally cause **apatite gout** but are so small they are difficult or impossible to see with brightfield microscopy and do not polarize light (they are nonbirefringent). Other crystal or crystal-like deposits seen are calcium oxalate, collagen fibrils, cartilage fragments, glove powder, metallic fragments after prosthetic arthroplasty, or corticosteroid esters. Glove powder or starch might be introduced into the specimen during the collection or processing of the specimen. Starch shows a Maltese cross appearance with polarized light and might be confused with lipid droplets of cholesterol, which also polarize (Fig. 7-5). Corticosteroid crystals can be deposited in joints of patients after treatment with this drug and can appear similar to other crystals such as monosodium urate (MSU) and calcium pyrophosphate dihydrate

Figure 7-4

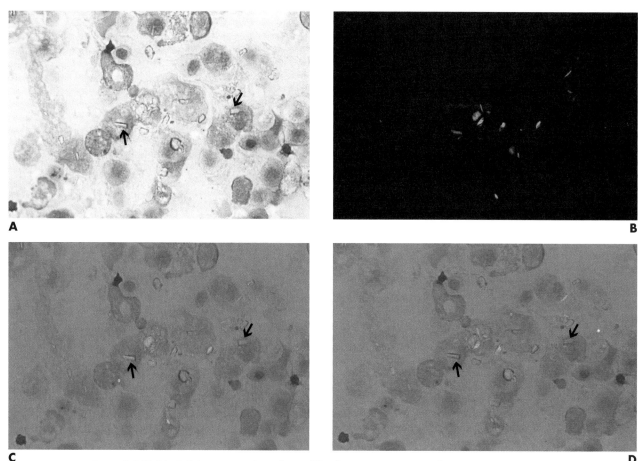

A B

C D

Synovial fluid. Calcium pyrophosphate dihydrate (CPPD) crystals in Cytospin preparation, Wright's stain, ×640. A, Brightfield illumination. Shows cells with intracellular chunky crystals (*arrows*) and some extracellular chunky crystals; crystals morphologically resemble CPPD. **B,** Same field with polarized light. Shows weakly birefringent crystals. **C,** Same field with compensated polarized light, slow wave orientation N-S. Shows cells with intracellular crystals (*arrows*) and extracellular crystals that are blue when the long axis of the crystal lies parallel to the direction of the slow wave vibration of the compensator. **D,** Same field with compensated polarized light, slow wave orientation E-W. Shows cells with intracellular cyrstals (*arrows*) and extracellular crystals that are yellow when the long axis of the crystal lies perpendicular to the direction of the slow wave vibration of the compensator.

(CPPD) (see Figs. 7-2 and 7-6). Steroid crystals generally are extracellular and appear in large numbers, greater than that typical of either MSU or CPPD deposits. The clinical history for the patient is especially important in these cases.

POLARIZED LIGHT MICROSCOPY AND USE OF COMPENSATED POLARIZED LIGHT. By using polarized light, more definitive microscopic examination may be done to assess the morphology of crystals deposited in synovial fluid. A polarizing microscope with a **first-order red com-**pensator (quartz compensator or filter) is used. This microscope is set up by placing a polarizing filter (also called a **polarizer**) between the light source (bulb) and the specimen. A second polarizing filter (also called an **analyzer**) is placed above the specimen, usually between the objective and the eyepiece. This analyzer can either be placed at some point in the microscope tube or in the eyepiece itself. One of the polarizing filters, usually the polarizer, is rotated until the two filters are at right angles to each other (crossed polariz-

Figure 7-5

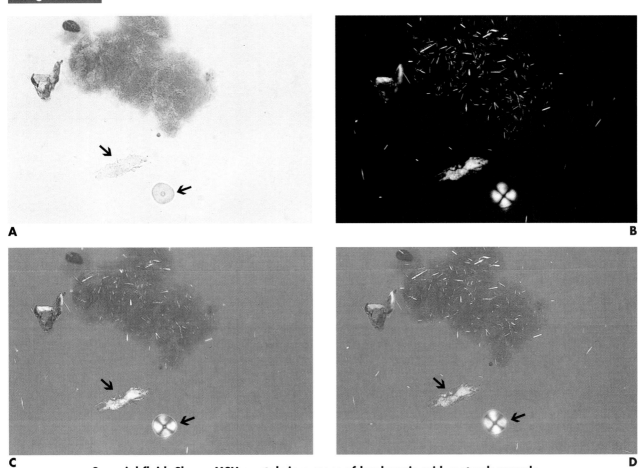

A

B

C

D

Synovial fluid. Shows MSU crystals in a mass of hyaluronic acid, a starch granule (contaminant: powder from gloves), and a fiber (also a contaminant). Cytospin preparation, Wright's stain, ×400. A, Brightfield illumination. Shows pink mass (crystals not well defined), starch granule (*right arrow*), and fiber (*left arrow*). B, Same field with polarized light. Many needle-shaped strongly birefringent crystals, morphologically resembling MSU, fiber polarizes (*left arrow*), starch granule polarizes and exhibits typical Maltese cross formation (*right arrow*). C, Same field with compensated polarized light, slow wave orientation N-S. Shows many extracellular crystals that are yellow when the long axis of the crystal lies parallel to the direction of the slow wave vibration of the compensator (N-S); starch granule (*right arrow*) shows a Maltese cross formation. D, Same field with compensated polarized light, slow wave orientation E-W. Shows many extracellular crystals that are blue when the long axis of the crystal lies perpendicular to the slow wave vibration of the compensator; starch granule (*arrow*) shows a Maltese cross formation.

ing filters). When looking through the microscope, one notices extinction of light seen as a black field because all light waves are canceled when the filters are at right angles to each other.

Certain structures or crystals have the ability to rotate or polarize light so they are visible when viewed through crossed polarizing filters. This property or ability is known as **crystal anisotropy** or **birefringence**.

Objects exhibiting this ability are termed weakly or strongly birefringent depending on how completely they polarize light. Objects that are strongly birefringent appear bright (white) against a dark background, whereas weakly birefringent objects appear less bright.

Using the polarizing microscope, MSU crystals appear as strongly birefringent with a needle or rod shape and are from 1 to 30 μm in length (see Fig. 7-2).

Figure 7-6

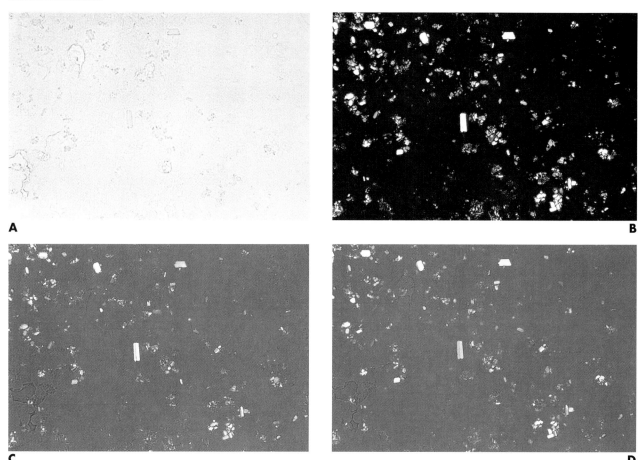

A

B

C

D

Synovial fluid from joint after injection with Aristocort® (triamcinolene diacetate)—a corticosteroid drug used as an intraarticular or intrasynovial injection, wet preparation, unstained, ×400. Example of contaminant causing confusing results where the overall morphology resembles CPPD and the sign of birefrigence is like that of MSU. **A,** Brightfield illumination. Many needle-shaped crystals, morphologically similar to CPPD. **B,** Polarized light. Shows many stongly birefringent crystals, resembling MSU. **C,** Compensated polarized light, slow wave orientation N-S. Crystals with their long axes lying parallel to the slow wave vibration of the compensator (N-S) are yellow; crystals are exhibiting characteristics similar to those of MSU. **D,** Compensated polarized light, slow wave orientation E-W. Crystals with their long axes perpendicular to the slow wave vibration of the compensator (E-W) are blue; crystals are exhibiting characteristics similar to those of MSU.

They may be intracellular or extracellular. This distinction is reported. The presence of intracellular MSU crystals is characteristic of acute urate gout. Monosodium urate crystals may also deposit in a stony growth or **tophus** around the joint area. Crystals from a tophus may be quite large in size.

With polarized light, crystals of CPPD appear as weakly birefringent and can be rod-shaped, rectangular, or rhomboid. They can occasionally be needle-shaped (see Fig. 7-4). They more often appear short and chunky, varying from 1 to 20 µm in length and up to about 4 µm in width. CPPD crystals are character-

istic findings in CPPD crystal-deposition disorders (pseudogout or pyrophosphate gout are examples).

By use of compensated polarized light, crystals of MSU and CPPD that have previously been identified with polarized light microscopy are further identified by adding a first-order red compensator. Morphology and intensity of birefringence alone are not enough to completely identify these crystals. With the addition of a first-order red compensator, birefringent crystals have different properties that aid in their identification. When the compensator is in place, the background appears magenta, rather than black, when looking through the microscope. The compensator may be inserted either above the analyzer or the polarizer and is inserted in such a way that the axis of the **slow vibration** of the compensator (referred to as the **slow wave**) is at an angle of 45 degrees to the crossed polarizers. In establishing the identity of the crystals observed under these conditions, it is necessary to know the direction of the slow wave. Crystals are identified by observation of the color of the long axis of the crystal and its relationship or orientation to the direction of the slow wave. MSU and CPPD have distinct, but opposite, characteristics when viewed with compensated polarized light (see Figs. 7-2 and 7-4).

Crystals of MSU appear yellow when the long axis of the crystal lies parallel to the slow wave of the red compensator. These same crystals appear blue when the long axis of the crystal lies perpendicular to the slow wave. This observation may be made by looking for crystals that have a particular orientation (as yellow when parallel to the slow wave) and then repositioning the slow wave at right angles to its original position. This crystal should then change its color to blue. If the microscope has a rotating stage, the stage may be moved so that the crystal is rotated 90 degrees. A useful reminder for MSU crystals is yellow parallel equals gout.

Crystals of MSU will appear yellow when parallel to the slow wave and blue when perpendicular to it (see Fig. 7-2). Crystals that exhibit this characteristic are termed negatively birefringent—the sign of birefringence is negative. This term is not used in the report to avoid any misinterpretation that the MSU crystal analysis itself is negative. Crystals are reported as being present or absent and are identified as to their type.

Crystals of CPPD appear blue when parallel to the slow wave and yellow when perpendicular to it (see Fig. 7-4). Crystals that exhibit this characteristic are termed positively birefringent—the sign of birefringence is positive. Positive birefringence is defined as occurring when the crystal appears blue when the long axis is parallel to the slow wave. With CPPD crystals, it may be difficult to determine what the long axis is; they often appear chunky and almost square in shape.

When crystals are examined using compensated polarized light for identification purposes, it is important that a **control preparation** be used to ensure the correct interpretation. Permanent cytocentrifuged slides or a wet preparation of known MSU crystals can be used. As an alternative, the birefringent properties of some corticosteroids, commonly used to treat joint disease, may be used as a control. A suspension of betamethasone acetate corticosteroid gives reactions very similar to that of MSU crystals when examined with compensated light (see Fig. 7-3). This suspension can be used as a wet preparation or in a more permanent cytocentrifuged slide preparation. Other control solutions are also available.

SEROUS FLUID ANALYSIS (PLEURAL, PERICARDIAL, AND PERITONEAL FLUIDS)

Pleural, pericardial or peritoneal (or ascitic) fluids are contained in the cavity or space between the two membranes lining the lungs (the pleural cavity), the heart (the pericardial cavity), and the viscera of the abdomen and pelvis (the peritoneal cavity). Each of these spaces or cavities normally contains only a small amount of fluid, which serves as a lubricant. These body cavities are each lined with two thin, mesothelium-lined membranes referred to as **serous membranes**. One membrane lines the cavity wall (the parietal membrane); the other covers the organ contained in the cavity (the visceral membrane), and there is normally very little space between the two. Collectively, the fluid contained in the space is known as **serous fluid**.

Normally there is only enough serous fluid to lubricate the surfaces of the membranes and organs as they move within the cavities: heart contraction and relaxation within the pericardial membrane, lung expansion and contraction within the pleural membrane, and movement of the viscera of the abdomen and pelvis within the peritoneal membrane. The normal fluid is an ultrafiltrate of plasma—a transudate— and is continuously produced and reabsorbed. It does not usually accumulate unless there is onset of disease or injury. The increased accumulation of serous fluid is known as a **serous effusion**. Fluid accumulating in the pleural space is **pleural effusion**, in the pericardial space is **pericardial effusion**, and in the peritoneal space is **peritoneal effusion** or **ascites**. The accumulation of serous fluid is most frequently caused by damage to the lining of the cavity associated with changes in the membrane permeability caused by an imbalance or disruption in homeostatic forces that control movement of fluid across the membrane, as from circulatory disturbances, infection, or malignancy. Formation depends on capillary hydrostatic pressure, plasma oncotic pressure, and capillary permeability. Under normal conditions, serum proteins exert colloidal osmotic pressure, which acts to retard the movement of fluid into the serous space. If the level of plasma protein decreases, the osmotic pressure drops. As more fluid moves into the serous space, the serous effusion develops. Serous effusions can develop when there is a decrease in osmotic pressure, an increase in hydrostatic pressure, an increase in capillary permeability, a decrease in lymphatic reabsorption, or an obstruction. The reason for the accumulation of excess fluid can usually be determined by various laboratory assays.

Aspiration of the accumulated fluid is indicated for any undiagnosed effusion, to confirm a prior diagnosis, or for therapeutic reasons when the excess fluid causes problems for the patient. Aspiration of pleural fluid is **thoracentesis**, of pericardial fluid is **pericardiocentesis**, and of peritoneal fluid (ascitic fluid) is **paracentesis**.

Transudates Versus Exudates

Effusions of serous fluid are either transudates, ultrafiltrates of plasma, or exudates. Classification of serous effusions as exudates or transudates is an important step in establishing a diagnosis for effusions with an unknown etiology.

Historically, transudates have been differentiated from exudates based on their specific gravity and their levels of total protein. Transudates are defined as fluids with a specific gravity less than 1.015 and a total protein less than 3.0 g/dL. Exudates have a specific gravity greater than 1.015 and a total protein level of 3.0 g/dL or greater (meeting either of these criteria makes the fluid an exudate). Because the procedure for specific gravity is considered unsafe (because of potential transmission of a pathogenic organism—a biohazard), it is no longer done on body fluids in most laboratories. Traditional parameters cannot always be followed, therefore, and other measures are used. The differentiation should be established in conjunction with a combination of test results and use of sound clinical judgment (Table 7-4). Systemic conditions such as congestive heart failure or cirrhosis of the liver usually result in the formation of a transudate. Transudates resemble clear, pale yellow tissue fluid, with a low protein content and few or no cells (the total protein is usually <1 g/dL). The classification of a serous fluid as a transudate usually defines it as a benign (nonmalignant) condition. If the effusion is found to be a transudate, generally no more diagnostic procedures are needed.

When the serous membranes are directly affected by a more localized condition such as an inflammatory, infectious, or malignant process the resulting effusion more likely is an exudate. In general, exudates contain more total protein and more cells, resulting in a higher specific gravity and requiring additional diagnostic procedures to elicit the cause of the effusion. These fluid exudates should be saved in the refrigerator for about 1 week in case further testing is necessary. When serous fluid is collected, a specimen of venous blood should be collected at the same time for blood chemistries. Specific chemistry tests performed to help differentiate an exudate from a transudate include total protein, lactate dehydrogenase, glucose, cholesterol, and possibly bilirubin. Total protein levels are necessary to establish the protein fluid:serum ratios; for pleural fluid, if the total protein level is greater than 50% of the serum total protein level, the fluid represents an exudate.

Table 7-4

DIFFERENTIATING EXUDATES FROM TRANSUDATES*		
Observation/ Test	Exudate	Transudate
Appearance	Cloudy, turbid, purulent, or bloody; may clot (may have high fibrinogen)	Watery, clear, pale yellow; does not clot
Leukocyte Count	0.5 - >1.0 × 10⁹/L with increased neutrophils; lymphocytes seen with tuberculosis or rheumatoid arthritis	Low <1.0 × 10⁹/L with more than 50% mononuclear cells (lymphocytes and monocytes)
Erythrocyte Count	>100.0 × 10⁹/L, especially with a malignancy	Low (unless from a traumatic tap)
Total protein	>3 g/dL (or greater than half the serum level)	<3 g/dL
Lactate Dehydrogenase	Raised (>60% of the serum level because of cellular debris)	Low
Glucose	Lower than serum level with some infections and high cell counts	Varies with serum level

*Note: Some values are variable between the two effusions. Clinical considerations must always be used in combination with the laboratory findings.

Pleural Fluid

There is normally about 1 to 15 mL of pleural fluid in the pleural space surrounding the lungs. In normal conditions, there is not a true pleural cavity. An abnormal accumulation of pleural fluid (pleural effusion) in the pleural space is seen in the presence of certain diseases—where an excess amount of fluid is formed, when there is decreased lymphatic resorption from the pleural cavity, or from a combination of these factors. This can be seen when inflammation occurs, when the plasma protein level drops, when congestive heart failure is present, or when there is decreased lymphatic drainage. Many pleural effusions result from congestive heart failure. Normal pleural fluid does not clot, but it is important that some of the specimen be collected into a tube with anticoagulant present (heparin) since abnormal fluids frequently contain fibrinogen that will result in the formation of a clot. Cell counts cannot be done accurately on a clotted specimen. The total protein level of pleural fluid can be used to distinguish transudates from exudates—normal pleural fluid total protein is about 1 to 2 g/dL. Pleural fluids with a total protein greater than 3.0 g/dL generally are classified as exudates, whereas fluids with a total protein less than 3.0 g/dL are classified as transudates. Other differentiating criteria for a pleural exudate are (1) pleural fluid/serum protein ratio greater than 0.5; (2) pleural fluid lactate dehydrogenase (LD) greater then 200 IU (upper normal limit for serum equal to 300 IU); (3) pleural fluid/serum LD ratio greater than 0.6; and (4) pleural fluid cholesterol greater than 60 mg/dL or with a ratio of pleural fluid/serum cholesterol greater than 0.3.[3]

Pericardial Fluid

The pericardial space surrounding the heart normally contains about 10 to 50 mL of a clear, straw colored tissue fluid, an ultrafiltrate of plasma called pericardial fluid. When an abnormal accumulation of this fluid occurs, it fills the space around the heart and can mechanically inhibit the normal activity of the heart. This mechanical interference must be relieved immediately by aspiration of the excess fluid. Pericardial effusion is most frequently caused by damage to the lining of the cavity. It is associated with changes in the permeability of the membranes caused by an infection (pericarditis), malignancy, or metabolic damage (uremia).

Peritoneal (Ascitic) Fluid

There is normally less than 100 mL of clear, straw colored tissue fluid present in the peritoneal space—the serous space surrounding the abdominal viscera. Much larger amounts of fluid can be removed to alleviate discomfort associated with massive ascites in some patients. This fluid is called peritoneal fluid or ascitic fluid. The accumulation of peritoneal fluid, or peritoneal effusion, signals that the patient has ascites. Ascites is seen with increased hydrostatic pressure of the systemic circulation (seen in congestive heart failure), with decreased plasma oncotic pressure (seen with hypoproteinemia), increased permeability of the capillaries in the peritoneum (seen with peritonitis), and decreased lymphatic absorption (seen in some neoplastic conditions).

Collection of Serous Fluid Specimen

It is important that serous fluids be collected and handled in an appropriate manner so that the interpretation of laboratory results be fully used for diagnostic purposes. Only when the specimen has been properly collected, preserved, handled, transported, and tested can the results be considered valid and useful information for diagnosis. The collection process requires close cooperation between the clinician and the laboratory. Appropriate procedures should be established for this collection process. Serous fluids are collected under strictly sterile conditions by using a needle inserted into the serous cavity and by aspirating the fluid. This collection is done for diagnostic purposes as well as to relieve the patient of symptoms such as difficult breathing due to excess fluid accumulating around the lungs or from massive ascites in the abdomen. A pleural effusion can compress the lungs, a pericardial fluid can compress the heart (cardiac tamponade), and peritoneal or ascitic effusion can elevate the diaphragm, compressing the lungs.

The fluid aspirated should be divided into several different tubes or containers for the various laboratory assays: ideally 5-7 mL into an EDTA (purple-topped) tube for gross appearance, cell counts, cell morphology and differential (with Wright's stained smears); 7-10 mL into a heparin (green-topped) tube for lactate dehydrogenase, total protein, glucose, amylase, or other chemistry assays; 7-10 mL into a sterile heparin (green-topped) tube for culture, Gram stain, acid-fast bacilli stain on spun sediment or cytocentrifuge smear; 2-3 mL in a heparin syringe for pH; and 25 mL or more in a heparin container for cytologic examination (Papanicolaou stain or cell blocks). Requirements for specific tests should be consulted when collecting and handling serous fluid specimens. Sequentially collected specimens can be collected and observed to establish a possible traumatic or bloody tap.

A **traumatic tap**, in which blood is introduced into the specimen as a result of the puncture itself, must be differentiated from the presence of blood in the specimen from other sources. In a traumatic, or bloody tap, the blood is usually not distributed in a homogeneous manner. Sequentially collected tubes will gradually clear as the collection continues; the first tube collected will appear more bloody than the last tube.

Laboratory Assays

The purpose of laboratory assays of most serous effusions is (1) to differentiate an exudate from a transudate, (2) to differentiate a malignancy from a non-malignancy in patients with serous exudates, and (3) to diagnose specific causes of a serous effusion (malignancy, infection, systemic lupus erythematosis). The most important diseases requiring laboratory assay of pleural exudates, for example, are infection and malignancy. For this reason, culture and cytologic studies are the most useful tests done using pleural fluid. Reference values for normal serous fluids are not generally known, because these fluids are normally present in only small volumes, and aspiration/collection is not done unless a disease process/trauma is suspected.

The usefulness and significance of specific assays varies depending on the serous fluid being evaluated. General laboratory assays performed on most serous fluids include gross examination, cytologic studies, stains and culture for organisms, and total protein assay. On selected fluids, cell counts (RBC, WBC), cell differential counts, or other chemistry tests as necessary are done. In establishing a diagnosis, results of laboratory assays must always be used in correlation with clinical findings, along with results of other specialized diagnostic procedures.

As stated previously, differentiation of exudates from transudates is important to determine which of the serous effusions require further laboratory evaluation. No single test can do this. Several observations or tests must be used in combination to assist in making this distinction (see Table 7-4).

In an exudate, when cellular debris is present in the fluid, tests for lactate dehydrogenase (LD) levels performed on the fluid are often raised. If the fluid LD level is greater than 50% of the serum level, the fluid is considered an exudate. Glucose levels done on serous fluid and blood collected simultaneously will show a fluid glucose level lower than the blood glucose with some infections and with high cell counts.

Tests done on exudates can include Gram stain and culture, cytology, WBC and cell differential studies, glucose, total protein, pH, enzymes, and tumor marker assays. As stated previously, if the effusion is a transudate, no further laboratory testing is usually necessary. To maintain proper quality assurance, it is important to establish a clear differential diagnosis before ordering any extra laboratory assays, when possible.

Gross Examination. The serous fluid is first observed for its appearance. This initial observation can be important in determining the pathogenesis of the effusion. Fluids that are transudates are usually clear and pale yellow and do not clot (no fibrinogen is present). Exudates are generally cloudy to purulent and often clot while standing because of fibrinogen in the specimen. The total volume of fluid collected should be estimated and the appearance (clarity and color) of the specimen noted.

APPEARANCE. Cloudy and purulent serous exudates are usually associated with an infectious condition. The presence of large numbers of cells, microorganisms, and debris, along with elevated protein levels, contribute to the cloudy appearance of the fluid. Hemorrhagic fluid can be present because of a traumatic tap or because of malignancies or trauma: in pleural fluid from a pulmonary infarction; in peritoneal fluid from intestinal infarction, ruptured liver or spleen, or pancreatitis. Some fluids take on characteristic colors caused by specific conditions. Bile-stained peritoneal fluid can be green when there has been perforation of the gallbladder or intestine or with duodenal ulcers. The presence of bile can be confirmed by performing a tablet test for urine bilirubin (such as Ictotest, Miles) on the specimen (see Procedure 4-4). Peritoneal fluid can also be green because of cholecystitis and acute pancreatitis. Milky white fluid can be caused by a chylous or pseudochylous effusion. True chylous fluid is lymph fluid that has leaked into the pleural or peritoneal cavities as a result of damage to or obstruction of the thoracic duct. The presence of chyle is indicative of neither a transudate nor an exudate. On occasion it is possible to have exudates that appear straw colored, much like the color of a transudate.

Clarity is reported as clear, cloudy, or bloody: color as colorless or yellow, for example. Turbidity can be further described as being slightly, moderately, or markedly cloudy.

CLOTTING. Serous fluids that are transudates do not clot, whereas exudates generally do clot. The ability to clot must be observed in a specimen collected in a container without anticoagulant. Clotting will occur when there is fibrinogen present in the fluid.

Microscopic Examination. Counting red and white cells in serous fluid by using a **manual counting chamber method** is the method of choice (Procedure 7-3). Cell counts on serous fluids are classically performed using the Improved Neubauer Hemocytometer (see Fig. 7-1). Based on the appearance of the fluid, the count is done on an undiluted or diluted sample. If the fluid is visibly cloudy, a dilution is probably needed. To identify the cells morphologically, a method is needed to concentrate the cells, ideally to yield a high recovery rate while preserving the cells intact. Use of the cytocentrifuge produces good cell recovery and preserves the cellular detail for most serous fluid specimens. Thus most smears of serous fluids for leukocyte cell differentials and general cytologic studies are made using stained cytocentrifuge preparations, if possible. Wright's stain is used for cell leukocyte differentials and Papanicolaou stain for cytologic studies. Other preparations of the specimen for morphologic examination can include recovery of sediment by use of a filtration or sedimentation technique, or by use of a general purpose laboratory centrifuge.

CELL COUNTS. The serous fluid should be examined for the presence of clots and fibrin strands. Their presence should be noted on the report since they may affect the results reported for the cell count. Completely clotted specimens cannot be used for cell counts.

Clear, well-mixed, anticoagulated specimens may be mounted undiluted in the hemocytometer and the cells counted (see Procedure 7-3). The technique for counting the cells in serous fluids is the same as that for counting leukocytes in CSF specimens (see Fig. 7-1). Usually leukocyte and erythrocyte counts can be done on the same chamber. Dilutions for higher counts, if needed, can be done using isotonic saline. Special diluents are also available. Glacial acetic acid is not used to dilute serous fluids (as is done for leukocyte counts in blood), because if fluids are high in protein, acetic acid will clump the leukocytes. Micropipetting devices can be used for the needed dilution. To count white cells in bloody fluids, the red cells must first be lysed. Turk's solution (a lysing and staining diluent) or an ammonium oxalate with methylene blue diluent can be used. It is important to know the limitations of the diluent being used. Turk's solution, for example, must not be used when the specimen has a high protein content; the acetic acid in

the diluent will cause the protein to clump, entrapping white cells.

Diluted samples are remounted and recounted in the hemocytometer, and the cells counted multiplied by the dilution factor used.

Total cell counts alone are not generally very useful in differential diagnosis using pleural and pericardial effusions. Leukocyte counts greater than 0.5×10^9/L are considered clinically significant. Generally, increased total leukocyte counts suggest an infectious process—as bacterial or tuberculous—and can also be used to distinguish transudates from exudates in many instances (see Table 7-4). Leukocyte counts greater than 1.0×10^9/L are suggestive of an exudate, whereas counts less than 1.0×10^9/L are suggestive of a transudate.

The total leukocyte count may be helpful in differentiating between a true peritoneal transudate (such as with cirrhosis) and fluid from a spontaneous bacterial peritonitis (SBP), which is caused by bacteria passing from the blood to the peritoneal/ascitic fluid. Leukocyte counts greater than 0.5×10^9/L in peritoneal fluid are consistent with patients with SBP. Properly anticoagulated specimens should be used for cell counts and cell differentials. If the specimen is completely clotted, cell counts cannot be done accurately. Cytologic studies for malignant cells can be done using clotted fluid, but an attempt should be made to break up the clots before making the smears. If a clotted specimen must be used for cell counts or other morphologic studies, this fact should be noted on the results report.

Procedure 7-3

MANUAL CELL COUNTS USING SEROUS FLUID

1. Mix the fluid for several minutes.

2. Using a disposable Pasteur pipette, mount the well-mixed fluid onto a clean hemocytometer with a coverglass in place by touching the pipette tip to the edge of the chamber. Mount both sides of the chamber. Discard the pipette in the appropriate biohazard waste container.

3. Using the 40× objective (high-power) of the microscope, count and classify the red and white blood cells (keeping each type as a separate count) in 10 square millimeters (see Fig. 7-1. If the cells are too numerous to count accurately, dilute the specimen with isotonic saline or other diluent, mix, mount, and recount. Apply dilution factor to result.)

4. Calculate cell count for each type of cell—white and red. To calculate, the following considerations apply:
   a. The number of cells counted
   b. The dilution factor, if needed
   c. The volume counted (depth of chamber—0.1 mm—× area counted)

Calculation formula:

$$\frac{\text{No. of cells counted} \times \text{dilution}}{\text{area counted} \times \text{depth}} = \text{cell count per } \mu L$$

Example: The fluid is diluted 1:10 before being counted. If a total of 50 white cells are counted in the 10 square millimeters of the hemocytometer,

$$\frac{50 \times 10}{10 \times 0.1} = \frac{500}{1} = 500 \text{ cells/}\mu L \text{ (or } 0.5 \text{ cells} \times 10^9\text{/L)}$$

EVALUATION OF CELL MORPHOLOGY (CELL DIFFERENTIAL). The accuracy and precision of the leukocyte differential count is greatly enhanced by using a Wright's stained cytocentrifuge preparation for the smear. The yield of cells, along with their preservation, is better than with ordinary centrifugation methods. In tuberculous pleural fluids, there is a moderately elevated leukocyte count with a predominance of lymphocytes, with some plasma cells also present. In many bacterial infections, the leukocyte count performed on pleural fluid is usually higher and neutrophils predominate such as in acute inflammatory conditions caused by pneumonia. Pulmonary infarct and pancreatitis also show a predominance of neutrophils in the pleural fluid. In malignant conditions, lymphocytes are frequently increased. In pericardial fluids, cell differentials are of little value in differential diagnosis. In patients with a true spontaneous bacterial peritonitis (SBP), 50% of the leukocytes in the peritoneal fluid are neutrophils. It is important to use cytologic studies for the presence of possible tumor cells in serous fluids. Any suspicious cells should always be referred to the appropriately trained cytologist for confirmation (see also Morphologic Characteristics of Cells Seen in Body Fluids).

Microbiologic Tests. For serous effusions of unknown etiology, a Gram stain and culture are done. These tests are positive in only a limited percentage of cases of infectious effusions, however. Special cultures are done when necessary.

Other Laboratory Tests. Specific chemistry tests used to distinguish transudates from exudates have already been discussed: total protein, lactate dehydrogenase, cholesterol, and bilirubin. Other tests necessary to diagnose or treat may be ordered.

■ SEMEN ANALYSIS

Seminal fluid (semen) consists of a combination of products of various male reproductive organs: testes and epididymis, seminal vesicles, prostate and bulbourethral and urethral glands. Each product or fraction varies in its individual composition, each contributing to the whole specimen. During ejaculation, the products are mixed in order to produce the normal viscous semen specimen or **ejaculate.**

Spermatozoa (sperm cells) are produced in the **testes** under the influence of testosterone; these mature in the epididymis. The seminal fluid serves to maintain the spermatozoa. The majority of the seminal fluid volume (60%) is produced by the seminal vesicles. The seminal fluid component produced in the seminal vesicles has a high content of flavin that contributes to the fluorescence of the fluid. Other characteristics of this fluid are high amounts of fructose, potassium, and

ascorbic acid. Fructose is the primary source of energy for the sperm's survival and motility. Some of the seminal fluid volume (20%) is produced by the prostate. This portion consists of a milky fluid containing acid phosphatase and coagulation and liquefaction enzymes. The remaining seminal fluid volume (10-15%) is produced by the **epididymides, vas deferentia, bulbourethral glands,** and **urethral glands.**

Ejaculated human semen appears as a viscous and yellow-gray fluid. It forms a fairly firm gel-like clot immediately after ejaculation. In vitro (at room temperature), this clot liquefies spontaneously and completely within 5 to 60 minutes. If the **liquefaction process** requires more than 1 hour, the specimen is considered abnormal. The entire collection represents a thorough mixture of coagulated seminal plasma with sperm trapped within its matrix. Until the liquefaction process is complete, sperm are effectively immobilized within this coagulum. The liquefaction process must be complete before any laboratory analyses can be done.

Analysis of semen is done for several reasons. These include assessment of fertility/infertility, forensic purposes, determination of the effectiveness of vasectomy, and determination of the suitability of semen for artificial insemination procedures.

Approximately 40% of diagnosed infertility can be attributed to male infertility, with another 40% attributed to the female partner. Infertility therefore must be considered as a factor involving both partners and investigated as such. If valid information is to be provided about the fertility of the male partner, semen analysis must be performed only by using properly standardized procedures.

Objective information on the qualitative and quantitative characteristics of the semen is perhaps the most important aspect of the laboratory diagnosis of male infertility. In cases of alleged rape, sexual crimes or sexual abuse, the collection and analysis of the semen specimen is an important step in establishing the chain of evidence needed in courts of law. Identification of a specimen such as semen (by presence of sperm) can be important in these forensic cases.

To evaluate male infertility, routine analytical assays of semen usually include physical measurements such as viscosity, coagulation and liquefaction, volume, pH, sperm concentration (sperm count), and sperm motility, morphology, and viability studies. When antisperm antibodies are detected, fertility potential can be compromised. These antibodies can interfere with sperm cell motility, viability, or the interaction of the sperm with the oocyte. Immunoassays are done to detect the presence of antisperm antibodies—there are several methods used. These antibodies can be present in the semen and on the sperm of an infertile male and/or in the serum circulating in the male and the female being evaluated.

Biochemical assays include measurements of the concentration of fructose, citric acid, acid phosphatase, zinc, and transferrin/lactoferrin.

In postvasectomy analyses, only the presence of sperm, viable or nonviable, is significant. After vasectomy, sterilization is not immediate—as many as six to ten ejaculations after the surgery may be necessary to render the ejaculate free of residual sperm cells. It is important that the patient have one or more semen analyses after the vasectomy to ensure that sterility has been achieved. To obtain an appropriate specimen for sperm counts after vasectomy, the patient should collect the specimen after 2 or 3 days of abstinence. The count is performed as for a routine semen analysis. A patient is considered sterile when two sperm counts, done on specimens collected 1 month apart, are negative for the presence of sperm cells.

When forensic examinations are requested, usually in cases of alleged rape or suspected homicide, it is extremely important that special precautions be employed in collecting the specimens to maintain the chain of evidence being constructed for the case. Proper specimen identification procedures are of special importance. The presence of sperm cells in vaginal washings or in fluids obtained by direct vaginal aspirations can be detected in examinations for forensic purposes. Direct smears can be prepared from the vaginal specimen and stained with Papanicolaou stain. It is possible to recover well-preserved sperm cells from the vagina even after several hours following coitus. Semen present on clothing or on other fabrics can also be analyzed for the presence of sperm cells.

Since a semen sample may contain biohazardous organisms—HIV and/or viruses causing hepatitis and herpes, for example—the same universal precautions should be taken in handling this specimen as for any other biologic sample being tested in the laboratory. Gloves should be worn and other barrier protection observed, if needed.

Collection of Semen Specimen

Because the quality of the specimen is critical to the quality of the analysis, proper collection and handling are essential. More errors in semen analysis results have occurred because of improper collection and handling than all other possibilities combined. The composition of the semen specimen varies between the fractions contained in the ejaculate, adding to the importance of maintaining strict collection protocol. Complete written or oral instructions must be given to the patient before collection so that the best possible specimen will be collected for analysis. These instructions must also include transport requirements for the specimen, if needed.

The sample, ideally, should be collected after a minimum of 48 hours, but not longer than 7 days, of sexual abstinence—a period of no sexual activity (Procedure 7-4). It is best if the semen sample is produced and collected in a private setting or room near the laboratory where the actual analyses will be done. The specimen container should be clean and free from contamination (trace detergents, for example) and wide mouthed to allow more ease in collection. Glass or plastic can be used, provided that the surface has no

SEMEN COLLECTION[6]

1. The name of patient, period of abstinence, date and time of collection, and interval of time between actual collection and laboratory analysis should be recorded on the request form submitted with the specimen. Appropriate similar information should be on the collection container itself.

2. Preferably, the sample should be collected on site, in privacy, near the laboratory. If this is not feasible, the sample must be delivered to the laboratory within 1 hour of collection, keeping it from temperature extremes as noted earlier.

3. The sample should be produced by masturbation and ejaculated into a labeled, clean (sterilized, if microbiologic studies are to be done), wide-mouthed glass or plastic container. The entire

ejaculate must be included in the collection for an accurate analysis. Incomplete samples should not be analyzed. The use of condoms is not advised when infertility studies are being done because of their possible detrimental effects on the viability of the sperm. Coitus interruptus is not acceptable because of the probability of loss of the first portion of the ejaculate, which usually contains the highest concentration of sperm. The container should be warmed to minimize the risk of cold shock, since extreme temperature changes can alter some laboratory results.

4. The sample must be transported to the laboratory as quickly as possible, within 1 hour of collection, for validity of the analyses.

spermicidal characteristics. Some laboratories use plastic bags for the collection, and some use special collection kits commercially available.

Temperature extremes and transportation time are important considerations. Decreased temperatures above freezing are not usually detrimental to semen specimens, but elevated temperatures are clearly detrimental (more than 40° C). Temperature fluctuations in either direction can alter motility characteristics measured during a routine semen analysis. Substantial sudden changes in temperature during handling or transportation of the specimen should be avoided. Sperm are susceptible to sudden temperature changes. Any specimen produced and collected away from the laboratory must be transported to the testing lab within 1 hour of collection and protected from temperature extremes during transport (transport temperature should be between 20°-40° C). The specimen should be transported at body temperature (kept next to the body), if at all possible.

For most routine infertility initial evaluations, two to three semen samples should be collected. The samples are collected at different times for analysis, because an individual's sperm output can vary considerably over time. The time interval between the collections vary, but generally no less than 7 days or more than 3 months. Generally, a 2-week interval provides a reliable initial evaluation for satisfactory baseline values. The patient should be informed about the need to collect more than one ejaculate before beginning the initial evaluation process. If the motility of the sperm is abnormally low, the time interval between collections should be kept as short as possible. If the results of the two or three assessments differ greatly, additional samples must be collected and studied. If sperm function tests are to be done, the sperm must be separated from the seminal plasma within 1 hour of ejaculation. For

determining the effectiveness of vasectomy, only the presence of sperm, viable or nonviable, is needed. Identification of a fluid as a semen sample, by the presence of spermatozoa, can be useful in forensic studies.

An appointment with the laboratory must be made in advance of any specimen collection. Any medications the patient is taking should be included with the information submitted with the sample.

Laboratory Assays

Analysis of the semen specimen cannot begin until the liquefaction process is complete. Assays ordered will vary, depending on the indication for analysis (infertility studies, postvasectomy effectiveness, forensic purposes, for example). Reference ranges for standard tests included in a semen analysis are given in Table 7-5.

Macroscopic Examination

LIQUEFACTION. The normal semen sample liquefies at room temperature usually within 30 minutes. Liquefaction of the normal highly viscous ejaculated semen usually occurs spontaneously within 10 to 20 minutes and forms a translucent but turbid viscous fluid. If this liquefaction does not occur within 60 minutes, this observation should be noted on the report. When liquefaction is complete, the sample may be analyzed for other constituents or parameters. Before any further testing is begun, the sample must be thoroughly mixed in the original container.

APPEARANCE. When liquefaction is complete or within 1 hour of ejaculation, the semen sample should be observed for its gross appearance. This observation should be done at room temperature and the results included on the report. A normal semen sample appears homogeneous, with a white-gray opalescence. It may appear red or brown if red blood cells are pre-

Table 7-5

REFERENCE RANGES FOR SEMEN ANALYSIS (STANDARD TESTS)[6]

Test Parameter	Reference Range
Volume	2.0 mL or more
pH	7.2-8.0
Sperm concentration	$>20 \times 10^6$ spermatozoa/mL
Total sperm count	$>40 \times 10^6$ spermatozoa per ejaculate
Morphology	>30% with normal forms
Vitality/viability	>75% live forms
White blood cells	$<1 \times 10^6$/mL
Red blood cells	none

sent (hematospermia) or less opaque if the concentration of sperm is abnormally low. A dense, white turbid appearance of the semen is seen with an inflammatory process in the urethra where there are large numbers of white blood cells.

VOLUME. Volume is measured either in a graduated cylinder or centrifuge tube or by aspirating the whole sample into a wide-mouth pipette using a mechanical device. Plastic disposable pipettes may also be used. Whatever the measuring device, it must be clean and completely free of contaminating water or detergent residue. The entire sample must be included in the measurement. Volumes are usually recorded to the nearest 0.1 mL, with a normal range being between 2 and 6 mL per ejaculation.

VISCOSITY OR CONSISTENCY. After the normal liquefaction process has taken place, the consistency of the sample can be observed. One method is to gently aspirate the liquefied sample into a 5-mL pipette and then allow the semen to drop by gravity while observing the length of the thread formed. The longer the thread formed, the more viscous the sample. A semen specimen with normal viscosity will be expelled from the pipette in distinct drops. Semen that is extremely viscous often cannot even be drawn into the pipette. The reported observation of viscosity can be made as normal, more viscous than normal, or very viscous. There are several specific methods used to establish this observation depending on the laboratory doing the analysis. The general relative ease or difficulty of semen flow is noted as part of this observation. If the viscosity of the sample is too high due to a high mucus content, determinations of various other semen characteristics can be affected, such as sperm motility and concentration.

pH. The hydrogen ion concentration of semen is an important determinant of sperm motility, viability, and other general metabolic parameters. Optimal pH for sperm survival is between 7.2 and 8.0. Both sperm motility and metabolism decline below the optimal pH of 7.2. A drop of semen can be spread evenly onto the pH paper (with a range of pH 6.1 to 10.0). The color of the impregnated zone should be uniform and is compared with the calibration color strip provided with the paper. Before use, the accuracy of the pH paper should first be checked against standards. The reference range for semen pH is between 7.2 and 8.0.

Microscopic Examination. The microscopic parameters routinely measured on semen include total white blood cell count, sperm count/mL, total sperm count, sperm morphology, and motility. For reference ranges for semen analyses, see Table 7-5. Motility and viability of the sperm decrease with time; therefore these observations must be performed within 1½ to 2 hours of collection after the liquefaction process is complete. The temperature at which these analyses are done—optimally, at 37° C—is very important.

Antisperm antibodies are also detected microscopically after treatment with a specific immunoassay reagent. Routinely, most sperm analyses are performed at room temperature, since sudden changes in room temperature can alter the results.

An ordinary light microscope with correctly reduced light can be used for unstained preparations. Use of a phase contrast microscope is strongly recommended for all examinations of unstained preparations of fresh semen or washed spermatozoa.

WET MOUNT ANALYSIS. Some subjective observations can be made by simply mounting a drop of well-mixed semen on a glass slide, coverslipping it, and looking at it under the microscope. This is known as the wet mount analysis, and it is used to determind the approximate sperm count (reported as few, several, many, numerous sperm/hpf). The wet mount analysis also can give information about sperm agglutination patterns, viability, motility, and morphology. The more accurate, objective sperm count must be done with a hemocytometer or counting chamber method where actual numbers of sperm are counted in the traditional fashion described in standard hematology textbooks.

PREPARATION OF SEMEN FOR INITIAL WET MOUNT ANALYSIS. The semen specimen must be thoroughly mixed before a drop of the undiluted semen is placed on a clean glass slide and coverslipped. It is important that the volume of semen delivered onto the slide and the dimensions of the coverslip are standardized so that the analyses are carried out using a preparation of a fixed depth. A standardized volume of 10 μL of semen is delivered onto the slide using a micro pipette, after which it is coverslipped with a 22 x 22 mm coverglass. These parameters will result in a preparation of a fixed depth of about 20 μm—a depth allowing the necessary observation to estimate sperm numbers, morphology, motility, and velocity. These are considered subjective observations. A freshly made preparation is allowed to stabilize for about 1 minute before any microscopic analysis is done. For most estimated observations using microscopic analyses, 10-20 microscopic fields are observed using an objective between 40× to 60× (high power).

In normal semen specimens, mature sperm cells make up the greatest percentage of cells seen. Other cells typically seen are epithelial cells arising from the male genital tract, immature germ cells, and white blood cells. Many epithelial cells may be present in men with urethritis. Percentages of the various types of cells seen should be determined and reported. Abnormal gross bacteria or the presence of other microorganisms such as Trichomonas or Candida should be reported. If the numbers of sperm vary considerably from field to field, the sample may not have been properly mixed before pipetting. The sample should be mixed thoroughly and another sample pipetted onto the glass slide. Lack of uniformity can also be caused by abnormal liquefaction, from sperm agglutination or aggregation, or from semen with an abnormal consistency.

MOTILITY. The relative percentage of motile sperm is determined while estimating the sperm count subjectively in 10-20 high-power microscopic fields—part of the wet mount analysis. Only semen without stain can be observed for sperm motility. One reasonably accurate method to determine sperm motility is to actually count the motile and nonmotile sperm in at least five different microscopic fields (counting at least 200 total sperm) and then calculate the percentage of motile sperm from these counts:

% motility =

(total sperm − nonmotile sperm)/total sperm × 100

In normal semen, 50% or more of the sperm should be motile. Less than 50% motility can increase the risk of infertility.

AGGLUTINATION. Agglutination of sperm is reported when motile sperm stick to each other in an associated, definite pattern. These patterns include head-to-head, head-to-tail, or tail-to-tail. Several high-power fields should be observed to establish the presence of patterns of sperm association. The clumping of sperm, with no definite pattern of association, is different from sperm agglutination. Agglutination of nonmotile sperm is usually nonspecific and is not usually noted in the report. The presence of agglutination can indicate an immunological cause of infertility.

VIABILITY. The viability of sperm cells can be determined by using a supravital staining method. Many of these methods use eosin or a combination of eosin and nigrosin. The percentage of sperm cells that appear alive and those that appear dead can be determined based on their color reaction to the staining method used. The membranes of the sperm cells that are dead or are dying take up the stain, whereas the cells that are alive (viable) do not. These techniques make it possible to distinguish sperm cells that are nonmotile but still alive from those that are dead. It is important to compare the results of viability observations with the estimate of motility for the sperm sample. The percentage of dead or nonviable sperm cells should not significantly exceed the percentage of nonmotile sperm cells.

SPERM MORPHOLOGY. Characteristics of sperm morphology can be observed by performing a differential cell count on a smear of the semen specimen (Fig. 7-7). Smears can be made using a technique similar to that for making blood smears. Several different stains may be employed. Spermatozoa are classified as morphologically normal, immature, or abnormal. When fewer than 30% of the sperm are normal and mature, there is an associated increased risk of infertility.

PREPARATION OF SMEAR. A smear of semen is prepared and stained using, most often, hematoxylin and eosin,

Figure 7-7

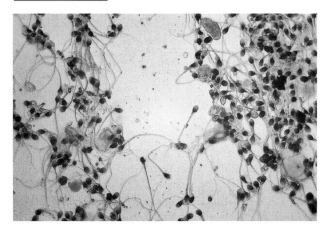

Sperm in semen smear. Wright's stain, brightfield, ×400.

Papanicolaou, or Wright's stain. The smear of semen on the slide must not be too thick, or it will be difficult to see and evaluate the morphology of the sperm cells. There are several methods for preparing the specimen on the slide. The traditional "feathering" technique uses the edge of a second slide to drag a drop of semen along the surface of the slide, a technique used for preparation of blood smears. As an alternative, a drop of semen can be placed in the middle of a slide and a second slide placed on top of it so the semen spreads between the two slides, and then gently pulling the two slides apart using a sliding action to make two smears simultaneously. Each method requires practice.

MICROSCOPIC EVALUATION OF SPERMATOZOAN MORPHOLOGY. The outline of all parts of the sperm cells should be easily seen, and only recognizable cells are classified. It is best to count and classify a total of 200 sperm cells, although sometimes only 100 are counted. Sperm morphologic characteristics include the head region, the midpiece, the principal tailpiece, and the endpiece. Sperm cells can exhibit alterations in either the head or the tail. The most common morphologic aberrations of the head include absence or an abnormal shape of the head, double-headed sperm, micro (small) or megalo (large) sperm. Tail abnormalities include coiled, kinked, or lengthened tailpieces. Morphologic conclusions can be given in percentages of normal, immature, or abnormal sperm seen for the cells counted.

BACTERIA IN SEMEN. In addition to the morphologic evaluation of the sperm cells, the presence of bacteria, white blood cells, or red blood cells should be recorded. Cultures can be done for a variety of microorganisms.

SPERM COUNT (OBJECTIVE). The objective counting of sperm, the sperm count, is routinely done using a hemocytometer or counting chamber method. Two commonly used manual counting methods are the improved Neubauer Hemocytometer and the Makler Counting Chamber® (Sefi-Medical Instruments, Israel, available in the U.S. from Zygotek Systems, Inc., Springfield, Mass) (see Procedure 7-5). Use of the Neubauer Hemocytometer is discussed in detail in most traditional hematology textbooks. The use of **computer assisted semen analysis (CASA)** increases accuracy and reproducibility of sperm counts and motility studies and has also allowed measurement of speed and direction of travel for the sperm in the specimen being studied.

Fewer than 20 million (20×10^6) spermatozoa/mL is a significantly decreased number (**oligospermia**) and is associated with a significantly increased risk of infertility. If absence of sperm cells is noted (**azoospermia**), a fructose measurement should be ordered to verify the integrity of the vas deferens and the seminal vesicles. Fructose is generally necessary for sperm cell survival.

PREPARATION OF SEMEN FOR SPERM COUNT (Procedure 7-5). Using the improved Neubauer Hemocytometer method, the well-mixed liquefied semen sample is diluted 1:20 with a staining solution (sodium bicarbonate, formalin, and a stain of trypan blue or saturated aqueous gentian violet is one diluent that can be used). If a phase-contrast microscope is used, the stain may be omitted. Many laboratories have found that distilled water as a diluent is adequate and also convenient. A drop of the diluted semen is added to the prepared, coverglassed hemocytometer. Using this method, any sperm present are immobilized by the diluent.

Improved Neubauer Hemocytometer Method. After the diluted semen is transferred to each side of the chamber, it is allowed to settle for a few minutes for easier counting (Fig. 7-8). Sperm are counted in the central square millimeter of the hemocytometer grid, which contains 25 large squares (where red blood cells are counted); Each large square is $\frac{1}{25}$ mm square. Each $\frac{1}{25}$ mm square is divided into 16 small squares (see Figs. 7-9 and 7-10). For samples with fewer than 10 spermatozoa counted per large square ($\frac{1}{25}$ mm square), the whole grid of 25 large squares (1 mm square) should be counted; for samples with 10-40 spermatozoa per large square, 10 large squares (10 $\frac{1}{25}$ mm squares) should be counted; and for samples with greater than 40 spermatozoa per large square, 5 large squares (5 $\frac{1}{25}$ mm squares) should be counted. Five large squares (5 $\frac{1}{25}$ mm squares) are counted when the sperm count is being done for the first time. It is important that the same cell not be counted twice. To provide a systematic procedure for doing this, if a cell lies on the line dividing two adjacent squares, it should be counted only if it is touching the upper or left lines of the square being assessed.

CALCULATION OF SPERM COUNT (SPERM/ML SEMEN). To determine the concentration of spermatozoa in the original semen sample in millions/mL, a conversion calculation must be applied. This calculation is based on the area counted, the dilution factor used to prepare the fluid used in the chamber, the depth of the area counted, and the average of the numbers of sperm counted in the two sides of the hemocytometer. It is

SPERM COUNT USING IMPROVED NEUBAUER HEMOCYTOMETER METHOD[6]

1. Thoroughly mix specimen and dilute 1:20 with diluent. (To obtain this dilution, dilute 50 µL of liquefied semen with 950 µL of diluent using a micropipette (a positive-displacement type of pipette is best.)

2. Thoroughly mix diluted specimen and allow a drop (10-20 µL) to flow into each side of the hemocytometer covered with a coverglass.

3. Allow chamber to stand for about 5 minutes in a humid container to prevent drying. During this period, the cells settle and can be more easily counted.

4. After cells have settled, place chamber under phase contrast microscope (preferably), using a 40× objective.

5. Count spermatozoa present in 5 $\frac{1}{25}$ mm squares in center square millimeter on both sides of the hemocytometer (Figs. 7-9 and 7-10). Calculate the average count. Each side should be tallied separately. The difference between the two sides should not vary more than 10%. If there is more than 10% variation between the two sides, another chamber must be prepared and the count redone. Only morphologically mature germinal cells with tails are counted. "Pin-heads" or tailless heads are not counted.

6. Apply dilution factor and report result in millions of spermatozoa per mL of original semen specimen. If the total sperm count is to be reported, multiply the count per mL by the volume of the ejaculate collected.

Figure 7-8

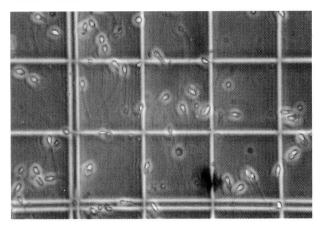

Sperm in counting chamber. Semen has been diluted for the sperm count. Shows a portion of one square. Phase contrast, ×400.

Figure 7-9

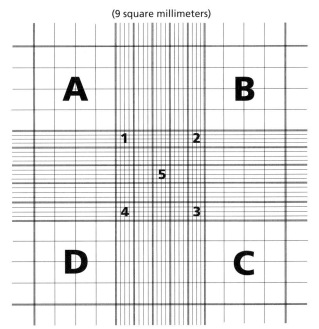

White blood cells in blood are counted in areas A, B, C, and D (4 sq. mm)
Red blood cells are counted in areas 1, 2, 3, 4, and 5 (80/400 sq. mm.)

Improved Neubauer ruling for one counting chamber area (9 mm square). Spermatozoa are counted in areas 1, 2, 3, 4, and 5 in center square millimeter.
(From Linne JJ, Ringsrud KM: *Basic techniques in clinical laboratory science*, ed 3, St. Louis, 1992, Mosby.)

important to note that when any of the variables change, the count correction factor will change.

If the usual 1:20 dilution has been made and sperm counted in five of the large squares (five $\frac{1}{25}$ mm squares), by adding six zeros to the number of sperm counted (an average of the count from the two sides of the chamber), the total sperm count (in millions of sperm/mL semen) is:

Example: If 64 sperm are counted in 5 large squares;
Add six zeros = 64,000,000 or
64×10^6 sperm/mL semen.

For other dilutions and areas counted, see Table 7-6. To use this table, the following information must be known: number of large squares ($\frac{1}{25}$ mm squares) counted on the hemocytometer (5, 10, or 25, for example), average count of spermatozoa counted in that area, and dilution factor used to prepare the specimen placed in the hemocytometer. When using the improved Neubauer Hemocytometer, the depth factor is constant at 0.1 mm. As an example, using the table, if the sample has been diluted 1:20, and 60 and 68 spermatozoa (cells) have been counted in five large squares (areas 1, 2, 3, 4, and 5 in Fig. 7-10) on each side of the chamber (or an average of 64 cells), the concentration of spermatozoa in the original semen sample is 64×10^6 spermatozoa/mL (64 divided by 1). This sperm count is within the reference range for normal seminal fluid.

The total sperm count for the sample is calculated by multiplying the count per mL by the volume (in mL) of the ejaculate collected.

The Makler Counting Chamber has been specially designed for counting sperm and for estimating sperm motility; it does not require any specimen dilution, but the specimen itself must be pretreated before sampling.

Figure 7-10

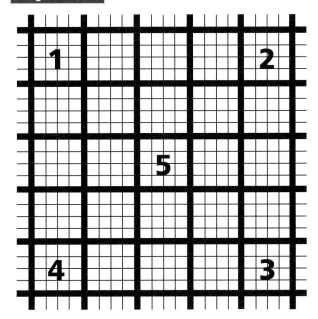

Area where sperm are counted in hemocytometer (center square millimeter). Squares 1, 2, 3, 4, and 5 are examples of area usually counted; each is $\frac{1}{25}$ mm square. (From Linne JJ, Ringsrud KM: *Basic techniques in clinical laboratory science*, ed 3, St. Louis, 1992, Mosby.)

Table 7-6

**HEMOCYTOMETRY CORRECTION FACTORS
(USING IMPROVED NEUBAUER HEMOCYTOMETER)[6]**

Dilution of semen	Number of $^1/_{25}$ mm squares counted		
and diluent	25	10	5
1:10	10	4	2
1:20	5	2	1
1:50	2	0.8	0.4

The Makler Counting Chamber has a well-defined and constant depth allowing sperm to be visualized in a single plane.

Sperm Antibody Assay

A variety of methods are used to detect the presence of antisperm antibodies either on the sperm cells or circulating in the serum. One commonly used methodology involves the use of immunobead assays available commercially. In these tests IgG, IgA, or IgM molecules are bound to polystyrene beads in the commercially available reagent and, when these beads are mixed with sperm, they will adhere to any sperm cells that are antibody coated. Any beads binding sperm are detected by microscopic observation, and the percentage of human sperm bound can also be determined. The presence of IgG, IgA, or IgM antibodies can be assessed simultaneously using this method. In using the immunobead assays, sperm cells are washed free of seminal fluid and then mixed with a suspension of Immunobeads in the reagent. As the sperm cells move through the suspension, the Immunobeads adhere to the motile sperm that have surface-bound antibodies. The reaction can be seen microscopically.

Different sets of immunobeads are available for distinguishing between the IgG, IgA, and IgM immunoglobulins. The percentage of sperm cells with surface antibodies is determined. A positive test is defined when 20% or more of the motile sperm cells have Immunobead binding. Antisperm antibodies can also be detected by use of enzyme-linked immunosorbent assay (ELISA) or by flow cytometry.

AMNIOTIC FLUID ANALYSIS

Amniotic fluid is present in the amniotic cavity which surrounds the embryo or fetus. The inner membrane of the cavity in contact with the amniotic fluid is called the amnion. It has a single layer of cuboidal epithelial cells lying on a basement membrane. The fluid serves to (1) protect the fetus, (2) allow fetal movement and growth, (3) maintain an even temperature, and (4) participate in fetal biochemical homeostasis. During growth of the fetus in utero, the amniotic cavity enlarges and fills with fluid that contains both living and nonviable cells. The fluid is produced by the amniotic membrane, the fetal cord, and the fetal gastrointestinal, respiratory, and renal systems.

The major source of amniotic fluid is probably fetal urine after the first trimester. The volume is balanced by the amount of urine produced and how much the fetus swallows: the normal fetus swallows from 200 to 500 mL of amniotic fluid each day. There is a total volume of 0.5 to 1.5 L of amniotic fluid by the end of the normal 40 weeks of gestation.

Aspiration of amniotic fluid, **amniocentesis**, can be carried out safely by the fourteenth week of gestation. The collection of amniotic fluid for most clinical examinations is done during the second and third trimesters. Amniocentesis is usually done during the second trimester to diagnose genetic and developmental conditions. During the third trimester, it is done to assess severity of erythroblastosis fetalis and to predict neonatal respiratory distress.

Collection of the Amniotic Fluid Specimen

Before amniocentesis is performed, an **ultrasound** examination should be done. The ultrasound examination confirms gestational age, detects gross fetal anomalies, verifies fetal cardiac activity, determines location of the placenta, determines the volume of the amniotic fluid, determines number of gestational sacks, and determines the correct abdominal puncture site for the amniocentesis procedure.

Amniocentesis is usually performed transabdominally, but it can be done vaginally. Transabdominal amniocentesis is the preferred method, since vaginal amniocentesis carries an increased risk of infection. The earliest the procedure can be safely performed is

16 weeks from the last menstrual period or the fourteenth week of gestation. Ideally, an amniocentesis done under sterile conditions will provide a clean sample of amniotic fluid without damage to the fetus or placenta. No more than 30 mL should be removed as more may precipitate premature labor or spontaneous rupture of the membranes. The first 1 to 2 mL removed should be discarded because it might be contaminated with blood or maternal cells. Clear fluid should be obtained, if possible.

The major risks for the amniocentesis procedure is trauma to the fetus, umbilical cord, or placenta; infection, spontaneous abortion, a prematurely ruptured membrane, preterm labor, hemorrhage, and alloimmunization of the mother.

The specimen should be labeled and sent to the laboratory for processing and testing immediately to preserve the biochemical constituents. The appearance of the specimen should be noted on the report.

Laboratory Assays

The indications for examination of amniotic fluid vary, depending on the gestational age. Amniotic fluid from the 16th or 17th week of gestation is used for genetic karyotyping to detect possible genetic defects, to measure alpha-fetoprotein to detect neural tube defects, or to measure certain enzymes in patients who have a high risk for enzyme-deficient diseases (such as Tay-Sachs disease). Fluid collected later in the pregnancy can be examined to determine **fetal lung maturity,** to diagnose infectious conditions, or to assess the severity of an Rh isoimmunization condition.

The specific specimen requirements for each test must be followed to give valid information. Specimen handling requirements vary for different tests; for example, the specimen must be kept on ice, protected from light, refrigerated, kept at room temperature, or separated by centrifugation, for the specific test results to be valid and meaningful. For cytogenic studies, the cells in the fluid must be kept alive so they can be cultured in the laboratory. For most tests, the specimen must be processed soon after removal from the amniotic cavity. Centrifugation is usually done first, with the appearance of the specimen being noted before and after centrifugation. It is especially important to note the appearance of any blood or discoloration in the fluid.

Appearance of Amniotic Fluid. The gross appearance of the amniotic fluid can indicate the well-being of the fetus. The color of normal amniotic fluid is colorless to pale straw. Some blood can appear in the fluid because of a traumatic or bloody tap. Usually this blood is of maternal origin. If the blood is of maternal origin, the patient should be watched for a short while and maternal vital signs and fetal heart rate monitored. If the blood is of fetal origin, immediate delivery or careful monitoring is essential. It is important to differentiate between the presence of **fetal red cells** or **maternal red cells** in the fluid. Laboratory examination of the mother's blood for evidence of fetomaternal hemorrhage can be done following trauma to the abdomen or pelvis during pregnancy. Other obstetrical manipulations can potentially also cause a fetomaternal hemorrhage. When a test for alpha-fetoprotein (AFP) is ordered, accurate identification of the origin of the red cells in the fluid is important, because there is a significant false-positive rate of AFP caused by the contamination of the amniotic fluid with fetal red cells. A green-stained amniotic fluid is caused by the presence of **meconium,** a mixture of fluids found in the intestine of the fetus.

KLEIHAUER-BETKE STAIN. Fetal hemorrhage can be identified by use of a **Kleihauer-Betke stain.** This stain identifies the presence of fetal red blood cells, including the percentage of red cells that contain hemoglobin F. Fetal red cells will appear red and refractile, whereas the maternal red cells will appear as ghosts on the blood film when stained with the Kleihauer-Betke stain. Fetal red cells can also be identified using hemoglobin electrophoresis or flow cytometry.

MECONIUM. The dark green mixture of secretions of fetal intestinal glands and amniotic fluid will give a green-stained color to the amniotic fluid. The intensity of the green color can be classified as thin (light), moderate, or thick (heavy). Presence of heavy meconium is associated with an increased risk of meconium aspiration syndrome. The presence of light meconium does not usually indicate a poor fetal outcome.

Chemistry Assays. As pregnancy progresses, the concentration of the various analytes present in amniotic fluid changes. Any interpretation of these analyte levels depends on gestational age, the amount of amniotic fluid present in the amniotic sac, and the accuracy of the analyte measurements. New technologies applied to biochemical, immunological, and microbiological methods have allowed more available information about the conditions in utero using analysis of the amniotic fluid. Information about fetal lung maturity, neural tube defects, and the many inherited metabolic disorders can be obtained from these assays.

LECITHIN-SPHINGOMYELIN RATIO (L/S RATIO). One of the most frequent complications of early delivery is that of fetal immaturity. The maturation of the fetal lung is identified by the production of a substance called surfactant, a lipid compound, detergent-like substance that forms a film on the surface of the alveoli. A measurement of surfactant can determine the maturity of the fetal lungs. About 75% of the surfactant consists of lecithin, another 10% is phosphatidyl glycerol, and the remainder is other phospholipids and sphingomyelin.

The laboratory assay routinely used to assess the maturity level of the fetal lungs is the **lecithin-sphin-go-myelin ratio** or **L/S ratio**. The amount of sphingomyelin produced is constant throughout gestation and is used as a control on which to base the ratio of the two components, lecithin and sphingomyelin. The amount of lecithin produced increases noticeably at weeks 35 and 36 of gestation. At this time the fetal lung alveoli have stabilized, and a preterm delivery can safely be considered. When the L/S ratio is less than 2.0, the fetal lung is still immature; a ratio between 2.1 and 3.0 indicates a borderline mature lung, and a ratio greater than 3.1 indicates a mature lung.

ALPHA-FETOPROTEIN (**AFP**). Alpha-fetoprotein is produced in the fetal liver and yolk sac. A small amount is normally present in the amniotic fluid. Its presence is increased when there is increased diffusion from the fetal serum through **open neural tube defects**, such as anencephaly, spina bifida, or hydrocephaly. There are other disorders that are also associated with increased amniotic AFP levels. Tests for the presence of amniotic AFP are usually done following a positive maternal serum AFP test but can also be done in patients undergoing amniotic cytogenetic analyses. The specimen for this test is collected during the middle of the third trimester.

MICROSCOPIC EXAMINATION. The identification of the types of cells present in amniotic fluid is of limited clinical value as compared with the other tests discussed. A microscopic test, the Fern test for estrogen/progesterone, can be used to diagnose ruptured membranes. There are many false-positive results with this test, however. A more reliable test is to determine the type of amniotic cells found in the vagina by cytologic examination.

For the Fern test, mucus aspirated from the cervix is spread on a glass slide and allowed to dry for a few minutes. The slide is examined microscopically for a characteristic ferning pattern. From about the seventh day of the menstrual cycle to about the eighteenth day, there is normally a characteristic fern-like pattern of the dried cervical mucus seen, described as a palm-leaf pattern. The pattern seen depends on the stage of the ovarian cycle and the presence or absence of pregnancy—progesterone secretion in large amounts. A beaded or cellular pattern is seen after approximately the twenty-first day; the fern-like pattern does not develop. This beaded pattern is usually seen in pregnancy. The test has been used for many years and is still used in clinics and physicians offices because it is easy and quick.

MORPHOLOGIC CHARACTERISTICS OF CELLS SEEN IN BODY FLUIDS[1]

The following descriptions are included for those cells commonly found in body fluids when prepared by cytocentrifugation, air-dried, and stained with Wright-Giemsa. The many blood cells from the erythroid, lymphoid, and myeloid series are not specifically included in this description, although they may often be seen in body fluid specimens. Some pertinent material on blood cells will be included.

Cells from Peripheral Blood

Most blood cells found in body fluids still maintain some of their typical features as described in standard hematology textbooks. It should be kept in mind, however, that blood cells found in body fluids often lose some of their cytologic features. Processing fluids with the cytocentrifuge can also alter some of the cellular features compared with the same cells as seen on blood smears. As an example, the segmented lobes of the neutrophil nucleus can appear eccentrically situated on a cytocentrifuged smear. Blast cells are especially susceptible to distortion from cytocentrifugation.

Erythrocytes. The presence of red blood cells in body fluids is usually derived from contamination of the fluid during the collection process but can be a sign of hemorrhage. Determination of the origin of the red cells from hemorrhage or traumatic tap is important.

Eosinophils. Eosinophils can be recognized in body fluids because of their characteristic red-pink granules. Eosinophils can be seen in cerebrospinal fluids with ventricular shunts or in pleural fluids following pneumothorax. In nasal fluids, the identification of eosinophils is an important finding to distinguish an allergic rhinitis from a nonallergic, infectious process.

NASAL SMEARS. A relatively thin smear of nasal fluid is usually examined. After air-drying, the smear is stained for eosinophils, using Wright's, Hansel's, or eosin and methylene blue stain (see also Chapter 6). The entire slide must be examined, since eosinophils may be distributed in uneven streaks or clumps. Finding a predominance of eosinophils in the nasal fluid will correlate with an allergic discharge. A nasal discharge caused by a "runny nose," a nonallergic condition, will show a predominance of neutrophils or acellular mucus.

Phagocytic (Mononuclear) Cells

Macrophage/Monocyte. Macrophages engage in active phagocytosis. Specific macrophages will be described when the material ingested is unique or of some importance diagnostically. Any pigment appearing in the macrophage should be distinguished from bacteria and yeast, which have a characteristic shape.

Macrophages are large cells (15 to 30 microns) with an abundant cytoplasm that shows evidence of active phagocytosis (ingested material, postingestion vacuoles, remnants of digested products). One or more round to oval nuclei are present. There is a single large vacuole in some cells, displacing the nucleus, that replaces the cytoplasm in those cells. This gives the appearance of a "signet ring," as seen in some tumor cells. **Alveolar macrophages** are the predominating cells seen in **bronchial lavage washings** (cells are obtained by instilling sterile saline into the alveolar spaces by use of a fiberoptic bronchoscope). These cells have an eccentric, round nucleus, light blue cytoplasm, a variable number of azurophilic granules in their cytoplasm, and appear similar to the macrophages seen in pleural or peritoneal fluids. Blue-black carbon particles can be seen in the cytoplasm of cells originating from the lungs of persons who inhale smoke.

Monocytes show a variable range of descriptions for their appearance in body fluids. They are usually quite large (14 to 24 microns) with an abundant blue cytoplasm containing sparse azurophilic granules. The nucleus is round to oval, and it may be indented, giving it a horseshoe or kidney bean shape. Small nucleoli are present, and the cytoplasm appears lacy.

Lipophage. Macrophages that contain fat are called lipophage cells. The fat is usually in small vacuoles that completely fill the cytoplasm of the cell. These inclusions may originate from extracellular fatty material or from membranes of ingested cells. Lipophages may be seen in cerebrospinal fluid following a cerebral infarct, pneumoencephalography, or chemotherapy, irradiation, dye procedures into the intrathecal areas of the spinal cord, or in pleural fluids associated with a chylothorax or with extensive cell destruction.

Erythrophage. Macrophages that have ingested red blood cells are called erythrophages.

Siderophage. Macrophages containing large brown-black hemosiderin granules (seen when stained with Prussian blue) arise from the iron of ingested red blood cells. Hemosiderin granules are seen in the cytoplasm of the macrophages. These cells are seen approximately 48 hours after there has been a hemorrhage into the cerebrospinal fluid and can remain for up to 4 months. Finding hemosiderin granules in macrophages (a siderophage) is diagnostic of a true hemorrhage as differentiated from blood in the fluid from a traumatic tap.

Neutrophage. Macrophages containing one or more phagocytized neutrophils is called a neutrophage. Initially, the segmented nucleus of the neutrophil is seen, surrounded by a clear zone of cytoplasm. As the process continues, the nucleus becomes round and pyknotic. Finally the remnants of the digested nucleus may appear as small, purple inclusions.

These remnant inclusions found in the neutrophage must be differentiated from the smaller azurophilic lysosomal granules characteristic of macrophages. Macrophages are called neutrophages only when the phagocytized material in the cell can be clearly identified as originating from a segmented neutrophil.

Lining Cells

Mesothelial Cell. The large mesothelial cell (12 to 20 microns) lines the pleural, peritoneal, and pericardial cavities. These cells can be shed individually or in clusters. The nucleus is round to ovoid with a definitive nuclear membrane and regular contour. The nucleus is often eccentrically placed, and the nuclear to cytoplasmic ratio is small—the nucleus is usually less than half the size of the cytoplasm. The cytoplasm is usually light to dark blue. In a chronic effusion, the mesothelial cells can proliferate. When these cells appear in clusters or in pairs, they frequently have articulated or coupled cell borders with "windows" between many of the cells. They may degenerate and show vacuolization, with the large vacuoles occurring in the cell periphery, although small vacuoles may be present. The vacuoles in the normal mesothelial cells are poorly defined and have an irregular shape as contrasted to vacuoles seen in malignant cells where the vacuole represents a synthesized product. Mesothelial cells can be phagocytic and can transform into macrophages. Mesothelial cells can resemble plasma cells but are usually larger than the plasma cells.

Synoviocytes. Lining cells from the synovial membrane that lines the joint capsule are called synoviocytes. These cells appear identical to mesothelial cells found in serous fluids. The nuclei are round to oval and are eccentrically placed. There is abundant cytoplasm that is light to deep in color. Forms with multiple nuclei may occur. Their presence in synovial fluid does not have any diagnostic specificity.

Ependymal or Choroid Cells. Cells that line the ventricles of the brain (ependymal cells) or the choroid plexus (choroid plexus cells) may be shed into the cerebrospinal fluid. This can occur particularly in neonates or in the presence of a ventricular shunt. These cells appear singly or in clumps. Their nuclei are round to oval with a definite smooth nuclear membrane. The chromatin is distributed evenly and appears finely granular or hyperchromic. Nucleoli are not present. The nucleus usually is eccentrically located and may appear pyknotic. The cytoplasm is abundant and blue, pink, or amphophilic (a combination of both pink and blue) and grainy. Only the bare nuclei may be seen when there has been degeneration of the choroidal and ependymal cells. The presence of these cells is not diagnostically significant, but they must be differentiated from any malignant cells that might be present.

Leptomeningeal Cells. Cells lining the subarachnoid space are called leptomeningeal cells. They rarely slough off into the cerebrospinal fluid. Leptomeningeal cells may appear in clusters, with spindle-shaped nuclei and a moderate amount of blue gray cytoplasm. Hemosiderin pigment may be present in the cytoplasm. Giant arachnoid cover cells with large, oval nuclei with fine chromatin and nucleoli also may be seen. These cells have abundant pink or blue cytoplasm and appear cracked or brittle. There may be a pigment in the cytoplasm. As these cells degenerate, only bare oval nuclei are left.

Bronchial Lining Cells. Cells with cilia may be seen as a contaminant in fluids obtained from bronchial lavage. This implies that bronchial, rather than alveolar cells have been sampled. These cells from the bronchial lining have a unique appearance, showing an extremely eccentric nucleus and a tuft of amphophilic (pink-blue) cytoplasm, terminating in a row of cilia.

Miscellaneous Cells

Squamous Epithelial Cells. In rare instances, these cells can be found in fluids, particularly cerebrospinal fluids, when there has been contamination from the skin. These cells have a low nuclear to cytoplasmic ratio; a small, round nucleus with fairly dense chromatin; often abundant, elongated cytoplasm that may show keratinization. It is important to contrast these cells with squamous carcinoma cells. The contaminant squamous epithelial cells lack nuclear atypia.

Megakaryocytes. These cells can rarely be accidentally obtained, particularly during the collection of cerebrospinal fluid. They are hematopoietic components of bone marrow and appear as large cells with a multilobulated nucleus and a distinctly granular cytoplasm.

Cartilage Cells (Chondrocytes). These cells can be accidently obtained during lumbar puncture for cerebrospinal fluid collection. They have round, dark nuclei and dense, wine-red cytoplasm. Occasionally, these cells are also seen in synovial fluid from patients with osteoarthritis or after trauma.

LE Cells. Lupus Erythematosus (LE) cells can be found in pleural and synovial fluids. Characteristically, these cells appear as an intact neutrophil containing a large, homogeneous, pink inclusion (degenerated nuclear material) that distends the cytoplasm and displaces the nucleus.

Malignant Cells. A variety of neoplastic cells may be found in the various body fluids. Malignant cells are rarely found in synovial fluid, however. The morphology varies with the underlying malignancy. In primary tumors of the central nervous system, tumor cells may be found in cerebrospinal fluid. Metastatic carcinoma and melanoma may also result in malignant cells being found in the cerebrospinal fluid. Almost any neoplasm can invade the serous cavities, resulting in malignant cells being found in the fluids collected from these cavities. Identification of the various malignant cells found in body fluids must be done by an experienced cytologist.

Miscellaneous Other Findings

Microorganisms. Organisms such as yeast and bacteria may be found in body fluids especially during acute phases of infections. Both intracellular and extracellular forms may be seen. These organisms tend to be uniform in structure and in their staining characteristics. They should be differentiated from nonspecific phagocytic debris commonly found in neutrophils and macrophages and from stain that has precipitated. There also may be a wide variety of parasites found in body fluids; their features are usually characteristic. These parasites include *Echinococcus*, tapeworm, schistosomes, roundworms, *Giardia*, and *Trichomonas*.

Crystals. A variety of crystals may be found in body fluids. These can include monosodium urate (MSU), calcium pyrophosphate dihydrate (CPPD), cholesterol, starch granules from gloves, and hematin.

The differentiation of MSU from CPPD in synovial fluids is done by use of polarized, light microscopy (see Synovial Fluid Analysis). Rarely, fragments of degenerate cartilage, "foreign" material from prosthetic devices (usually silicone or polyester), betamethasone (a steroid drug whose appearance resembles MSU) or other corticosteroids may also be found in synovial fluid.

Hematin crystals may be seen in macrophages found in cerebrospinal fluid approximately 2 weeks after a central nervous system hemorrhage. Hematin crystals are golden and refractile and often parallelogram shaped.

REVIEW QUESTIONS

CEREBROSPINAL FLUID

1 Lumbar puncture for cerebrospinal fluid analysis is most essential to diagnose which of the following conditions?
   a. Subarachnoid hemorrhage
   b. A malignancy of the central nervous system
   c. Meningitis
   d. Multiple sclerosis

2 What are the routine laboratory tests usually included in analysis of cerebrospinal fluid?

3 In observing blood in a sequential collection of cerebrospinal fluid from a traumatic tap, the last tube collected would usually appear (There may be more than one correct response for this question):
   a. Less red than the first tube
   b. More red than the first tube
   c. The same degree of redness as the first tube
   d. Clear

4 The centrifuged supernatant cerebrospinal fluid from a subarachnoid hemorrhage usually appears:
   a. Clear
   b. Faint pink or yellowish

5 In a cytocentrifuged spinal fluid, a predominance of neutrophils usually indicates which etiology for an infection?
   a. Viral
   b. Bacterial
   c. Fungal
   d. Mycobacterial

SYNOVIAL FLUID -joint cavity.

6 In synovial fluid, the most characteristic microscopic finding in gouty arthritis is:
   a. Monosodium urate crystals
   b. Calcium pyrophosphate dihydrate crystals
   c. Cartilage debris
   d. Intracellular microorganisms

7 Crystals in synovial fluid that appear chunky or rhomboid-like and are blue when their long axes lie parallel to the direction of the slow wave vibration of the compensated polarized light are:
   a. Monosodium urate
   b. Corticosteroid
   c. Hydroxyapatite
   d. Calcium pyrophosphate dihydrate

8 Crystals in synovial fluid that appear needle-like and are yellow when their long axes lie parallel to the direction of the slow wave vibration of the compensated polarized light are:
   a. Monosodium urate
   b. Corticosteroid
   c. Hydroxyapatite
   d. Calcium pyrophosphate dihydrate

9 To definitively identify crystals found in synovial fluid specimens, the best microscopy technique employs the use of a:
   a. Brightfield microscope
   b. Phase contrast microscope
   c. Polarized light microscope
   d. Compensated polarized light microscope

10 What is the component present in synovial fluid that provides its normal viscosity?
   hyaluronic acid.

11 What tests on synovial fluid are important in establishing a differential diagnosis for the type of arthritis present in a patient?
   Microscopic analysis of crystal, Gram Stain Culture!

SEROUS FLUIDS →Visceral memb and Parietal memb

12 An effusion formed as a result of direct injury or change to the serous membranes themselves is known as a/an:
   a. Exudate
   b. Transudate

13 The increased accumulation of fluid in the pleural cavity is known as a: Pleural effusion

14 To establish a diagnosis for an effusion of serous fluid with an unknown etiology, the tests done are primarily used to differentiate it as:
   Exudate or a Transudate

15 To differentiate a serous fluid as an exudate, the following test results would be expected (There may be more than one correct response for this question):
   a. Small numbers of cells present
   b. Total protein level of 3.0 g/dL or greater
   c. Large numbers of cells present
   d. Appearance: pale yellow and clear

SEMINAL FLUID

16 After semen is collected, which process must occur before any testing is begun?

17 What are some of the tests usually done on semen to evaluate male infertility?

18 In a normal semen sample, which of the following cells are seen? (There may be more than one correct response for this question.)
   a. White blood cells
   b. Bacteria
   c. Mature sperm cells
   d. Epithelial lining cells

19 In normal semen, which percentage of the sperm cells seen should be motile?
   a. 25%
   b. 50%
   c. 75%
   d. 100%

AMNIOTIC FLUID

20 In amniotic fluid, the laboratory measurement used to assess fetal lung maturity is:
   a. Alpha-fetoprotein
   b. Lecithin/sphingomyelin ratio
   c. Meconium
   d. Fetal red blood cells

21 The chemistry procedure performed on a specimen of amniotic fluid to determine the possible presence of a neural tube defect is:
   a. Lecithin/sphingomyelin ratio
   b. Amniotic fluid creatinine
   c. Alpha-fetoprotein
   d. Surfactant level

22 To determine if the red blood cells present in a specimen of amniotic fluid originate in the fetus, as opposed to being of maternal origin, which of the following tests can be used? (There may be more than one correct response for this question.)
   a. Kleihauer-Betke stain
   b. Hemoglobin electrophoresis
   c. Direct antiglobulin test
   d. Wright's stain

◆ CASE #1

A 50-year-old man is seen by the physician because of the sudden onset of a swollen, painful, red, warm knee joint. He has a history of joint pain and swelling in a big toe associated with elevated serum uric acid level. Synovial fluid is aspirated from the knee joint by arthrocentesis. The fluid collected is pale yellow and has a cloudy and watery appearance, not the expected viscosity of raw egg white. While crystal-induced inflammation is suspected, infection must be considered also.

The synovial fluid specimen is sent to the laboratory for Gram stain and culture, cell count and leukocyte differential, and microscopic examination for crystals. After the analyses are completed, the following results are reported:

Microbiology: Gram stain and culture: no organisms reported on Gram stain; culture subsequently sterile

Microscopic Examination:

Cell counts
WBC: 10×10^9/L
Leukocyte differential (on cytocentrifuged slide, Wright stain): 76% neutrophils, 19% monocytes and macrophages, 5% lymphocytes
(Reference value = WBC: 0.15×10^9/L with more than 25% neutrophils)

Crystals:
Brightfield illumination—crystals appear as long, thin needles; many are seen inside the neutrophils and occasionally in the monocytes/macrophages; a few crystals are seen outside the cells.
Compensated polarized light—birefringent crystals appear yellow when the long axis of the crystal is parallel to the slow wave of the red compensator and blue when the long axis is perpendicular to the slow wave.
A differential diagnosis of the condition affecting the patient's joint is needed: inflammatory, infectious, degenerative, hemorrhagic, or a combination of diagnostic conditions, so that treatment may be started.

1. What is the term for the abnormal accumulation of joint fluid?
2. The results of which laboratory assays help rule out an acute bacterial infectious arthritis for this patient?
3. Turbidity in the specimen can be caused by the presence of which constituents?
4. The presence of which microscopic cellular constituents suggest a possible acute inflammatory condition?
5. The findings reported for this case suggest which type of condition?
6. Why have you selected this diagnosis?

CASE #2

A 20-year-old female university student living in a dormitory complains of fever, chills, and headache. She feels nauseated and has vomited early in the morning before going to see a physician. On examination, she is febrile and has neck rigidity and back pain. Blood is drawn for **hematology tests (CBC)** and for a **glucose level**. A lumbar puncture is done and the cerebrospinal fluid (CSF) is collected into three sterile tubes and sent to the laboratory for routine examination. **All CSF tubes appear cloudy** but do not appear bloody.

After the analyses are completed, the following results are reported:

Blood:
Hematology: WBC 22.0 × 10⁹/L, white cell differential 85% neutrophils (cells show toxic changes and increased band forms), 10% lymphocytes, 5% monocytes.
Chemistry: Glucose 95 mg/dL
(Reference value: 70-100 mg/dL)

Cerebrospinal Fluid:
CSF pressure 250 mm water (Reference value = 50-185 mm)
Glucose level 15 mg/dL (Reference value: 50-80 mg/dL); compare with blood level)

Total protein level 160 mg/dL (Reference value = up to 60 mg/dL)
WBC: 0.90 × 10⁹/L (Reference value: 0.0-0.005 × 10⁹/L mononuclear cells—lymphocytes and monocytes)
WBC differential: (cytocentrifuged slide, stained with Wright's stain) 90% neutrophils (Reference value: 90% mononuclear cells—lymphocytes and monocytes)
Gram stain: gram-negative cocci in pairs, some intracellular, and many neutrophils. (probable organism is *Neisseria meningitidis*)

1. Considering the patient's clinical findings, what are the routine tests usually included in examination of this CSF?
2. Does a Gram stain report "no organisms seen" rule out a bacterial infection?
3. Which of the findings in the blood and spinal fluid (exclusive of the Gram stain) substantiate a bacterial rather than a viral infection?
4. Which concentrating method is preferred for preparation of a slide for differentiation of cells in spinal fluid?
5. What is the reference range for white cells in normal cerebrospinal fluid?
6. Why is the difference in the blood and cerebrospinal fluid glucose levels an important clinical finding in this patient?
7. What is a probable tentative diagnosis for this patient?

 CASE #3

A 60-year-old man with a history of several bouts of pneumonia presents to his physician with possible congestive heart failure. There is an accumulation of fluid noted around the base of his lungs—a pleural effusion. Thoracentesis is performed, and a pleural fluid specimen collected. The fluid appears **very pale yellow, watery, and just slightly cloudy**. The pleural fluid is sent to the laboratory for examination: **total protein level, cell counts and differential, Gram stain and culture**. A **serum protein level** is also ordered.

After the analyses are completed, the following results are reported:

Pleural fluid:
Total protein 1.8 g/dL (Reference value: 1-2 g/dL)
Cell count: WBC: 0.450 × 10⁹/L with lymphocytes, monocytes, a few neutrophils, and a few red cells seen on cytocentrifuged slide, Wright stain (Reference value: <0.50 × 10⁹/L)

Gram stain and culture: no organisms reported on gram stain; culture sterile.
Blood: Serum total protein 6.2 g/dL (Reference value: 6.0-7.8 g/dL)

1. Using the serum and pleural fluid protein levels, is this pleural fluid classified as an exudate or a transudate?
2. Which of the other laboratory results or observations would also define a pleural fluid as a **transudate**?
3. Following an **infectious process** involving the lungs, is an associated pleural effusion likely to be an exudate or a transudate?
4. With **congestive heart failure**, an accumulation of fluid in the pleural cavity (pleural effusion) is likely to be a transudate or an ultrafiltrate of the plasma. What causes the accumulation of pleural fluid with heart failure?

REFERENCES

1. College of American Pathologists: *Supplementary appendix, CSF and body fluids*, from 1993 Surveys manual, section II: hematology, coagulation, clinical microscopy, Chicago, 1993, CAP Press.
2. Fiechtner JJ, Simkin PA: *Urate spherulites in gouty arthritis, JAMA*, 245:1533, Apr. 17, 1981.
3. Henry JB: *Clinical diagnosis and management by laboratory methods*, ed 18, Philadelphia, 1991, WB Saunders.
4. Kjeldsberg C, Knight J: *Body fluids*, ed 3, Chicago, 1993, American Society of Clinical Pathologists.
5. McCarty DJ, ed: *Arthritis and allied conditions: a textbook of rheumatology*, ed 11, Philadelphia, 1989, Lea & Febiger.
6. World Health Organization: *WHO laboratory manual for the examination of human semen and sperm—cervical mucus interaction*, ed 3, New York, 1992, Cambridge University Press.

BIBLIOGRAPHY

Becan-McBride K, Ross DL: *Essentials for the small laboratory and physician's office*, Chicago, 1988, Year Book Medical Publishers.
Bradley M, ed: *University of Minnesota Hospital and Clinic laboratory handbook*, ed 2, Hudson, Ohio, 1992, Lexi-Comp.
Keel BA, Webster BW, eds: *CRC handbook of the laboratory diagnosis and treatment of infertility*, Boston, 1990, CRC Press.
Linne JJ, Ringsrud KM: *Basic techniques in clinical laboratory science*, ed 3, St. Louis, 1992, Mosby.
Schumacher RH, Jr, Reginato AJ: *Atlas of synovial fluid analysis and crystal identification*, Philadelphia, 1991, Lea & Febiger.
Tilton RC, Balows A., Hohnadel DC, Reiss RF: *Clinical laboratory medicine*, St. Louis, 1992, Mosby.

APPENDIX A

ANSWER KEYS

ANSWERS TO REVIEW QUESTIONS—CHAPTER 1

1. b
2. c
3. (1) waived, (2) moderately complex, (3) highly complex
4. to ensure that all laboratory workers are fully aware of possible hazardous situations present in their workplace that might be detrimental to their safety and well-being.
5. a, b, c, and d
6. to avoid direct contact with patient specimens in general—precautions used should recognize the infectious potential of any patient specimen.
7. Hepatitis B vaccine and the vaccination series of injections.
8. handwashing
9. The Material Safety Data Sheet (MSDS) for the particular chemical must be consulted. This information includes specific details about the chemical—hazardous ingredients, physical data, fire and explosion data, and health hazard and protection information. The MSDS is provided by all chemical manufacturers and suppliers about each chemical that they sell or manufacture and must be available in the laboratory where the chemicals are in use in the event that this information is needed.
10. to confine or isolate any possible hazardous waste from all workers—laboratory personnel, custodial or housekeeping personnel.
11. b, c, d
12. E   accuracy
    I   control specimen
    F   precision
    D   proficiency testing (PT)
    A, B   quality assurance (QA)
    C   quality control (QC)
    G   reliability
    H   variance
13. two control specimens (negative/normal and positive/increased) run in every 24-hour period when patient specimens are run.

ANSWERS TO REVIEW QUESTIONS—CHAPTER 2

1. a. diagnosis of disease
   b. screening of asymptomatic, congenital, or hereditary disease (monitor wellness)
   c. monitor disease progress
   d. monitor therapy/effectiveness and complications
2. a. physical properties
   b. chemical screen
   c. microscopic examination of the urine sediment
3. a. kidney and urinary tract (renal)
   b. metabolic disorders (nonrenal)
4. a. test principle
   b. limitations/sensitivity and specificity.
   c. interferences—false positive and also negative.
   d. any critical steps
   e. clinical application
   f. additional or confirmatory tests needed
5. a. kidney (2)
   b. ureters (2)
   c. bladder
   d. urethra
6. c
7. a. salt (sodium and some potassium chloride)
   b. urea
8. a
9. growth of bacteria
10. refrigeration

ANSWERS TO REVIEW QUESTIONS—CHAPTER 3

1. d
2. generally inverse—the darker the color, the smaller the volume; the paler the color the greater the volume.
3. J   blood or heme-related pigment
   A   concentrated urine
   I   dilute urine
   D   hemoglobin
   B   homogentisic acid, melanin
   C (also A) jaundice/bilirubin
   G   myoglobin
   F   porphobilinogen (porphyrin)
   E   red blood cells
   H   urobilinogen (urobilin)

4. b
5. A   abundant vivid yellow foam
   C   abundant white foam
   B   small amount of white foam which dissipates
6. inverse relationship—the higher the specific gravity, the smaller the urine volume; the lower the specific gravity, the greater the volume.
7. b
8. A and B   measures all dissolved substances
   C   measures ionizable substances only
   A   values affected by temperature of the urine specimen
   A, B, and C values affected by the presence of protein
   A and B   values affected by the presence of glucose
   A and B   values affected by the presence of radiographic contrast media
   A   measurement requires relative large urine volume

ANSWERS TO REVIEW QUESTIONS— CHAPTER 4

1. I   copper reduction test
   A, E, F, and K diazo reaction
   G   double pH indicator system
   C   double sequential enzyme reaction based on glucose oxidase
   K   Ehrlich's aldehyde reaction
   B   peroxidase activity of heme resulting in oxidation of chromogen on reagent strip
   J pK_a change of polyelectrolytes in relation to ionic concentration
   H   protein error of pH indicators
   D   reaction with sodium nitroprusside (Legal's test)
2. d
3. a. kidney status
   b. state of hydration
4. d
5. a
6. d
7. a
8. To avoid false negative reactions. Intact red cells must come in contact with the reagent strip and be lysed in order to show a reaction.
9. a
10. d (a and c)
11. d
12. diabetes mellitus
13. Specificity: Reagent strips are specific for glucose. Copper reduction tests are non-specific and react with glucose and non–glucose-reducing substances.
   Sensitivity: Reagent strips are significantly more sensitive to glucose than is the copper reduction test.
14. a
15. b
16. a. acetone
    b. acetoacetic (diacetic) acid
    c. β-hydroxybutyric acid

17. a. diabetes mellitus (uncontrolled)
    b. starvation
18. c
19. d (a and b)
20. c
21. b
22. e (c and d)
23. e (a, c, and d)
24. a
25. a

ANSWERS TO REVIEW QUESTIONS— CHAPTER 5

1. a. urine volume
   b. time of centrifugation
   c. speed of centrifugation
   d. concentration of sediment
   e. volume of sediment examined
   f. reporting format
2. b
3. c
4. birefringence
5. d

ANSWERS TO REVIEW QUESTIONS— CHAPTER 6

Cells

1. b
2. Distorted or misshapen red cells. Indicate glomerular damage.
3. Remaining red cell membrane after hemolysis (rrelease of hemoglobin). Occurs in dilute or hypotonic urine, especially when alkaline. Very difficult to visualize with brightfield microscopy.
4. d
5. b
6. Swollen neutrophils showing Brownian motion in the cytoplasm. Indicate dilute urine with a specific gravity of 1.010 or less.
7. b
8. d
9. Sqamous epithelial cells of vaginal origin encrusted with a coccobacilli, *Gardnerella vaginalis*. Indicates vaginitis due to *G. vaginalis*.
10. b
11. a
12. Fat-filled renal tubular epithelial cells (aka renal tubular fat [RTF]). The nephrotic syndrome.
13. c
14. e.
15. A   bacteria
    D   cholesterol
    B   eosinophils
    E   hemosiderin
    F   neutral fat/triglycerides
    D and E oval fat bodies
    C   Trichomonas
    A   yeast

Casts

1. a
2. Hyaline cast with one end tapering off to a tail or point. Significance is equivalent to a hyaline cast.
3. c
4. G   acute glomerulonephritis
   A and I acute pyelonephritis
   H   chronic renal disease/renal failure
   B   heavy metal/nephrotoxic poisoning
   C   nephrotic syndrome
   F   severe crushing injury
   D   severe hemolytic episode
   E   strenuous exercise
5. a
6. e

Crystals

1. a
2. calcium oxalate
   diaper fibers
   cholesterol
   uric acid
   triple phosphate
   radiographic contrast media
   calcium carbonate
   sulfonamides
   starch
3. a. uric acid
   b. calcium oxalate
4. a
5. c
6. a
7. a

Contaminants

1. a
2. e
3. a

ANSWERS TO REVIEW QUESTIONS— CHAPTER 7

Cerebrospinal Fluid

1. c
2. Cell counts, leukocyte differential, glucose level, protein level.
3. a and d
4. b
5. b

Synovial Fluid

6. a
7. d
8. a
9. d
10. Hyaluronic acid (hyaluronate)
11. Microscopic analysis for cells and crystals; Gram stain and culture.

Serous Fluid

12. a
13. pleural effusion
14. an exudate or a transudate
15. b and c

Seminal Fluid

16. liquefaction
17. Viscosity, coagulation, liquefaction, volume, pH, sperm count, sperm motility, morphology, and viability.
18. a, c, d
19. b

Amniotic Fluid

20. b
21. c
22. a, b

ANSWERS TO CASE #1—CHAPTER 4

1. Abnormal: hazy transparency, 30 mg/dL/1+ protein, positive leukocyte esterase, 10-25 white blood cells, moderate bacteria.
   Discrepant: none.
2. Because of the positive protein and leukocyte esterase tests and abnormal physical appearance (hazy transparency).
3. No. If the urine is to be cultured, it should be a clean-catch, midstream collection. Using aseptic technique, urine is first removed for culture and Gram stain if requested. It may then be used for urinalysis. In this case, the collection was not a clean-catch, and the specimen was potentially contaminated by the routine urinalysis procedure.
4. In this case, the bacteria was found to be a gram-positive cocci, *enterococcus* sp. In order for the nitrite test to be positive, the organism must be able to reduce urinary nitrate to nitrite. Gram-positive organisms such as *Enterococcus* do not have this ability.
5. Lower. The degree of proteinuria is low (30/mg/dL – 1+ SSA), there are no casts present, and the patient is asymptomatic.

ANSWERS TO CASE #2—CHAPTER 4

1. The low hemoglobin value, marked rouleaux, and extremely high ESR.
2. The reagent strip test for protein is most sensitive to albumin, whereas the SSA test will precipitate all urinary proteins (albumin and globulins). In this case an abnormal monoclonal protein (globulin) is suspected based on the urine protein tests, rouleaux, and ESR value.
3. To rule out a possible discrepancy in the protein values caused by the presence of an nonionizable chemical such as radiographic media. In this case the specific gravity values are essentially the same (within the error of the method by reagent strip) and suggest that the discrepancy in the protein tests is due to a protein other than albumin, and not another chemical or drug.
4. To further rule out the presence of a compound such as radiographic media rather than protein. In this case, the precipitate was seen as a fine lacy precipitate, which did not polarize light. This is consistent with the appearance of protein which has been precipitated by sulfosalicylic acid. This is not a usual procedure, but may be helpful in difficult cases.

5. Serum and urine electrophoresis. In this case a monoclonal spike of globulin was found in the urine and the patient was eventually diagnosed as having multiple myeloma.

ANSWERS TO CASE #3—CHAPTER 4

1. Patient has diabetes mellitus and is in coma (unconscious) caused by ketoacidosis.
2. Acetone, one of the ketone bodies evidenced by the positive urine ketone reaction. The odor is similar to that after ingestion of alcohol.
3. The reagent strip measures ionic compounds, or substances that ionize. The refractometer measures any dissolved substances. Glucose is a nonionizing dissolved substance, that raises the specific gravity .004 for each gram/dL. At this rate, the urine probably contains $1.030 − 1.010 = 0.020 + 4$, or 5 g/dL (5000 mg/dL). This is a significant amount of glucose in the urine, consistent with diabetes mellitus.
4. To differentiate coma, which results from extremely high blood glucose, from shock, the result of very low blood glucose. With coma, the patient is given insulin to reduce the blood glucose and prevent further accumulation of ketones; with shock, the patient is given glucose to raise the blood glucose. Both ketosis and very low blood glucose are damaging to the brain and eventually incompatible with life.

ANSWERS TO CASE #4—CHAPTER 4

1. Color of urine and foam suggest presence of bilirubin. Presence of bilirubin in urine is abnormal.
2. The presence of yellow sclera (whites of the eyes) indicates an increased concentration of bilirubin in the blood (jaundice). The lack of color in the stool specimens indicates a blockage (obstruction) to the normal excretion of bilirubin from the liver into the intestine (with intermediate storage in the gall bladder). Since the water-soluble form of bilirubin (conjugated bilirubin diglucuronide that is formed in the liver) is unable to enter the intestine, it is regurgitated back into the liver and bloodstream and eliminated from the body by way of the urine.
3. Since the reagent strip test for bilirubin is significantly less sensitive for bilirubin than the tablet test, many laboratories routinely test all urine specimens suspected of containing bilirubin on the basis of color and clinical history with the more sensitive tablet test for bilirubin. In addition, the tablet test is used as a confirmatory test for the reagent strip test, which is subject to masked and false-positive reactions.
4. c. probably caused by the presence of a gallstone in the common bile duct.

ANSWERS TO CASE #5—CHAPTER 4

1. To rule out the presence of other Ehrlich-reactive substances in addition to urobilinogen. The diazo reaction is specific for urobilinogen. If this test is negative and a reagent strip test based on the Ehrlich aldehyde reaction is positive, the presence of porphobilinogen or other Ehrlich-reactive substances is indicated.

2. The Hoesch test is specific for porphobilinogen and, if positive, indicates its presence.
3. As a further confirmatory test. The Watson-Schwartz test will differentiate between urobilinogen, porphobilinogen, and other Ehrlich-reactive substances. Performance of this test is avoided because of the use of chloroform, a known carcinogen, in the procedure.
4. Porphobilin. An oxidation product of porphobilinogen, which is a colorless compound. Unfortunately, the common tests for porphobilinogen will not detect porphobilin; therefore the urine specimen should be absolutely fresh when tested for porphobilinogen.
5. Surgery is no longer necessary, since the abdominal pain may be explained by the presence of porphobilinogen. In addition, persons with this condition are likely to have very adverse reactions to anesthetics, especially barbiturates.
6. Most likely acute intermittent porphyria. Variegate porphyria and hereditary coproporphyria also result in excretion of porphobilinogen.

ANSWERS TO CASE #6—CHAPTER 4

1. Abnormal: amber (orange-red) color, 8 EU urobilinogen. Discrepant: none
2. To rule out the presence of porphobilinogen or another Ehrlich-reactive compound. In this case both strips give the same reaction, indicating the presence of urobilinogen. A negative Hoesch test for porphobilinogen would further confirm the absence of porphobilinogen.
3. The hemoglobin that is formed from excess hemolysis is converted to bilirubin and eliminated from the body by the usual pathway.
4. In chronic hemolytic anemia, the liver is functioning normally. Therefore the excess bilirubin that is formed is conjugated to bilirubin diglucuronide in the liver and passed into the intestine for conversion to urobilinogen and elimination by way of the feces.
5. Because of the excess destruction of red cells and production of bilirubin, there is an excess production of urobilinogen in the intestine. Half of this production is recirculated to the liver for re-excretion into the intestine. However, the excess production of urobilinogen results in increased concentration of urobilinogen in the blood. This is filtered through the glomerulus and eliminated via the urine.
6. Urobilin, an orange-red pigment. The oxidation product of urobilinogen that is colorless.
7. a

ANSWERS TO CASE #1—CHAPTER 6

1. Abnormal: red/red-brown color, cloudy transparency, 300 mg/dL/3+SSA protein, large blood, 10-25 red blood cells/hpf (and dysmorphic forms), 2-5 red blood cell casts/lpf.
   Discrepant: none
2. An indication of glomerular damage.
3. a. 1
   b. 1, 2, and 3
4. An indication of acute glomerular disease (if blood or blood pigment casts were present, a more chronic condition would be indicated).

5. This is not an active infection; rather, it is a immune complex sequele of a past infection.
6. Acute poststreptococcal glomerulonephritis.

ANSWERS TO CASE #2—CHAPTER 6

1. Abnormal results: pale color, hazy transparency, large quantity of white foam, >2000 mg/dL/4+ protein, 2-5 fatty casts, 5-10 hyaline casts, moderate oval fat bodies, few renal epithelial cells, fat globules.
   Discrepant results: none
2. The extremely large amount of albumin shown by the reagent strip and SSA protein results.
3. Massive amounts of protein are being lost into the urine, which results in decreased plasma protein. This decreased plasma protein results in a decreased oncotic pressure, which together with sodium retention, is seen as edema, or an accumulation of fluid in all of the tissues of the body.
4. Renal epithelial cells, which are filled with fat (lipid) droplets. These, together with massive proteinuria, fatty casts, and fat globules, indicate severe renal dysfunction of glomerular origin.
5. The nephrotic syndrome.

ANSWERS TO CASE #3—CHAPTER 6

1. Abnormal: cloudy transparency, 100 mg/dL/2+ protein, positive nitrite, positive leukocyte esterase, 25-50 white blood (and glitter) cells, 5-10 granular and 2-5 cellular casts, many bacteria.
   Discrepant: none
2. Upper. The presence of casts places the infection within the kidney. The level of proteinuria also suggests kidney involvement.
3. Neutrophils. Leukocyte esterase is positive—cells must be granulocytes (primarily neutrophils) to react. Glitter cells are special neutrophils exhibiting Brownian motion of their cytoplasmic granules and are seen in dilute urine of specific gravity 1.010 or less.
4. White cells, more specifically neutrophils. The urine contains many white cells (probably neutrophils) and bacteria. It is assumed that these are the origin of the cells contained within the cellular casts.
5. b. Actually it is a tubulo-interstitial disease.

ANSWERS TO CASE #4—CHAPTER 6

1. Abnormal: Cloudy transparency, alkaline pH (with other findings), trace protein, positive nitrite, positive leukocyte esterase, 10-25 white blood cells/hpf, moderate transitional epithelial cells, many bacteria.
   Discrepant: none
2. Lower. There are no casts present. The degree of proteinuria is also more consistent with a lower urinary tract (bladder) infection.
3. Neutrophils. The presence of nitrite indicates a bacterial infection. This is confirmed by the presence of bacteria in the sediment. The presence of leukocyte esterase is consistent with neutrophils, which are present in response to the bacterial infection.
4. With an infection of the bladder, the bladder epithelium, which consists of transitional epithelial cells, may be infected and sloughed off into the urine. In addition, the specimen was collected by catheterization, a process that often results in the presence of transitional epithelial cells in the urine caused by mechanical disruption of the epithelium by the catheter.
5. The original source of infection is fecal contamination from the patient's own intestinal flora. In this case, the patient is incontinent and retains residual urine in the bladder caused by his enlarged prostate. This results in a continuing infection, since the patient is unable to completely void upon urination. Such infections begin in the bladder but have a risk of ascending into the kidney.

ANSWERS TO CASE #5—CHAPTER 6

1. Abnormal: pink color, cloudy, trace protein, large blood, 10-25 red cells, 5-10 cystine crystals.
   Discrepant: none
2. Cystine. This patient suffers from cystinuria, an inherited condition in which the amino acids cystine, ornithine, lysine, and arginine (COLA) are not reabsorbed by the renal tubules as normally happens. As a result, cystine precipitates out of solution and forms renal stones. These may be extremely large, blocking the entire renal pelvis, as shown on the radiograph of this patient.
3. Red cells are the result of bleeding into the tubules because of abrasion by the stones that are formed and passed through the renal tubules.
4. Cystine crystals are typically found in urine of an acid pH. The specific gravity is high, representing a concentrated urine specimen. This favors stone formation, caused by increased concentration of solutes (in this case increased concentration of cystine). Persons with cystinuria should be well hydrated at all times to prevent stone formation.
5. An unusual hexagonal (six-sided) form of uric acid may resemble cystine. Uric acid crystals tend to show a yellow to yellow-brown color, whereas cystine crystals are colorless. Cystine crystals are typically layered, uric acid may be. Uric acid is strongly birefringent. Thin cystine crystals fail to polarize light, although thicker forms may show the presence of birefringence. The nitroprusside reaction should be used to differentiate uric acid from cystine crystals before the presence of cystine crystals is reported.

ANSWERS TO CASE #6—CHAPTER 6

1. Abnormal: cloudy transparency.
   Discrepant: negative blood and 10-25 red cells/hpf.
2. Because of the abnormal transparency—cloudy.
3. Note normal color (yellow) and lack of protein. Test for ascorbic acid (negative) to rule out a false-negative reaction for blood caused by ascorbic acid. Ensure yeast are not being mistaken for red cells by observing morphologically for variation in size and budding forms. Further investigation might include adding glacial acetic acid to lyse red cells, supravital staining, and Gram staining.
   Observe sediment with polarized and compensated polarized light. Rare ovoid forms of calcium oxalate resembling red blood cells will polarize light—red cells and yeast will not. Most probable discrepancy in this example.

ANSWERS TO CASE #1—CHAPTER 7

1. effusion, caused by an inflammatory exudate
2. negative Gram stain and culture, no microorganisms reported; rules out acute bacterial infections—staphylococcus, gonococcus.
3. cells, crystals, microorganisms
4. many white blood cells with a high percentage of phagocytic neutrophils; monocytes and macrophages are also present; turbidity increases with the degree of inflammation present; the presence of a few red blood cells is a normal finding.
5. an acute inflammatory arthritis—acute crystal-induced urate gout—gouty arthritis
6. The fluid appears watery and cloudy, it has a high WBC—with most of the cells being neutrophils. When using compensated polarized light, the cells show *intracellular*, needle-shaped crystals that are yellow when the long axis of the crystal is lying parallel to the direction of the slow wave vibration of the compensator and blue when the long axis of the crystal is lying perpendicular to the direction of the slow wave vibration. The morphologic appearance of the crystals is consistent with monosodium urate (MSU). MSU crystals can be seen in a patient with both urate gout and an infectious arthritis—seeing crystals does not rule out a concurrent infection. In this patient, however, the negative Gram stain and culture would generally rule out an infection.

ANSWERS TO CASE #2—CHAPTER 7

1. White cell count and differential count, glucose level and total protein level, Gram stain and culture. For suspected infections of the meninges, Gram stain and culture are done to aid in the diagnosis.
2. No, the Gram stain lacks sensitivity. Specific screening tests for *antigens* released from bacteria and yeast can be done if a specific organism is suspected and Gram stain and cultures are negative. This is especially useful when antibiotics have been used.
3. Blood: increased WBC with an increase of neutrophils—polymorphonuclear leukocytes—PMNs.
   Cerebrospinal fluid: increased WBC with an increase of neutrophils; glucose level is low compared with blood glucose (cells and bacteria have utilized the glucose); protein level is increased indicating inflamed meninges. Generally, increased neutrophils are seen with bacterial infection, whereas increased lymphocytes are seen with viral infections.
4. Cytocentrifugation followed by Wright stain for blood cell morphology.
5. 0-0.005 × 10⁹/L mononuclear cells (lymphocytes and monocytes); a rare neutrophil is seen with the cytospin method.
6. It serves to substantiate other findings. Bacteria and increased presence of leukocytes have been reported. The glucose level in the spinal fluid is low because the bacteria and leukocytes present utilize the glucose. For this reason, when glucose assays are done on spinal fluid, blood is also drawn for plasma glucose levels for comparison purposes. The cerebrospinal fluid glucose level should be about 60% of the plasma glucose level.
7. Acute bacterial meningitis (probably *N. meningitidis*). This is the most probable organism considering the patient's age and circumstance. The organism is disseminated in crowded living quarters like military camps and dormitories.

ANSWERS TO CASE #3—CHAPTER 7

1. Transudate. A total protein level of 3 g/dL is often used as a cutoff between a transudate and an exudate; a transudate has low protein levels. A pleural fluid protein to serum protein ratio can also be calculated:

$$\frac{1.8}{6.2} = 0.29$$

When the ratio of pleural fluid protein to serum protein is less than 0.5, the fluid is considered to be a transudate (a ratio greater than 0.5 would be an exudate). This ratio can be helpful in differentiating effusions as exudates or transudates. (Note: Specific gravity measurements of pleural or other serous fluids are unsafe, unsatisfactory, and are no longer used.)
2. The fluid is very pale yellow and translucent. The WBC is not increased, and lymphocytes are seen. Gram stain and culture show no organisms.
3. An exudate. Because of the dilation and increased small blood vessel permeability associated with the infectious process, there is exudation of fluid, plasma proteins, and cells into the pleural cavity. The accumulated fluid is called an exudate and sometimes resembles pus. (Generally, pleural exudates are defined as having a total protein level greater than 3 g/dL with the ratio of pleural fluid protein to serum protein being greater than 0.5.) There is also an increase in the number of neutrophils in the fluid.
4. A transudate is a noninflammatory (noninfectious) accumulation of fluid with a low protein and cell content precipitated by an increase in hydrostatic pressure in the lung blood vessels resulting from poor heart pumping function with poor circulatory return of blood to the heart from the lung.

APPENDIX B

ABBREVIATIONS

ADH	antidiuretic hormone
AFP	alpha-fetoprotein
AGN	acute glomerulonephritis
AIDS	acquired immune deficiency syndrome
ASCLS	American Society for Clinical Laboratory Science (formerly ASMT, American Society for Medical Technology)
ASCP	American Society of Clinical Pathologists
AST	aspartate aminotransferase
ATN	acute tubular necrosis
CAP	College of American Pathologists
CASA	computer assisted semen analysis
CDC	Centers for Disease Control and Prevention
CK	creatine kinase
CLIA '67	Clinical Laboratory Improvement Act of 1967
CLIA '88	Clinical Laboratory Improvement Amendments of 1988
COLA	Commission on Office Laboratory Accreditation
CPPD	calcium pyrophosphate dihydrate
CQI	continuous quality improvement
CSF	cerebrospinal fluid
EDTA	ethylenediamine tetraacetic acid
ELISA	enzyme-linked immunosorbent assay
EPA	Environmental Protection Agency
FDA	Food and Drug Administration
HBV	Hepatitis B virus
HCFA	Health Care Financing Administration
HHS	Health and Human Services, US Department of
HIV	human immunodeficiency virus
HPF, hpf	high power field
IDDM	insulin-dependent diabetes mellitus
Ig	immunoglobulin

JCAHO	Joint Commission for the Accreditation of Healthcare Organizations
L	liter
L/S ratio	lecithin-sphingomyelin ratio
LD	lactate dehydrogenase
LPF, lpf	low power field
MBP	myelin basic protein
mL	milliliter
mol	mole
MSDS	material safety data sheets
MSU	monosodium urate
NCCLS	National Committee for Clinical Laboratory Standards
NIDDM	non–insulin-dependent diabetes mellitus
NS	nephrotic syndrome
OFB	oval fat body
OSHA	Occupational Safety and Health Act
OSHA	Occupational Safety and Health Administration
PEL	permissible exposure limits
PMN	polymorphonuclear neutrophil
POC	point-of-care (testing)
POL	Physician Office Laboratory
PPE	personal protective equipment
PPM	physician performed microscopy
PT	proficiency testing
QA	quality assurance
QC	quality control
RTE	renal tubular epithelium
RTF	renal tubular fat
TQM	total quality management
TTAT	total turnaround time
UBBST	universal blood and body substance technique
UTI	urinary tract infection

GLOSSARY

accuracy The correctness of a test result; freedom from error or how close a test result is to the "true" or actual value.

action levels (for hazardous substances) There are exposures to specific hazardous chemicals that while below the permissible exposure limit, still require that certain action take place—under specific conditions, medical surveillance or monitoring of the workplace be done.

active reabsorption Reabsorption that requires an expenditure of energy for the analyte to be reabsorbed—usually against a concentration gradient from a region of lower to one of higher concentration.

acute glomerulonephritis (AGN), postinfectious glomerulonephritis The acute form of glomerulonephritis that may occur 1 to 6 weeks after a streptococcal (usually Group A, β-hemolytic) infection. Characterized by hematuria, oliguria, edema, and proteinuria with red cell and/or granular casts.

acute tubular necrosis (ATN) Sudden failure of the kidney tubules, commonly caused by an interruption of the blood supply to the tubules, resulting in ischemia.

aerosols Infectious particles that are airborne; fine mist in which particles are dispersed.

albuminuria Presence of albumin in urine. Also called **proteinuria**.

aldosterone A mineral corticosteroid hormone released from the adrenal medulla that stimulates active absorption of sodium ion in exchange for potassium ion that is excreted by renal tubular cells (the sodium/potassium pump).

amber Term used to describe urine color; a dark yellow or orange-red color that may indicate a very concentrated urine specimen, or the presence of bilirubin or urobilin pigment.

amniocentesis Needle aspiration of amniotic fluid.

amorphous material Crystalline material seen in the urine sediment as granules, without shape or form.

antidiuretic hormone (ADH) A pituitary hormone that decreases the production of urine by increasing the reabsorption of water by the renal tubules. Also called **vasopressin**.

arthritis Inflammation of a joint.

arthrocentesis Needle aspiration of synovial fluid from the joint space.

ascites Abnormal accumulation of peritoneal fluid.

ascorbic acid, vitamin C. A strong reducing agent; ascorbic acid acts as an interfering substance (resulting in delayed or false negative results) in many reagent strip tests that utilize the release of oxygen and subsequent oxidation of a chromogen.

azoospermia Absence of sperm cells.

barrier precautions Personal protective devices (gloves, gowns) placed between blood or other potentially infectious body fluid specimen and the person handling the specimen to prevent transmission of the pathogenic agents borne by the specimen.

Bence Jones protein A light chain immunoglobulin seen almost exclusively in urine of patients with multiple myeloma, which coagulates at temperatures of 45° to 55°C and redissolves completely or partially on boiling.

Benedict's test Copper reduction test for reducing substances based on the reduction of cupric (copper II) ions to cuprous (copper I) ions in the presence of alkali and heat.

bilirubin Vivid yellow pigment; major by-product of normal red blood cell destruction. See also **conjugated bilirubin, free (unconjugated) bilirubin**.

biohazard A potential risk to the health of persons from contact, either directly or through the environment, with an infectious agent or material; is designated by means of a specific universal biohazard symbol or written term.

biohazard container A special container to be used for disposal of all potentially infectious materials—blood, other body fluids and tissues, and disposable materials contaminated with them; containers should be tagged "biohazard" or bear the universal biohazard symbol.

birefringence Ability of some crystals or objects to rotate or polarize light so they are visible when viewed with crossed polarizing filters. Also, **anisotropy**.

bladder (urinary) Muscular membranous sac that stores urine for discharge through the urethra. It is located in the pelvis, connected anteriorly with the two ureters and posteriorly with the urethra.

blood-brain barrier Prevents passage of certain plasma constituents from the blood to the brain.

body cavity fluid Fluid normally found in varying amounts in various cavities or body spaces (e.g., cerebrospinal, amniotic, pleural, abdominal, pericardial, peritoneal, synovial); in certain conditions this fluid is aspirated (collected) and assayed.

Bowman's capsule See **glomerular capsule.**

brightfield microscope Illumination system used in the common clinical microscope.

calculus (urinary) Stone or deposit of mineral salts formed and found in the urinary tract.

casts Structures that result from solidification of Tamm-Horsfall mucoprotein in the lumen of the kidney tubules; they form a mold, or cast, of the tubule and trap other material that may be present when formed. Several types exist. They represent a biopsy of the kidney and are clinically significant.

catheterized urine specimen Urine specimen obtained by the introduction of a catheter into the urinary bladder by way of the urethra.

Centers for Disease Control and Prevention (CDC) A part of the U.S. Department of Health and Human Services' (HHS) Public Health Service.

cerebrospinal fluid (CSF) Formed by the choroid plexus in the ventricles of the brain and found within the subarachnoid spaces, the central canal of the spinal cord and the ventricles of the brain.

Chemical Hygiene Plan Mandated as part of the OSHA hazard communication standard. This plan must be in place in the laboratory to inform workers and carry out implementation of safety practices necessary to protect the workers from potential health hazards associated with laboratory chemicals in use.

clean-catch (midstream) urine specimen Urine specimen collected during the middle of a flow of urine, after the urinary opening has been carefully cleansed. The type of urine collection used for bacterial culture.

Clinical Laboratory Improvement Act of 1967 (CLIA '67) Act providing for the licensing of laboratories that accept specimens for testing from across state lines (interstate commerce), generally large hospital and reference laboratories.

Clinical Laboratory Improvement Amendments of 1988 (CLIA '88) Standards set for all laboratories to ensure quality patient care; provisions include requirements for quality control and assurance, for the use of proficiency tests, and for certain levels of personnel to perform and supervise work done in all clinical laboratories. Applies to any entity that performs testing on material derived from humans for the purpose of diagnosis, assessment, or treatment. Under CLIA '88, laboratory tests are designated and laboratories licensed as waived, moderately complex, or highly complex.

Clue cell Squamous epithelial cells covered (encrusted) with *Gardnerella vaginalis*; indicates bacterial vaginitis.

collecting tubules The relatively large, straight renal tubules after the distal convoluted tubules of the nephron which connect individual nephrons at various intervals and funnel urine into the renal pelvis. The site of final concentration of urine under the control of ADH (vasopressin).

College of American Pathologists (CAP) This professional organization of pathologists provides services, guidance, and information to its members and to others. It develops programs, publications, and services that span the entire field of pathology; special attention is given to areas of laboratory improvement and quality control and laboratory planning and administration. Survey programs in laboratory improvement and quality assurance offer a wide range of interlaboratory comparison and proficiency testing programs, meeting the requirements set by CLIA '88, JCAHO, and most state regulatory agencies.

compensated polarized light Modification of the normal brightfield microscope in which two crossed polarizing filters plus a first-order red compensator or filter are inserted to observe the presence or absence and type of birefringence. Especially useful in identification of synovial fluid crystals in the clinical laboratory.

condenser Part of the microscope that directs and focuses the beam of light from the light source onto the material under examination; positioned just under the stage and can be raised and lowered by means of an adjustment knob.

confirmatory test A test used to confirm the accuracy or correctness of a procedure. An alternative method with at least the same or better specificity, based on a different principle, with equal or better sensitivity than the original test.

conjugated bilirubin, bilirubin glucuronide, direct bilirubin Bilirubin that has been made water soluble by conjugation with glucuronide by the Kupffer cells of the liver. Once conjugated, increased levels of bilirubin in the blood can be filtered through the kidney and found in the urine.

continuous quality improvement (CQI) A continual process to ensure that quality outcomes are attained to satisfy the needs of the patient; involves the philosophy of TQM. See also, **Total Quality Management.**

control specimen (solution) Material or solution with a known concentration of the analyte(s) being measured; used for quality control in which the test result for the control specimen must be within certain limits in order for the unknown values run in the same "batch" or time frame to be considered reportable.

cortex (renal) The outer layer of the kidney, made up of the glomerular portions of the nephron and the proximal convoluted tubules.

crenated (red cells) Red cells showing spicules or projections on the surface; this notched, shriveled surface results from loss of fluid from the red cell into the urine caused by hypertonicity.

critical (panic) value Dangerously abnormal test results (high or low) that are used to guide emergency notification of clinical teams. Accrediting agencies such as CAP require that clinical laboratories establish a list of critical limits to suit their needs and to develop formal notification policies with documentation of such communication. These values reflect medical decision levels for emergency patient evaluation and optimization points for critical care.

crystalluria The presence of crystals in the urine sediment.

crystals, abnormal Urinary crystals of metabolic or iatrogenic origin that are generally of pathologic significance and require further (if possible chemical) confirmation.

crystals, normal Urinary crystals that may be found in normal urine specimens of an acid or alkaline pH; generally they are not pathologic and can be reported on the basis of morphologic appearance.

cylindroid Hyaline cast with one end that tapers off into a tail or point; clinically equivalent to and reported as a hyaline cast.

cystitis Inflammatory condition of the urinary bladder and ureters, characterized by pain, urgency and frequency of urination, and hematuria. May be caused by a bacterial infection, calculus, or tumor.

cytocentrifugation Special slow centrifugation method used to prepare permanent microscope slides of fluids (e.g., urine, other body fluids), resulting in better morphologic preservation than by other centrifugation or preparation methods.

decontamination Process of eliminating something that has become contaminated or mixed with something that makes it impure; in the laboratory, the process of cleaning up a spill of an infectious specimen or general cleaning of the working surfaces after handling patient specimens.

Department of Health and Human Services (HHS) Department of the U.S. government under which the Health Care Financing Administration (HCFA) functions; is responsible for implementation of laws and writing of regulations that provide details of how various laws are to be carried out; publishes details of proposed and final regulations in the *Federal Register*, an official government document.

diabetes mellitus Chronic metabolic syndrome of impaired carbohydrate, fat, and protein metabolism that is secondary to insufficiency of insulin secretion or to the inhibition of the activity of insulin; characterized by increased concentration of glucose in the blood and urine.

diazo reaction Coupling of a diazonium salt with another aromatic ring to give an azo dye.

direct bilirubin See **conjugated bilirubin.**

distal convoluted tubule Convoluted tubules of the nephron furthest from the glomerulus where final reabsorption of sodium (maintaining water and electrolyte balance) and removal of excess acid (maintaining acid-base balance) occurs.

documentation A written record. In the laboratory this includes all personnel records, policies and procedures, quality assurance measures, incidents, and corrective actions.

dysmorphic (red cells) Distorted, irregular, or misshapen red cells, indicative of glomerular bleeding, especially when accompanied by proteinuria and red cell casts.

edema Abnormal accumulation of fluid in interstitial spaces of tissues.

effusion Abnormal accumulation of any of the extracellular fluids. Fluid moves from the blood or lymphatic vessels into the tissues of body cavities (e.g., pleural, pericardial, or peritoneal fluid) or the joints (synovial fluid).

Ehrlich's aldehyde reaction Reaction of urobilinogen, porphobilinogen, and other Ehrlich-reactive compounds with *p*-dimethylaminobenzaldehyde in concentrated hydrochloric acid to form a colored aldehyde.

ejaculate Viscous sample of semen; collected for assay.

erythrophagia Ingestion of red blood cells by macrophages.

exfoliate To peel or slough off, such as the process by which epithelial cells lining the urinary system are continually sloughed off and replaced.

exogenous Coming from or being introduced into a specimen from the outside, as contaminants from powder in gloves.

extravascular fluid Body fluid other than blood or urine.

exudate Effusion that results from inflammatory conditions such as infections and malignancies that directly affect the membranes lining a cavity; an effusion with a total protein greater than 3.0 g/dL, and increased cell count, is usually classified as an exudate.

Federal Register Official government document that publishes details of proposed and final regulations on how various laws are to be carried out; it is in the *Federal Register* that the final details on regulations for CLIA '88 and OSHA have been published, for example.

fern test Presence of characteristic "ferning" pattern of dried cervical mucus on a glass microscope slide; depends on the stage of the ovarian cycle and the presence or absence of pregnancy (i.e., progesterone secretion in large amounts.)

first morning urine specimen First urine voided in the morning. It is generally the most concentrated specimen of the day because less fluid or water is excreted during the night, yet the kidney has maintained excretion of a constant concentration of solid or dissolved substances.

fistula Abnormal connection such as a fistula between the colon and urinary tract.

free bilirubin, unconjugated bilirubin Water-insoluble form of bilirubin that must be carried through the bloodstream as a bilirubin-albumin complex. Because of its insolubility, this form of bilirubin cannot be excreted by the kidney and is not found in the urine.

galactosemia Inherited, autosomal recessive disorder of galactose metabolism, characterized by a deficiency of the enzyme galactose-1-phosphate uridyl transferase, resulting in increased levels of galactose in the blood and urine. Results in permanent physical and mental deterioration that may be controlled by early detection and dietary restriction of galactose.

ghost or shadow cell Red cells that have burst, releasing hemoglobin, leaving only the red cell membrane; visualization enhanced by phase contrast microscopy.

glitter cells Swollen neutrophil with cytoplasmic granules in constant Brownian motion; seen in dilute urine. Also known as Sternheimer-Malbin positive cells.

glomerular (Bowman's) capsule Cup-shaped end of the renal nephron that contains the glomerulus.

glomerular filtrate Ultrafiltrate of blood formed as blood is filtered through the glomerular capillaries of the glomerulus into Bowman's capsule. First step in urine formation, basically blood plasma without protein or fat.

glomerulonephritis Inflammation of the glomerulus of the kidney, characterized by proteinuria, hematuria, decreased urine production, and edema. Includes acute (poststreptococcal) glomerulonephritis, chronic glomerulonephritis, and subacute glomerulonephritis.

glomerulus Tuft or cluster of blood vessels, found in the renal nephron. Urine formation begins at the glomerulus.

glucose oxidase Enzyme that oxidizes glucose to gluconic acid while reducing atmospheric oxygen to hydrogen peroxide.

glucosuria, glycosuria Presence of measurable glucose in urine.

Gram staining reaction Using the Gram staining method, microorganisms retaining the violet (purple) color of the primary stain (crystal violet-iodine complex) are considered Gram "positive"; microorganisms having the red-pink color of the counterstain (safranin) are considered Gram "negative." Use of these properties serves to classify or differentiate organisms; it is a differential stain.

Hansel's stain Stain containing methylene blue and eosin-Y in methanol; used to stain for the presence of eosinophils.

haptoglobin Plasma protein that binds and carries free hemoglobin in the bloodstream. When haptoglobin is saturated, free hemoglobin is filtered into the urine.

hazard identification system Symbol that provides, at a glance, information about potential health, flammability, and chemical reactivity for potential hazards from materials used in the laboratory; a larger diamond-shaped figure made up of four smaller diamonds, one red, one blue, one yellow and one white, each indicating the particular hazardous information pertaining to the chemical in question.

Health Care Financing Administration (HCFA) Agency of the U.S. Department of Health and Human Services (HHS); regulates and administers funding for various legislative acts—CLIA '88 and the Health Insurance for the Aged Act of 1965 (Medicare), for example; HCFA coordinates its regulatory functions with the Centers for Disease Control and Prevention (CDC).

hemarthrosis Bleeding into a joint.

hematuria The presence of red blood cells in urine.

hemocytometer Counting chamber used to perform manual cell counts.

hemoglobinuria Presence of free hemoglobin in urine.

hemolytic jaundice, prehepatic jaundice Jaundice that results from increased destruction of red cells in the blood (intravascular hemolysis).

hemosiderin Iron-rich pigment that is a product of red cell hemolysis; storage form of iron in the bone marrow. In urine, hemosiderin is seen as iron-containing granules that may occur after a hemolytic episode. Stain blue with Prussian blue stain for iron (Rous test).

hepatic jaundice, hepatocellular jaundice Jaundice resulting from conditions that affect the liver cells directly, such as viral or toxic hepatitis.

hepatitis B virus (HBV) Virus that can be directly transmitted by blood or other body fluids, causing hepatitis, an acute viral illness. Recovery is usually complete, although some patients remain carriers or can develop chronic hepatitis conditions.

high power examination Usually a 40× magnification objective and 10× ocular giving a total magnification of 400 times; used for more detailed examination of wet preparations such as the urine sediment.

Hoesch test An inverse Ehrlich's aldehyde reaction used to detect porphobilinogen in urine.

human immunodeficiency virus (HIV) A type of retrovirus transmitted by blood or other body fluids that causes HIV infection and acquired immune deficiency syndrome (AIDS).

hyaluronate (hyaluronic acid) High molecular weight mucopolysaccharide polymer present in synovial fluid differentiating it from other body fluids; responsible for giving synovial fluid its viscosity; secreted by the synovial cells that line the joint cavity.

iatrogenic Caused by treatment or diagnostic procedures by medical personnel or through exposure to the environment of a health care facility. Also **nosocomial**; of or pertaining to a hospital.

infection control A program set in place in the healthcare facility to protect the workers from being exposed to possible pathogenic agents present in the workplace.

insulin Hormone that has the effect of lowering the blood glucose concentration by promoting transport and entry of glucose into muscle cells and other tissues.

interstitial nephritis Inflammation of the interstitial tissue of the kidney, including the tubules. May be acute or chronic. **Acute interstitial nephritis** is an immunologic, adverse reaction to certain drugs, often sulfonamide or methicillin.

iris diaphragm Part of the microscope located at the bottom of the Abbé condenser, under the lens but within the condenser body; controls the amount of light passing through the material under observation; can be opened or closed to adjust contrast.

jaundice Increase in the concentration of free or conjugated bilirubin in the blood (serum) with accumulation of bilirubin in the body tissues. See also **hemolytic jaundice**, **hepatic jaundice**, and **obstructive jaundice**.

Joint Commission for the Accreditation of Healthcare Organizations (JCAHO) Voluntary organization made up of representatives from various healthcare associations (hospital, physician, dentist)—not a governmental agency. Mission of JCAHO is to enhance the quality of healthcare provided to the public, and the organization is dedicated to improving the process to carry out this mission. One important function of JCAHO is the accreditation of U.S. hospitals. Hospital standards and guidelines are set, and accreditation is carried out and monitored, through a continual process of site visits, surveys, and reports. Site visits include visits to the clinical laboratories of the healthcare facilities seeking accreditation.

ketogenic diet Diet that consists of more than 1.5 g of fat per 1.0 g of carbohydrate; results in ketosis.

ketosis Increased concentration of ketones in the blood (**ketonemia**) and urine (**ketonuria**).

leukocyte esterase Enzyme present in the azurophilic or primary granules of the granulocytic leukocytes; presence of this enzyme in urine indicates urinary tract infection or inflammation.

lipiduria Presence of fat of biologic origin in urine; may be cholesterol or triglyceride (neutral fat).

liquefaction Process in which the ejaculated viscous semen specimen becomes liquid.

lithiasis Kidney stone (calculus) formation.

Loop of Henle The U-shaped portion of the nephron between the proximal and distal convoluted tubules, consisting of a thin descending (concentrating) limb and a thick ascending (diluting) limb.

low power examination Usually a 10× magnification objective and 10× ocular, giving a total magnification of 100 times; used for the initial scanning and observation in most clinical microscopic work.

lower urinary tract Portion of the urinary tract excluding the kidney (e.g., the ureters, bladder, and urethra). **Lower urinary tract infections** are generally infections of the bladder, also known as **cystitis.**

lumbar puncture Needle aspiration of CSF by puncture in one of the spaces between the third, fourth, or fifth lumbar vertebrae (depending on the age of the patient).

maltese cross White cross on a black background, characteristic of cholesterol ester droplets in urine or other body fluids, viewed with polarized light. Must not be confused with granules of starch.

material safety data sheets (MSDS) Information about the hazards of each chemical are provided by the supplier or manufacturer of the chemical; any hazardous chemicals used in the laboratory should be accompanied by this information.

meconium Dark green-black, thick, sticky mixture of amniotic fluid, biliary and intestinal secretions, epithelial cells, and other intrauterine debris passed from intestine of newborn as the first stools; presence of meconium in amniotic fluid during delivery can indicate fetal distress.

medulla (renal) A part of the parenchyma of the kidney, beneath the cortex, including the renal pyramids and columns. Includes the loop of Henle and collecting tubules.

meninges Covering of the brain and spinal cord.

meningitis Inflammation of the meninges; can be bacterial, viral, mycobacterial, or fungal in etiology.

microalbuminuria The consistent passage of very small amounts of protein as albumin into the urine.

midstream urine specimen Urine specimen collected during the middle of a flow of urine; used for routine urinalysis.

myoglobin Muscle hemoglobin; consists of one heme molecule, containing one iron molecule attached to a single globulin chain. A red-brown pigment, responsible for the red color of muscle and its ability to store oxygen.

myoglobinuria The presence of myoglobin in urine.

National Committee for Clinical Laboratory Standards (NCCLS) Nonprofit educational organization that sets voluntary consensus standards for all areas of the clinical laboratory.

nephron Working unit of the kidney, where urine is formed; includes the glomerulus, Bowman's capsule, proximal and distal convoluted tubules, and loops of Henle.

nephrotic syndrome (NS) A clinical syndrome characterized by massive proteinuria (with hypoalbuminemia and edema) and lipiduria; an abnormal kidney condition.

nidus The point or origin, focus or nucleus; such as the nidus for urinary stone formation.

obstructive jaundice, posthepatic jaundice Jaundice resulting from blockage of the normal outflow of conjugated bilirubin from the liver into the intestine.

occult blood Hidden blood; not observable by the naked eye, but requires use of a chemical test to be detected.

Occupational Safety and Health Act Legislation of 1970 that set a system of safeguards for the health and safety of workers in the United States; it is regulated by the Occupational Health and Safety Administration.

Occupational Safety and Health Administration (OSHA) Agency within the U.S. Department of Labor that regulates levels of safety and health in the workplace for all workers in the United States; carries out the mandate set by the Occupational Health and Safety Act of 1970.

oligospermia Number of sperm cells significantly decreased.

organized sediment Biologic portion of the urine sediment including cells derived from blood, epithelial cells, other cell forms, and fat of biologic origin.

OSHA safety standards Include provisions for warning labels to alert workers to potential hazards, availability of personal protective equipment, exposure control procedures being in place, implementation of training and educational programs to disseminate the available information to all workers.

OSHA standard: exposure to bloodborne pathogens Mandates use of universal precautions when handling patient specimens to prevent transmission of pathogenic agents borne by blood or other body fluids being tested in the laboratory; it mandates the use of barrier controls, safe work practices, use of personal protective equipment, and training and education for the healthcare workers.

OSHA standard: hazard communication Designed to ensure that all laboratory workers are fully aware of possible hazardous situations present in their workplace—includes the implementation of a Chemical Hygiene Plan. This is also known as the "right to know" rule.

osmolality A measure of the number of solute particles per unit of solvent; number of osmoles of solute per liter of solution.

oval fat bodies; renal tubular fat Renal epithelial cells (also macrophages or histiocytes) filled with fat droplets (cholesterol or neutral fat); associated with the presence of free fat globules and fatty casts.

paracentesis Needle aspiration of peritoneal fluid.

passive reabsorption Reabsorption that does not require the expenditure of energy; the analyte moves passively down a concentration gradient, from a region of higher to a region of lower concentration. Or, an analyte can move passively along with another analyte that may be actively reabsorbed such as the passive reabsorption of water with active reabsorption of sodium ions.

pericardial cavity Space between two serous membranes lining the heart; contains pericardial fluid.

pericardial fluid Extravascular fluid that surrounds the heart; forms in the pericardial cavity.

pericardiocentesis Needle aspiration of pericardial fluid.

perineal contamination Contamination originating from the perineum; generally from the foreskin, vagina, or anus.

peritoneal cavity Space between two serous membranes lining the abdomen; contains peritoneal fluid or ascitic fluid.

peritoneal fluid Extravascular fluid that surrounds the abdominal and pelvic cavities; forms within the peritoneal cavity.

permissible exposure limits (PEL) As designated by OSHA, laboratory workers must not be exposed to hazardous chemical substances in excess of certain levels—the PEL; this information must be part of the Chemical Hygiene Plan for the laboratory, and the workers must be informed about the permissible exposure levels for the various hazardous chemicals being used.

peroxidase Enzyme that catalyzes release of free oxygen from hydrogen peroxide. Peroxidase activity of the heme portion of the hemoglobin molecule is the basis of the reagent strip test for blood.

personal protective equipment (PPE) Specialized clothing or protective barriers worn or used for protection against a hazardous substance or agent.

phase contrast microscope Microscope illumination system that uses a special condenser with an annular diaphragm with a matched absorption ring in the corresponding objective. Used to give additional contrast in wet preparations; especially useful for observing the urine sediment.

phenazopyridine (Pyridium) Azo-containing compound often used as a urine analgesic to reduce pain in cystitis or other urinary tract infections. Azo-containing compounds are a common cause of interference (masking or false-positive reactions) in urine reagent strip tests.

physical properties In urinalysis, includes color, transparency (or clarity), odor, foam, volume, and specific gravity of a urine specimen.

pleural cavity Space between two serous membranes lining the lungs; contains pleural fluid.

pleural fluid Extravascular fluid that surrounds the lungs; forms within the pleural cavity.

Point-of-Care testing (POC testing) Tests that can be performed at the patient's bedside or patient care unit, thus giving a result more quickly by eliminating time for specimen handling and transportation to a distant centralized laboratory site. Generally the tests that can be completed within a 5-minute total turnaround time (TTAT) are candidates for POC testing (see **Total Turnaround Time**).

polarized light Light that is propagated in such a way that the radiation waves occur in only one direction in the vibration plane and not at random. In the microscope, light is polarized by adding a polarizing filter.

polarizing microscope Microscope illumination system that employs two polarizing lenses, which are crossed, extinguishing passage of light through the microscope; used to detect objects or crystals that bend or polarize light, making them visible when viewed with crossed polarizing filters.

porphobilinogen Colorless precursor of the porphyrins, a group of compounds utilized in the synthesis of hemoglobin.

postinfectious glomerulonephritis. See **acute glomerulonephritis** and **glomerulonephritis**.

precision The repeatability or reproducibility of a test result. A measure of the closeness of repeated test results on the same sample.

proficiency testing (PT) Program under which samples are sent to a group of laboratories for analysis; results are compared with those of other laboratories participating in the program. Included as a component of quality assurance programs to establish quality control between laboratories. Participation in a proficiency testing program is required under CLIA '88.

protein error of pH indicators Phenomenon in which at a fixed pH, certain pH indicators will show one color in the presence of protein and another color in its absence.

proteinuria Presence of protein, usually albumin, in urine.

proximal convoluted tubule Convoluted tubules of the nephron closest to the glomerular capsule in which about 80% of the fluid and electrolytes filtered through the glomerulus are reabsorbed.

pseudocast Variety of structures that resemble casts.

pseudogout (pyrophosphate gout) Arthritis in which calcium pyrophosphate dihydrate crystals (CPPD) are deposited in the synovial fluid.

pseudohyphae Elongated cell forms of yeast such as *Candida* sp. that resemble mycelia (hyphae), the threadlike filaments that make up most fungi.

pyelonephritis A diffuse pyogenic infection of the pelvis and parenchyma of the kidney. **Acute pyelonephritis** is usually the result of an infection that ascends from the lower urinary tract to the kidney. **Chronic pyelonephritis** develops slowly after bacterial infection of the kidney (usually associated with obstruction) and may progress to renal failure.

Pyridium See **phenazopyridine**.

pyuria The presence of white blood cells in the urine; a sign of inflammation or infection.

quality assurance (QA) Comprehensive set of policies, procedures, and practices in place and used to make certain that the laboratory's reported results are reliable and can be used by the physician to diagnose or treat the patient. QA includes all aspects of the laboratory (technical and nontechnical) to prevent errors and ensure accuracy of test results. It includes pre-analytical, analytical, and post-analytical factors such as record keeping, calibration and maintenance of equipment, quality control, proficiency testing, and training.

quality assurance program Plan to carry out policies and practices necessary to comply with quality assurance standards set by accreditation agencies to make certain that the laboratory's results are reliable and that these results are used in the best interest of the patient.

quality control (QC) A part of quality assurance utilizing a set of laboratory procedures designed to ensure that a test method is working properly and meets the diagnostic needs of the physician. QC makes use of control solutions or specimens and includes testing of control samples, charting the results, and analyzing them statistically.

random voided urine specimen A voided urine specimen obtained at any point of a 24-hour period.

refractive index Measure of dissolved substances in solution; the ratio of the velocity of light in air to the velocity of light in solution. Varies and corresponds with specific gravity.

refractometer Temperature-compensated instrument used to measure refractive index; in urinalysis, values are expressed as specific gravity.

reliability Ability of a laboratory assay to produce consistent results when testing is repeated successively. Includes accuracy and precision.

renal epithelial cells, renal tubular epithelium (RTE) Epithelial cells originating from (lining) the tubules of the kidney from the proximal to the collecting tubules; appearance varies and depends on actual site of origin.

renal epithelial fragment Fragment of renal epithelial cells originating from the collecting duct; three or more attached renal cells of collecting duct origin.

renal failure cast Synonym for waxy cast; clinically represents serious pathology.

renal plasma threshold The concentration of an analyte that can be completely reabsorbed from the glomerular filtrate. When the plasma concentration of an analyte exceeds this value, it will remain in the glomerular filtrate and be excreted in the urine.

renal tubular fat See **oval fat bodies**.

rhabdomyolysis Acute destruction of muscle fibers.

right to know rule OSHA standard whereby all persons working in the area must be made fully aware of possible hazardous situations present in their workplace that might be detrimental to their safety and well-being.

Rous test Wet staining procedure for hemosiderin granules in urine sediment utilizing a Prussian blue reaction for iron.

safety manual A manual readily available to all persons working in the laboratory that includes current information about all safety practices and precautions; anything that could pose a potential safety hazard for persons in the laboratory must be described in this manual and each worker in the laboratory must be familiar with its contents.

semen Viscous specimen produced from a combination of products from the testes, epididymis, seminal vesicles, and prostate produced by ejaculation; normally contains the spermatozoa (see also **ejaculate**).

sensitivity The minimum detectable level of an analyte in a given laboratory procedure or test. Statistically, the proportion of subjects with a positive diagnostic test result in a diseased population, expressed as a percentage.

sequential collection Samples are collected in order (sequence) with the order of collection noted on the specimen container (e.g., No. 1 is indicated on the first sample collected).

serous fluid Fluid found within the closed cavities of the body (pleural, pericardial, peritoneal).

serous membranes Two thin membranes that line body cavities such as pleural, pericardial, or peritoneal—the space between the two membranes containing the serous fluid.

sharps container Used disposable needles or other sharp objects must be safely discarded into these containers, which are made of rigid plastic, metal, or stiff paperboard. The containers must be conveniently located, easily recognized, and marked as a biohazard. All skin lancets, needles, scalpel blades, broken glassware, and anything else that is sharp must be discarded properly into a sharps container.

specific gravity A measure of the amount of dissolved substances present in a solution. Ratio of the density of a solution compared with the density of an equal volume of pure, solute-free water at a constant temperature; depends on the mass and number of particles in a solution.

specificity Refers to what is actually being measured in a given laboratory test. Statistically, the proportion of subjects with a negative diagnostic test in a population without the disease, expressed as a percentage.

squamous epithelial cells Large, flat, scalelike epithelial cells that line the female urethra and trigone, distal portion of the male urethra, and female vagina.

staghorn calculi Urinary calculi (stones) that fill the renal collecting system; especially characteristic of cystine, struvite (triple phosphate), and uric acid.

starch In urine sediment, refers to cornstarch a carbohydrate that is commonly used to line surgical or barrier protective gloves; a common urinary contaminant sometimes referred to, but different from, talc. Polarizes as a maltese cross.

stercobilin Pigment derived from bilirubin; responsible for normal color of the feces.

Sternheimer-Malbin stain An all-purpose, supravital stain, consisting of crystal violet and safranin O; useful in the brightfield examination of urine sediment. Available commercially as Sedi-Stain and KOVA stain.

struvite Triple phosphate; ammonium magnesium phosphate.

subarachnoid space Space between arachnoid mater and pia mater where CSF is found.

synovial fluid Extravascular fluid that surrounds the joints of the body.

talc, talcum Hydrated magnesium silicate; a chunky, irregular crystal formerly used to line surgical gloves; a possible urinary contaminant. Talc is not starch.

Tamm-Horsfall protein Glycoprotein (mucoprotein) secreted by the renal tubular cells and not derived from the blood plasma. This protein forms the matrix of urinary casts.

telescoped sediment Urine sediment seen after a period of renal shutdown, where a range of casts from hyaline to waxy with intermediate stages are seen.

thoracentesis Needle aspiration of pleural fluid.

toluidine blue A nuclear stain that is easily prepared in the laboratory; useful in the brightfield examination of urine sediment.

Total (or Therapeutic) Turnaround Time (TTAT) Time starting with that point where the physician determines a need for a particular laboratory value for a diagnosis or treatment plan to when the physician has the value in hand on which to act.

Total Quality Management (TQM) Design of systems and procedures used to ensure that quality is attained throughout an institution—it emphasizes teamwork or performance, rather than individual or departmental performance. Patient satisfaction is the goal for a healthcare institution—for the clinical laboratory, an example of TQM is the improvement of reporting results of tests so they have a greater impact on patient care.

transitional epithelial cells, urothelial cells Stratified epithelial lining of the urinary tract from the pelvis of the kidney to the base of the bladder (trigone) in females and the proximal part of the urethra in males. In the urinary tract, urothelial cells originate in structures located between structures lined by squamous and renal epithelial cells.

transparency In urinalysis, an assessment of the degree of clarity, or cloudiness of a urine specimen; a description of the amount of solid material suspended in the urine.

transudate Formation of an effusion as the result of filtration through a membrane; an ultrafiltrate of plasma with a low total protein, few or no cells, and a specific gravity usually less than 1.015, is generally classified as a transudate.

traumatic (bloody) tap Trauma to blood vessels during collection of specimen, resulting in the presence of blood in the specimen.

Trichomonas A motile protozoan parasite that may infect the vagina, urethra, periurethral glands, bladder, and prostate. May be seen in the urine sediment, but usually searched for in wet preparation of direct swabs from the vagina or urethra.

trigone A triangular structure; the base of the urinary bladder.

turnaround time For the physician, the time between which a laboratory test is first desired, ordered, or collected, and results are obtained. For the laboratory, generally the time between receipt of the specimen in the laboratory, and reporting of results. See also, **total turnaround time.**

ultrafiltrate of plasma Filtrate of plasma across a membrane, where extremely small particles such as proteins are restricted or not filtered—essentially the filtrate contains the same composition as the plasma.

unconjugated bilirubin See **free bilirubin.**

universal precautions Includes a system of recommended safety practices and policies (infection control) used for handling all biologic (patient) specimens; potential infectivity of any patient's body fluids including blood is unknown and therefore all blood and body fluid specimens are considered equally infectious (also known as universal blood and body fluid precautions).

unorganized sediment The chemical portion of the urine sediment, consisting of crystals and amorphous deposits of chemicals.

upper urinary tract Generally the kidney and renal pelvis. **Upper urinary tract infections** are infections of the kidney.

urate gout Arthritis in which monosodium urate crystals (MSU) are deposited in the synovial fluid.

urea The primary end product of protein metabolism—the result of amino acid and protein breakdown.

ureter The tubes that carry urine from the kidney to the bladder. Each kidney has one ureter.

urethra A small tubular structure that drains urine from the bladder. In men, the urethra serves as a passageway for semen during ejaculation, as well as a canal for urine during voiding.

urinalysis (routine) According to NCCLS, the testing of urine with procedures commonly performed in an expeditious, reliable, and cost-effective manner in clinical laboratories. Includes the physical, chemical, and microscopic analysis of urine.

urinary system Consists of two kidneys and two ureters plus the bladder and urethra.

urine sediment Any solid material that is suspended in the voided urine specimen. Includes cells, casts and crystals, and amorphous deposits of chemicals.

urinometer A specialized hydrometer calibrated to measure specific gravity of urine at a given temperature. Measurement of specific gravity by urinometer is considered inaccurate and discouraged by NCCLS.

urobilin An orange-red or orange-brown pigment; an oxidation product of urobilinogen present in small amounts in normal urine, and increased quantities in urine containing increased blood urobilinogen concentrations.

urobilinogen Group of colorless chromogens formed in the intestine by the reduction of bilirubin by bacteria present in the normal bacterial flora; normal product of bilirubin metabolism.

urochrome A yellow pigment; the primary pigment in normal urine.

uroerythrin A red pigment; present in small amounts in normal urine.

urothelial cells See **transitional epithelial cells.**

variance, error. A general term describing the factors or fluctuations that affect the measurement of a substance.

Vitamin C See **ascorbic acid.**

waived (waivered) tests A list of eight specific tests and methodologies under CLIA '88 that are exempt from proficiency testing regulations. Laboratories performing only waived tests must obtain a Certificate of Waiver from HHS.

xanthochromasia A faint pink, orange, or yellow color caused by release of hemoglobin from hemolyzed red blood cells; indicates presence of previous hemorrhage. Strictly speaking, xanthochromia produces a yellow color; however, the term is applied to pale pink to orange or yellow when describing color of specimen appearance.

INDEX

Italicized number denotes a page with an illustration; *italicized T* a page with a table.

Italicized number denotes a page with an illustration; *italicized T* a page with a table.

241

Italicized number denotes a page with an illustration; *italicized T* a page with a table.

Myelin basic protein
 cerebrospinal fluid
  multiple sclerosis, 190
Myoglobin in urine, 55*T*, 56
 effect on color of abnormal urine, 36
Myoglobinuria, 56

N

Narrow casts, 125
National Committee for Clinical Laboratory Standards. *See* NCCLS
NCCLS, 4
 decision to perform microscopic examination, 83
 definition of urinalysis, 23–24
 guidelines for urine containers, 29
 guidelines on laboratory procedure manuals, 13–14
 guidelines on standardized systems, 83–84
 recommendation on refractometers, 39–49
 recommendation on use of polarizing microscopy, 86
 recommendations on staining, 86
Nephrons, 25
Nephrotic syndrome, 112–113
Neutrophages, 216
Neutrophilic leukocytes. *See* White blood cells in urine, neutrophils
Neutrophils. *See also* White blood cells in urine, neutrophils
 cerebrospinal fluid
  indicator of bacterial infection, 188
NGRS. *See* Nonglucose-reducing substances in urine
Nitrite in urine
 clinical importance, 57
 reagent strip tests, 57–58
Nitroprusside reaction
 cystine confirmatory test, 162
 ketone bodies, 63
Nonglucose-reducing substances in urine, 61
Noninflammatory synovial fluid, 192

O

Obstructive jaundice. *See* Jaundice, obstructive
Occult blood
 detection by reagent strip tests, 55
Occupational Safety and Health Act of 1970, 5
Occupational Safety and Health Administration. *See* OSHA
Odor of urine, 37–38
 foul or putrid, 38
 fruity or sweet, 38
Oil droplets
 urine sediment, 169, *170*
  confused with red blood cells, 99
  fat of exogenous origin, *170*
Oligospermia, 211
Open neural tube defects, 215
Organized sediment. *See* Urine sediment, organized
Orthostatic proteinuria. *See* Proteinuria, orthostatic
OSHA, 3, 4
 hazard communication standard, 5, 8–9
 safety manual, 5
 standard on exposure to bloodborne pathogens, 5
 standards for clinical laboratories, 5
Osmometers
 measurement of urine solute concentration, 38

Italicized number denotes a page with an illustration; *italicized T* a page with a table.

Oval fat bodies, 113–114
 urine sediment, *112*, 112–114
  cytocentrifuged, *113*
  with free fat, *113*, *115*
  phase contrast, *113*
  polarized and compensated polarized light
   Maltese cross formation, *114*
  polarized light
   Maltese cross formation, *114*

P

Parasites
 body fluids, 217
 Trichomonas, 121–122
 urine sediment, 122–123
Pericardial effusion, 201
Pericardial fluid, 203
Perineal contamination, 117
Peritoneal effusion, 201
Peritoneal fluid, 192
Peroxidase activity
 reagent strip tests for blood, 56
Personal protective equipment
 role in infection control, 6
Personnel
 safety policies for clinical laboratories, 10–11
pH of body fluids
 seminal fluid, 209
pH of urine
 clinical importance, 48
Phase contrast microscopy, 85
 synovial fluid
  calcium pyrophosphate dihydrate crystals, 197
  crystals, 196
  monosodium urate crystals, 197
Phenazopyridine
 drug pigment casts, 143
 effect on color of abnormal urine, 36
Physical properties of urine, 34–40, 35*T*
Physician office laboratories
 federal regulation of, 3–4
Physician performed microscopies, 4
Pigmented casts
 urine sediment, 143
Pleural effusion, 201
Pleural fluid, 203
PMNs. *See* White blood cells in urine: neutrophils
Polarized light, 86
Polarized light microscopy, 86
 crystals in synovial fluid, 196–197, 198–210
Pollen grains
 urine sediment, 170, *171*
POLs. *See* Physician office laboratories
Polymorphonuclear neutrophils. *See* White blood cells in urine: neutrophils
Porphobilinogen in urine
 clinical importance, 68
 Hoesch test, 72, *72*
 reagent strip tests, 68–70
 Watson-Schwartz qualitative test, 70–72, *71*
Porphyria, 68
Porphyrins
 effect on color of abnormal urine, 36
Posthepatic jaundice. *See* Jaundice, obstructive
Potassium chloride
 component of urine, 27
Precipitation tests
 protein in urine, 51, 52–54

Italicized number denotes a page with an illustration; *italicized T* a page with a table.

Italicized number denotes a page with an illustration; *italicized T* a page with a table.